Student Study Guide

to accompany

Human Physiology

Sixth Edition

Stuart Ira Fox
Pierce College

Prepared by
Laurence G. Thouin, Jr.
Pierce College

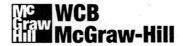

Boston   Burr Ridge, IL   Dubuque, IA   Madison, WI   New York   San Francisco   St. Louis
Bangkok   Bogotá   Caracas   Lisbon   London   Madrid
Mexico City   Milan   New Delhi   Seoul   Singapore   Sydney   Taipei   Toronto

WCB/McGraw-Hill

*A Division of The **McGraw·Hill** Companies*

Student Study Guide to accompany
HUMAN PHYSIOLOGY, SIXTH EDITION

Copyright ©1999 by The McGraw-Hill Companies, Inc. All rights reserved.
Printed in the United States of America.

The contents of, or parts thereof, may be reproduced for use with
HUMAN PHYSIOLOGY by Stuart Ira Fox, provided such reproductions bear
copyright notice and may not be reproduced in any form for any other purpose
without permission of the publisher.

1 2 3 4 5 6 7 8 9 0 QPD/QPD 9 0 9 8

ISBN 0-697-34220-4

www.mhhe.com

CONTENTS

Introduction

1. The Study of Body Function *1*
2. Chemical Composition of the Body *12*
3. Cell Structure and Genetic Control *22*
4. Enzymes and Energy *32*
5. Cell Respiration and Metabolism *40*
6. Membrane Transport and the Membrane Potential *50*
7. The Nervous System: Neurons and Synapses *61*
8. The Central Nervous System *73*
9. The Autonomic Nervous System *86*
10. Sensory Physiology *97*
11. Endocrine Glands: Secretion and Action of Hormones *109*
12. Muscle: Mechanisms of Contraction and Neural Control *123*
13. Heart and Circulation *135*
14. Cardiac Output, Blood Flow, and Blood Pressure *150*
15. The Immune System *166*
16. Respiratory Physiology *178*
17. Physiology of the Kidneys *194*
18. The Digestive System *207*
19. Regulation of Metabolism *219*
20. Reproduction *234*

Introduction
To The Student

Greetings! My name is Laurence G. Thouin, Jr., Ph.D. and I will serve as your guide through this wonderful story of the human body in action. This study guide is designed to improve the comprehension and performance of all students beginning the study of human physiology, and particularly those using the text entitled **Human Physiology,** by Stuart I. Fox, Ph.d. You do not have to be failing your course to benefit from the exercises I have laid out for you. Indeed, most students who use this study guide tell me that not only did they learn more about "how the body works", but also that they "had fun while earning better grades". Right now you probably feel frustrated, confused, or perhaps, intimidated by the enormous amount of information presented in the text. My hope is that I can help guide you through the text so that first, you might enjoy physiology more and yet also provide you with the tools necessary to achieve the goals you have set for yourself.

As a physiology instructor for almost 20 years, I have learned many valuable lessons from my students. They have pointed out many of their problem areas and have related to me many of the difficulties experienced by the beginning student. With their feedback in mind, I have selected the more important concepts presented in the text and have asked you to respond to a variety of questions from your reading. These exercises have been designed to challenge your reading comprehension and to supplement the text by giving you various perspectives of the many concepts being presented. Nevertheless, I hope to satisfy those students whose backgrounds and specific learning skills may differ quite widely and yet make this manual practical and enjoyable for each of you.

Your consistent use (daily, if possible) of this study guide will serve as an important interactive learning experience with immediate feedback. It should also represent a practical blend of your lectures, the textbook, the laboratory, and all examinations. Many of the questions in this study guide have been answered by my students either in a laboratory quiz or lecture examination. It is possible that they may represent questions similar to those you will face. Keep in mind that the focus of these exercises is on emphasizing the important physiological details (the "trees") while keeping track of the major concepts (the "forest") as well.

Each chapter in this study guide follows the textbook closely and incorporates a number of features for your benefit. Look for the:

- **Chapter SCOPE.** Each chapter begins with a brief "scope" of the chapter that highlights the essential features of each chapter and weaves them into the tapestry of the book. This feature should familiarize you with the current chapter and explain how it relates to other chapters, both those discussed earlier and those that follow.
- **Multiple Choice Questions.** These are "standard" scantron format questions which should help prepare you for exams. The arrangement or the wording of the questions and/or the choices may vary from question to question. I feel this variety in the questions will broaden your experience and develop your test-taking skills further. Answers follow each chapter.
- **True/False-Edit Questions.** These questions are also commonly seen on examinations, especially large scantron format exams. However, in this study guide you will be asked to correct or "edit" all false statements and then check your work against the answers I have provided at the end of each chapter.
- **Sequencer Questions.** In physiology, many body functions follow a definite "sequence" of events that are frequently found illustrated as flow diagrams in the text. These questions will feature a scrambled list of such events (such as in the contraction of a muscle fiber) which you are asked to place in the proper numerical order.
- **Match and Spell.** These are match-the-item questions with an extra feature. In addition to finding the correct match from a list of terms, you will be provided with a blank space in which you are asked to write the term out in your own handwriting. Although it will take a few extra seconds to do this, many of my students seem to have better recall of these terms if they write them out. Be sure you have spelled the terms correctly.

- **Draw and Label or Label the Figure.** These exercises are figures taken directly from the text with the terms replaced by blank answer lines for you to complete, or are blank spaces for you to draw, freehand, a figure or diagram complete with correct labels.
- **Completion or Fill-in Questions.** These are written statements or paragraphs, usually adapted from the summary at the end of each chapter of the text, with key words replaced by blank answer lines. You are asked to read these statements and compete or fill-in the blank spaces with the appropriate word(s).
- **Essay Tutorial.** This is a feature unique to this study guide. Like many instructors, I feel that essay or short-answer type questions play a vital role in the success of students learning physiology. Many of my students actually ENJOY these essay questions! They often request them in favor of scantron questions because they feel able to express themselves more clearly and therefore, are not as frustrated when confronted by difficult questions. Furthermore, like most professors, I reward effort with partial credit.

Also unique to this section is the **Essay Tutorial.** In response to question 1. Of each chapter of the text, I have provided one sample essay. I also include tips and suggestions for formatting and answering these types of questions. A few of my own essay questions have been added for you to try.

- **Chapter Review**—Each chapter concludes with a series of exercises which summarize the entire chapter.
- **Crossword Puzzles**—Most of the chapters have a crossword puzzle composed of important terms and concepts from the chapter just completed. Not only are these puzzles fun to complete, they will help you learn *definitions* and the correct *spelling* of many important words.

OVERVIEW OF THE TEXTBOOK FOR STUDENTS

There are 20 chapters in the Human Physiology textbook by Stuart I. Fox. The first 6 chapters organize and expand upon important topics in physiology you may have already been introduced to in general science, biology, anatomy or chemistry courses. These initial chapters will focus on the living cell, featuring reviews of basic cell types, their structures and the important functions they carry out. In this unit we will learn how the DNA or genetic material we inherit from our parents controls not only the chemical makeup of the cell—such as those unique protein and phospholipid molecules needed to construct the mitochondria or the cell membrane—but also how DNA controls the function of the cell through the metabolism of energy-rich fuels. This gene control over metabolism is assisted by custom-made enzymes. Conscientious study here will provide you with many fundamental concepts needed for complete understanding of metabolism and physiological principles presented in the remaining chapters.

The next 4 chapters (7-10) reveal the complex workings of the **nervous system** with a complete description of the rapid communication signals known as nerve impulses. These impulses travel along designated electrochemical pathways to and from the brain and spinal cord. The brain and spinal cord make up the central nervous system which quickly receive these messages from sensors around the body, interpret them and usually command a response.

The second form of communication used by the body is much slower, utilizing chemical messengers or hormones which are secreted by glands of the **endocrine system** (chapter 11). Chapter 12 is devoted to muscle tissue and the sequence of electrical, chemical and mechanical events which must take place during contraction of skeletal, cardiac and smooth muscle.

The organ system that most immediately represents the subject of physiology is the **cardiovascular system.** Chapter 13 begins this section with descriptions of the beating heart as the pump for the circulation of blood through vessels around the body, providing oxygen and nutrients to the cells and carrying away wastes for elimination. Chapter 14 defines arterial blood pressure as the product of characteristics from the beating heart and the constriction-dilation properties of the blood vessels.

The physiology of breathing and the exchange of oxygen for carbon dioxide at the lung alveolus and later, at each tissue cell is the subject of the **respiratory system** (chapter 15). The content of this chapter blends nicely with that of earlier cardiovascular system chapters especially when describing the role of the blood in oxygen and carbon dioxide transport. Here, we will also see how carbon dioxide in the blood can produce acid and thereby links the act of breathing to the important concept of acid-base balance in the body. Thus the lungs help prevent acidosis or alkalosis through control over the elimination of carbon dioxide from the lungs.

The **kidneys** (chapter 16) also play a vital role in acid-base balance while simultaneously filtering the blood at nephrons, reabsorbing substances from this filtrate that the body works to conserve and secreting other molecules into the urine that the body wishes to eliminate. The ultimate process of the **digestive system** (chapter 17), however, is absorption. We take in foods and fluid (ingestion), break them down into manageable pieces (digestion), which we then transport across our gastrointestinal membranes (absorption). In this way, nutrients and fluids can selectively enter the body. The nutritional fuels needed by the body and the various hormonal controls over **metabolism** of these fuels is described in chapter 18.

One of the latest physiological frontiers to be explored and, certainly one of the more exciting concepts in physiology is the **immune system** (chapter 19). In this chapter basic body defense mechanisms are presented. Topics presented here include the role of T and B-lymphocytes in the blood, antibody structure and function, and descriptions of tumors and various diseases of the immune system.

By tradition it seems that most physiology textbooks close, as this one does, with the female and male **reproductive systems** (chapter 20). This chapter is patterned after life itself, opening with control over sexuality in the embryo, leading through the hormone-directed events of puberty, the menstrual cycle, fertilization, pregnancy: and ending, with the physiological phenomena responsible for childbirth (parturition) and breast-feeding (lactation).

TO THE INSTRUCTOR

This is a study guide which should be of great assistance to you in your human physiology course. Each exercise follows the chapter in the text carefully, with objective and subjective questions related to each new topic. Many of the questions require writing from the student such as labels on a figure, spelling of terms, fill-in-the-blank statement or completion of written answers in an essay format. Each new chapter has a brief scope to introduce the subject and to give the student a feel for how it "fits in" or relates to the entire book. Each chapter has a variety of question formats with a chapter review to summarize the major concepts and challenge the student with various new exercises. In addition, there is an "essay tutorial" section which will answer the first essay question at the end of each chapter in the textbook and provide instruction in the approach to writing a good essay in physiology.

I have designed this study guide to be both a practical and fun learning experience for the beginning student of physiology. It is also tailored to be used with the Human Physiology textbook by Stuart I. Fox. I am responsible for the entire contents of this study guide. I would be very grateful for any comments or criticisms you may have which will improve the effectiveness of this manual as a learning aide.

I wish to acknowledge the help and friendship of Edmont Katz, whose many suggestions and experiments with different approaches to the education of physiology students made this study guide richer and more meaningful. I also wish to thank Colleen J. Nolan of St. Mary's University who devoted many hours in the review of this study guide.

CHAPTER 1
THE STUDY OF BODY FUNCTION

CHAPTER SCOPE

After introducing physiology, *chapter 1* presents a basic review of human organs, tissues, and control systems. Also featured here is a description of the biological methods of communication and controls that exist between these various organs, tissues, and systems in the body. The four primary **tissues** of the body — muscle, nerve, epithelium, and connective tissues — are all present in skin, an example of an **organ**. As you read the descriptions of how these tissues function independently, remember that they also perform in concert with other tissues in the body as smoothly operating **systems**. Most of these systems will be presented in the chapters that follow.

The underlying theme of any physiology course is summed up in the critical, but difficult-to-describe term ***homeostasis***. Homeostasis can be defined as the ability of the body to keep almost all internal body processes within normal limits, despite the many wide variety of forces and changes that occur externally. Each subsequent chapter will allude to, if not directly demonstrate, homeostasis at work. Operating through negative feedback mechanisms, homeostasis will oppose the initial stress on the body and conditions will return toward normal. Here, you will be introduced to the concept of homeostasis through examples of the **nervous** (electrical signals with neurotransmitter chemicals) system and the **endocrine** (hormone chemicals) system.

I. INTRODUCTION TO PHYSIOLOGY

Human physiology is the study of how the human body functions, with emphasis on specific cause-and-effect mechanisms. Knowledge of these mechanisms has been obtained experimentally through applications of the scientific method.

A. Multiple Choice

You will find multiple choice questions in each section of this study guide. Select the letter of the **best** choice to answer each of the following questions or to complete each phrase. Write that letter in the space provided. Answer all of the questions in each section, then check your work with the correct answers provided at the end of this chapter. Remember, if you are having difficulty, be sure to reread the corresponding section in your textbook before going on to the next set of questions. These exercises will help prepare you for similar questions you may see on "scantron"-type examinations. Good luck!

___ 1. Physiology is the study of
    a. biological function
    b. how the body works
    c. cause-and-effect sequences in the body
    d. observations that overlap many other sciences
    e. All of these are correct.

___ 2. Which of the following statements about physiology is *not* correct?
    a. The ultimate objective is to understand the normal functioning of the human body.
    b. Pathophysiology is a related science that complements normal physiology.
    c. The study of disease processes has helped our understanding of physiology.
    d. Because animals are so different from humans, the study of *comparative* physiology has very little direct application to *human* physiology.
    e. All of these statements are correct.

___ 3. According to scientific theory, all observations must be
    a. published
    b. reproducible
    c. clinical
    d. predictable
    e. None of these is correct.

___ 4. In the development of new pharmaceutical drugs, which phase of human or clinical trials is the drug tested on the *target* human population (for example, those with hypertension?)
   a. phase I clinical trials
   b. phase II clinical trials
   c. phase III clinical trials
   d. phase IV clinical trials

B. True or False/Edit

Decide whether the following statements are true or false. In the space provided write "**T**" if the statement is true and "**F**" if the statement is false. For statements that are **false, edit** (rewrite) the statement so that it now becomes **true.** As an example, the first statement is false and is edited for you. Notice that there are many ways to "edit" or rewrite the false statement to make it true. Always try the simplest method, and remember, that the answers and sample "edits" are provided for you at the end of each chapter.

___ 5. Physiology is the study of disease processes in the body.
   (**False/Edit:** Physiology is the study of how the body works normally at tasks essential for life [to maintain homeostasis].)
___ 6. The scientific method is based on a confidence in our rational ability, honesty, and humility.
___ 7. *Fact*: All athletes have lower resting pulse rates than sedentary people.
___ 8. Only 10% of all newly developed drugs are considered safe enough to advance from preliminary testing on experimental animals to clinical trials on humans.

II. HOMEOSTASIS AND FEEDBACK CONTROL

The regulatory mechanisms of the body can be understood in terms of a single, shared function: that of maintaining constancy of the internal environment. A state of relative constancy of the internal environment is known as homeostasis, and it is maintained by effectors that are regulated by sensory information from the internal environment.

A. Multiple Choice

___ 9. In homeostasis, the critical concept describing the body's response to any deviation from some particular setpoint (such as temperature rising when exercising), which results the activation of mechanisms to oppose that deviation (return temperature toward normal), is known as
   a. negative feedback
   b. the integrating center
   c. positive feedback
   d. *milieu interior*

___ 10. Which of the following mechanisms of homeostasis is analogous to the house thermostat setting that operates to regulate the temperature in the house?
   a. sensor
   b. the set point
   c. effector
   d. integrating center

___ 11. Arrange the following terms in the sequence that best reflects how the body maintains homeostasis (for example, during a fever). (1) effector activated; (2) integrating center process; (3) negative feedback loops activated; (4) sensor activated; (5) return to set point
   a. 2 4 3 1 5
   b. 5 3 2 4 1
   c. 4 3 1 5 2
   d. 4 2 1 3 5
   e. 1 2 4 5 3

___ 12. During homeostasis, increasing or decreasing the activity of particular effectors is the primary role of the
   a. integrating center
   b. sensor
   c. muscle or gland
   d. positive feedback loops
   e. negative feedback loops
___ 13. The term, *innervate* means to
   a. activate glands to release hormones
   b. inactivate glands
   c. activate nerve impulses in nerve fibers
   d. inactivate nerve fibers
   e. inactivate both glands and nerve fibers.
___ 14. Hormone secretion can result from stimulation of endocrine glands by
   a. nerves (releasing neurotransmitter chemicals)
   b. other specific body chemicals
   c. stimulation by other hormones
   d. a and c only
   e. All of these are correct.

B. True or False/Edit
___ 15. In medicine, illness occurs when the body is unable to maintain constancy within the internal environment.
___ 16. In homeostasis, the activation of effectors generally refers to the specific activation of muscles or bones.
___ 17. An initial rise in blood glucose level followed by a subsequent further increase in blood glucose is an example of *negative* feedback.
___ 18. Bleeding from a cut activates a *positive* feedback "cascade," whereas the subsequent formation of a blood clot represents the completion of a *negative* feedback loop.
___ 19. The regulation of homeostasis by messages sent from the nervous and endocrine systems to a target organs somewhere else in the body, is an example of *intrinsic* control.
___ 20. Although hormones are carried by the blood to all organs in the body, only those target organs displaying receptor proteins specific for those hormones will respond.

III. THE PRIMARY TISSUES

The organs of the body are composed of four different primary tissues each of which has its own characteristic structure and function. The activities and interactions of these tissues determine the physiology of the organs.

A. Multiple Choice
___ 21. Which primary tissue features *intercalated discs*?
   a. epithelial
   b. nervous
   c. muscle
   d. connective
   e. None of these is correct.
___ 22. Which of the following is *not* considered epithelial tissue?
   a. simple membranes
   b. exocrine glands
   c. endocrine glands
   d. brain and spinal cord
   e. All of these are considered epithelial tissue.

___ 23. The type of epithelium best adapted for diffusion and filtration is
   a. simple squamous
   b. simple cuboidal
   c. columnar
   d. ciliated columnar
___ 24. The type of epithelium that lines the ducts of exocrine glands and part of the tubules of the kidney nephron is
   a. simple squamous
   b. simple cuboidal
   c. columnar
   d. ciliated columnar
___ 25. Which of the following is *not* characteristic of epithelium?
   a. It may be simple or stratified.
   b. It may contain goblet cells.
   c. It may be keratinized (or cornified).
   d. It is constantly lost (exfoliated) and replaced.
   e. All of these are characteristic of epithelium.
___ 26. Which of the following is *not* an exocrine gland?
   a. liver
   b. pancreas
   c. spleen
   d. prostate
   e. sebaceous gland
___ 27. Tendons (muscle to bone) and ligaments (bone to bone) are examples of
   a. dense irregular connective tissue
   b. dense regular connective tissue
   c. loose (areolar) connective tissue
   d. cartilage
___ 28. Lamellae, lacunae, and canaliculi are characteristic of
   a. connective tissue proper
   b. cartilage
   c. bone
   d. blood

B. True or False/Edit

___ 29. Histology is the study of microscopic anatomy.
___ 30. Smooth and cardiac muscles are voluntarily controlled.
___ 31. Each skeletal muscle cell or fiber (myofiber) is controlled individually by nerve fibers so that the overall muscle strength of contraction can be varied or "graded."
___ 32. Intercalated discs couple myocardial cells mechanically and electrically.
___ 33. Heart muscle (myocardial) cells can be stimulated to contract individually, like skeletal muscle fibers.
___ 34. Peristalsis is a process requiring skeletal muscle contractions.
___ 35. Neuroglia are more numerous than neurons, do not conduct impulses, and are able to divide by mitosis throughout life.
___ 36. Columnar epithelial cells with projecting cilia are located in many respiratory passages and in the uterine (fallopian) tubes of females.
___ 37. Structures collectively called junctional complexes and the basement membrane are also features of epithelial tissues.
___ 38. The digestive tract is considered an outside or external body surface.
___ 39. The numerous *eccrine* (or *merocrine*) sweat glands secrete a dilute salt solution that evaporates and cools the skin during thermoregulation.

C. Matching

Match the **best** description on the right to the numbered terms on the left and write the corresponding letter in the space provided.

___ 40. tissue
___ 41. primary tissue
___ 42. organ
___ 43. system
___ 44. myofiber
___ 45. neuron
___ 46. neuroglia
___ 47. lumen
___ 48. endothelium

a. muscle cell
b. functioning unit made up of two or more primary tissues
c. cells that have similar function
d. simple squamous lining of blood vessels
e. organs grouped by function
f. examples are muscle, nervous, epithelial, and connective tissue
g. electrically active nerve cell
h. cavity of an organ or structure
i. supportive/nutritional cells for neuron

IV. ORGANS AND SYSTEMS

Organs are composed of two or more primary tissues that serve the different functions of the organ. The skin is an organ that has numerous functions provided by its constituent tissues.

A. Multiple Choice

___ 49. Which of the following glands is *not* exocrine?
    a. hair follicle
    b. apocrine sweat gland
    c. eccrine sweat gland
    d. sebaceous gland
    e. All of these are exocrine.

___ 50. The largest organ in the body in terms of its surface area, is the
    a. liver
    b. stomach
    c. skin
    d. brain
    e. heart

___ 51. Which of the following is *not* a cutaneous sensation?
    a. pain
    b. pressure
    c. heat/cold
    d. taste
    e. touch

___ 52. Which substance is a hormone secreted by the endocrine glands of the skin into the bloodstream?
    a. melanin
    b. vitamin D
    c. hemoglobin
    d. keratin
    e. collagen

B. True or False/Edit

___ 53. Sebaceous glands secrete oily sebum into hair follicles, which transport the sebum to the cornified surface of the skin to aid in lubrication.
___ 54. Both sensory and motor nerve fibers (neurons) are found in the skin.
___ 55. Blood flow to the skin is partially controlled by motor nerve fibers to smooth muscle in the walls of cutaneous blood vessels that regulate the degree of constriction or dilation.

C. Label the Figure and Application An Organ: The Skin

The skin is an excellent example of an **organ** that is composed of the four tissue types. Figure 1.1 is a diagram of the skin with structures numbered 56-68. Identify each structure and *write* the correct term in the space provided after the number in the figure. If you need help, see figure 1.20 in the text.

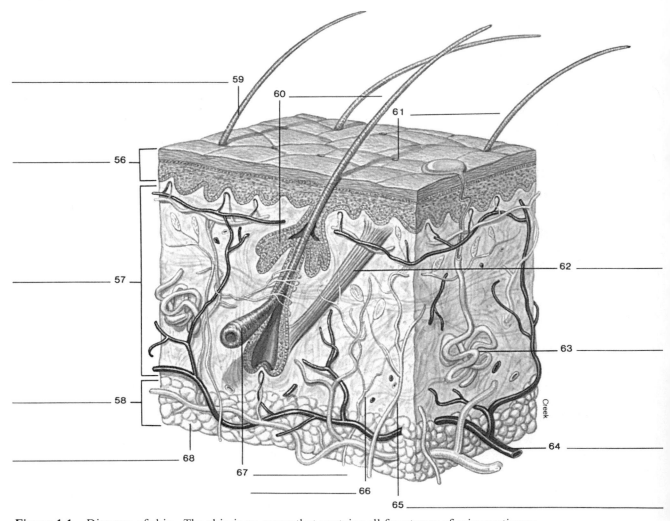

Figure 1.1 Diagram of skin. The skin is an organ that contains all four types of primary tissues.

Using Figure 1.1 as a reference, read questions 69-73 that follow and fill in the blanks with the correct word or phrase that applies to the skin.

69. The three examples of exocrine glands shown here are the _____ gland, which secretes sebum, the _____ gland, whose watery secretion cools the skin, and the _____ (two words).
70. The blood supply to skin arrives from the _____ tissue level, then branches into the layer, but does not enter the _____ layer of the skin, which is fed by diffusion.
71. Notice the ideal location of the Pacinian corpuscle for the sensation of _____.
72. The subcutaneous tissue, which contains adipose or _____ cells, nerves, and blood vessels, is also known as the _____.
73. Adipose tissue is a type of _____ (primary) tissue.

CHAPTER REVIEW

A. Completion

74. Physiology is the study of how the body works - from _____ to _____, to _____, to systems.
75. By asking questions beginning with "_____," scientists studying physiology discover answers that involve _____-and-_____ sequences during experiments.
76. The four primary tissues are _____, _____, _____, and _____.
77. The three types of muscle tissue are _____, _____, and _____; of which only _____ muscle is *not* striated.
78. Epithelial membranes provide a protective barrier of cells tightly joined by _____ _____ (two words), as they cover and line the body surfaces. These membranes may be simple or _____; and consist of _____, _____, or _____ cell shapes.
79. Invaginated epithelial tissue may form exocrine glands with _____, or form endocrine glands secreting _____ into the bloodstream.
80. Four types of connective tissue are _____ _____ _____, _____, _____, and _____.
81. Skin is a good example of a (an) _____.
82. Three exocrine glands found in the dermis of the skin are _____ _____, _____ _____, and _____ _____.
83. Also in the dermis of the skin are the _____ pili muscles and muscles constricting and dilating the walls of _____; *both* of these muscles are composed of _____ muscle fiber type.
84. Homeostasis is maintained through _____ feedback loops involving sensors, integrating centers, and _____, which communicate extrinsically through messengers of the _____ and _____ systems.
85. Both neurotransmitters and hormones bind with unique membrane _____ proteins and control specific _____ organs.

B. Crossword Puzzle — Tissues, Organs, and Control Systems

Across

1. Dense, regular type of connective tissue connecting muscle to bone
6. Maintaining a constant internal environment
9. Opposing a rise or fall in body temperature or blood glucose during homeostasis (2 words)
12. 37°C is an example of _____ point in homeostasis
13. Homeostasis strives to maintain all values at their _____ (2 words)
15. Adipose tissue of the hypodermis
16. Fibrous protein common to most connective tissue
19. Nerve fiber control over muscle or gland effector activity
21. Property of muscle in which the strength of its contraction can vary from weak to strong
22. The muscle or gland cell that receives nerve impulses
23. Single cytoplasmic extension of the neuron cell body
24. Connective tissue containing lamellae, lacunae, and canaliculi
25. Study of biological function emphasizing body mechanisms that involve cause-and-effect
26. Clusters of secretory ducts in exocrine glands that are squeezed by myoepithelial cells sequences
27. Rhythmic contractions of circular and longitudinal muscle, pushing food through the digestive tract
28. Oily secretion on hair follicles and cornified skin—prevents drying and cracking

Down

1. Watery secretion from lacrimal (exocrine) gland
2. The largest organ in the body
3. Homeostatic process that supports and worsens body changes rather than opposes and returns to normal
4. Cells of stomach or intestine that secrete mucus
5. Receiver of relayed sensory information to process and help maintain homeostasis (examples: brain and spinal cord)
7. Characteristic of exocrine glands
8. Water-resistant protein in dead cells of the cornified epidermis of the skin
10. Physiology seeks answers to help explain cause-and-_____ sequences
11. Study of microscopic anatomy
14. Physiology typically asks the question _____?
17. Cavity or space within an organ or structure—like the inner space within blood vessels or the stomach
18. Simple squamous membrane lining blood vessels; specifically adapted for diffusion and filtration
20. Cells that provide anatomical and functional support to the neuron

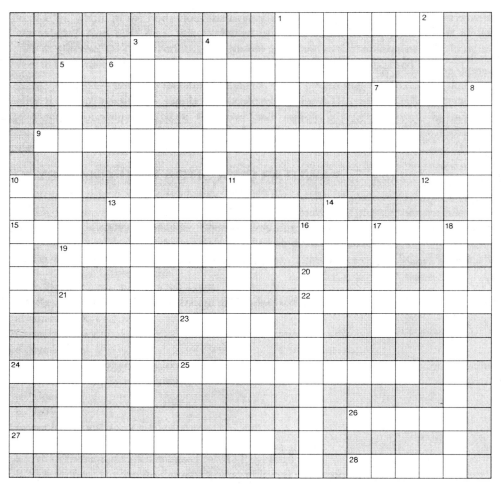

C. Essay

Essay Tutorial

This essay tutorial will answer the first essay question found in the "**Review Activities**" section of each chapter in your *Human Physiology* textbook. Please look for *essay question* 1. at the end of each text chapter, read it carefully, and let me guide you through one possible answer in this section. Watch for helpful tips and general suggestions on writing the essay or short-answer questions. Learn to spot key words in the questions such as those that I indicate in **bold-face** type, and to outline your ideas quickly on a separate piece of paper. This will help you organize your thoughts, express yourself clearly, and — since it will be easier to read — result in better scores! Using similar techniques, try the bonus essay questions I have written that follow. Enjoy!

86. Describe the **structure** of various **epithelial membranes,** and explain how their structures relate to their **functions.**

Answer. First, write the bold-faced key words as column headings. Next, list the membranes separately and then complete the descriptions of structure and function. Study Table 1.2 in your textbook for a sample table format.

Epithelial Membranes	**Structure**	**Function**
Simple squamous	Flat	Diffusion and filtration (endothelium)
Simple cuboidal	Cube	Line exocrine ducts and kidney tubules; → transport
Simple columnar	Tall	Stomach and intestinal lining (goblet cells) → barrier
Ciliated columnar	"Oars"	Uterine (fallopian) tubes and respiratory passages;→ movement and filtration
Stratified squamous (many layers)	Esophagus (nonkeratinized) Skin (keratinized)	→protection → protection
Glandular, exocrine	Ducts	Secretions to outside
Glandular, endocrine	No ducts	Hormone release into the blood

Note: Don't be frustrated if your answer didn't look like this at first. Be patient — and with practice, your skills will improve. Now, refer to the text for help in answering the remainder of these bonus essay questions, organize your thoughts based on key words in the question, then write your answer clearly and concisely. Good luck!

87. List and describe the structures of the skin that represent the four primary tissues. Include the function of each structure.

88. Blood levels of calcium are held constant (at a set point) by hormones. Parathyroid hormone is one hormone that helps raise the blood calcium concentration. Draw a flow diagram that shows how this hormone would act after you consumed a tall, frothy glass of calcium-rich milk (*hint*: similar to the glucose-insulin figure).

89. Draw a flow diagram showing how the parasympathetic nerve stimulation to the heart slows the heart rate, while sympathetic nerve stimulation speeds up the heart rate (*hint*: see figure 1.4 for help).

Answers — Chapter 1

I. Introduction
   A. 1. e, 2. d, 3. b, 4. b
   B. 5. F, 6. T, 7. F—Replace "fact" with "hypothesis," 8. T
II. Homeostasis and Feedback Control
   A. 9. a, 10. b, 11. d, 12. a, 13. c, 14. e
   B. 15. T, 16. F—Replace "bone" with "glands," 17. F—Replace "negative" with "positive," 18. T, 19. F—Replace "intrinsic" with "extrinsic," 20. T
III. The Primary Tissues
   A. 21. c, 22. d, 23. a, 24. b, 25. e, 26. c, 27. b, 28. c
   B. 29.T, 30. F—Replace "voluntarily" with "involuntarily," 31. T, 32. T, 33. F—Replace "can be" with "can*not* be," 34. F—Replace "skeletal" with "smooth," 35. T, 36. T, 37. T, 38. T, 39. T
   C. 40. c, 41. f, 42. b, 43. e, 44. a, 45. g, 46. i, 47. h, 48. d
IV. Organs and Systems
   A. 49. e, 50. c, 51. d, 52. b
   B. 53. T, 54. T, 55. T
   C. 56. epidermis, 57. dermis, 58. hypodermis, 59. hair, 60. sebaceous gland, 61. sweat pore, 62. arrector pili muscle, 63.sweat gland, 64. blood vessel (arteriole), 65. sensory nerve 66. motor nerve 67. hair bulb, 68. adipose tissue, 69. sebaceous; sudoriferous; hair follicle, 70. subcutaneous; dermis; epidermis, 71. pressure, 72. fat; hypodermis, 73. connective

Chapter Review
   A. 74. cells; tissues; organs, 75. how?; cause; effect, 76. connective; epithelial; nervous; muscle, 77. smooth; skeletal; cardiac; smooth, 78. junctional complexes; stratified, squamous; cuboidal; columnar, 79. ducts; hormones, 80. connective tissue proper; cartilage; bone; blood, 81. organ, 82. hair follicles; sweat glands; sebaceous glands, 83. arrector; blood vessels; smooth, 84. negative; effectors; endocrine; nervous, 85. receptor; target

B. Crossword Puzzle

									¹T	E	N	D	O	N	²S	
			³P		⁴G		E						K			
	⁵I		⁶H	O	M	E	O	S	T	A	S	I	S			I	
	N		S		B		R				⁷D		N		⁸K
	T		I		L						U				E
	⁹N	E	G	A	T	I	V	E	F	E	E	D	B	A	C	K		R
	G		I		T						T				A
¹⁰E	R		V			¹¹H							¹²S	E	T
F	A		¹³S	E	T	P	O	I	N	T	¹⁴H				I
¹⁵F	A	T		F		S			¹⁶C	O	L	¹⁷L	A	G	¹⁸E	N
E		¹⁹I	N	N	E	R	V	A	T	E		W		U		N
C		N		E			O		²⁰N			M			D
T		²¹G	R	A	D	E		L		²²E	F	F	E	C	T	O	R
		C		B		²³A	X	O	N		U			N		T
		E		A			G			R				H
²⁴B	O	N	E		C		²⁵P	H	Y	S	I	O	L	O	G	Y	E
		T		K			G					L
		E					L		²⁶A	C	I	N	I
²⁷P	E	R	I	S	T	A	L	S	I	S			U
								A		²⁸S	E	B	U	M

11

CHAPTER 2
CHEMICAL COMPOSITION OF THE BODY

CHAPTER SCOPE

To some students the prospect of studying chemistry in a biology or physiology class is frightening. However, it is possible to simplify the vast field of chemistry painlessly and to apply many of the basic chemical concepts directly to those in physiology. Chapter 2 does this well. Of the entire periodic table of elements, only the "big four" — **hydrogen** (H), **oxygen** (O), **carbon** (C), and **nitrogen** (N) must be well understood. Notice the role of *electrons* in chemical bonding; and the behavior of the **hydrogen ion** in regulation of acid-base balance (another example of homeostasis!). From the discussion of atoms the text continues with descriptions of the various types of chemical bonds and proceeds to construct the three major classes of organic molecules — carbohydrates, lipids, and proteins.

In succeeding chapters, the **carbohydrates** you assemble here will be digested and absorbed from foods we eat (digestion — chapter 17) and combusted by cells for energy (metabolism — chapter 5). Similarly, the **lipids** we build here will also be digested and absorbed as fuel for metabolism in these later chapters.

Within the lipid family of compounds are the *triglycerides*, perhaps best known as ordinary system such as estrogen, progesterone and testosterone-chapters 11 and 20); and the very exciting newest member of the lipid family, the *prostaglandins*. The **proteins** we consume, digest, and absorb into the body as individual amino acids will be used to construct new proteins in the cytoplasm of the cell. This assembly of proteins (protein synthesis — chapter 3) follows the DNA blueprints coded for by genes along the 46 chromosomes we inherited from our parents. Located in the nucleus, our genes dictate the construction of all proteins that range in specialty from microtubules, microfilaments, and active enzymes to the complex immune system complement proteins and antibodies.

I. ATOMS, IONS, AND CHEMICAL BONDS

The study of physiology requires some familiarity with the basic concepts and terminology of chemistry. A knowledge of atomic and molecular structure, the nature of chemical bonds, and the nature of pH and associated concepts provides the foundation for much of physiology.

A. Multiple Choice

___ 1. Approximately 65% to 75% of the body weight is composed of
   a. water (H_2O)
   b. proteins
   c. fat
   d. carbohydrates

___ 2. Which of the following is *not* an organic molecule?
   a. carbohydrate
   b. lipid
   c. protein
   d. nucleic acid
   e. All of these are organic molecules.

___ 3. The **atomic mass** of an atom is determined by the total mass of its
   a. protons and neutrons
   b. neutrons and electrons
   c. electrons and protons
   d. protons only
   e. electrons only

___ 4. The **atomic number** of an atom is given by the total number of its
   a. protons and neutrons
   b. neutrons and electrons
   c. electrons and protons
   d. protons only
   e. electrons only

___ 5. The second energy shell, or orbital, of an atom contains a maximum of _____ electrons.
  a. two
  b. four
  c. six
  d. eight
  e. eighteen
___ 6. The bond between two *adjacent* water molecules is a (an)
  a. hydrogen bond
  b. polar covalent bond
  c. nonpolar covalent bond
  d. ionic bond
___ 7. Solution A has a pH of 10 and solution B has a pH of 2. Which of the following statements about these two solutions is **true**?
  a. Solution A has a higher H^+ concentration than solution B.
  b. Solution B is basic.
  c. Solution A is acidic.
  d. All of these statements are true.
  e. None of these statements is true.
___ 8. The class of organic molecules featuring a **carbonyl** group within the carbon chain is known as a (an)
  a. organic acid
  b. aldehyde
  c. ketone
  d. alcohol

B. True or False/Edit

___ 9. By definition, organic molecules are those that must be composed of at least one hydrogen atom.
___ 10. The electrons of the outermost orbital, which participate in chemical reactions and form chemical bonds, are known as valence electrons.
___ 11. Atoms may exist as isotopes, which have the same atomic mass but a different atomic numbers.
___ 12. An atom that gains more electrons than it has protons becomes a negatively charged ion called a cation.
___ 13. In ionic bonds the electrons are *not* shared at all.
___ 14. A base is usually an anion which can combine with H^+, remove that H^+ from solution, and thus lower the pH value of the solution.
___ 15. Bicarbonate ion (HCO_3^-) is the major buffer of the blood.
___ 16. Hydroxyl groups are normally found on one end of the carbon chain (for example, an alcohol) rather than found near the middle of organic molecules.
___ 17. Enzymes in the cells of the body will only recognize D - amino acid and L - sugar stereoisomers during catalyzed reactions.

C. Matching

___ 18. water (H_2O)
___ 19. weak bond that dissociates in water
___ 20. atom that gains electrons when bonding
___ 21. equal sharing of electrons
___ 22. unequal sharing of electrons
___ 23. atom that loses electrons when bonding
___ 24. very weak bond — stabilizes proteins

a. nonpolar covalent bond
b. cation
c. polar covalent bond
d. polar solvent
e. hydrogen bond
f. ionic bond
g. anion

D. Label the Figure and Application Functional Groups of Organic Molecules

Here are the more important functional groups that are part of organic molecules. These groups appear often in various figures that follow. Study the structures of these functional groups and be able to recognize, categorize, and name them quickly, even when they appear as part of larger, more complex molecules. With practice, you will discover that new and different molecules will appear "friendlier" as you recognize familiar functional groups and learn how to predict their behavior in the body. Study figure 2.1 below and fill in the shaded boxed areas to the right with the correct functional group. (You can check your answers against figure 2.10 in the text.)

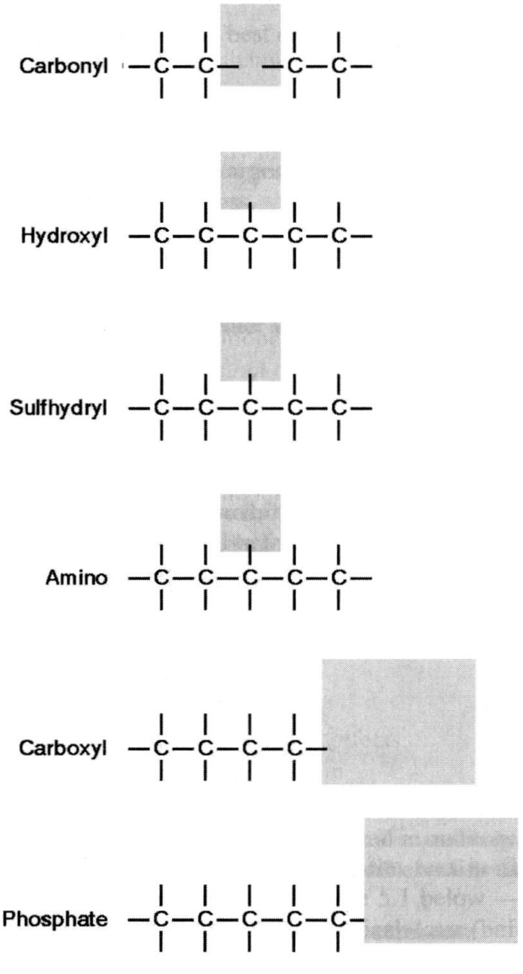

Figure 2.1 Various functional groups of organic molecules.

II. CARBOHYDRATES AND LIPIDS

Carbohydrates are a class of organic molecules that includes monosaccharides, disaccharides, and polysaccharides. All of these molecules are based on a characteristic ratio of carbon, hydrogen, and oxygen atoms. Lipids are a category of diverse organic molecules that share the physical property of being nonpolar and thus insoluble in water.

A. Multiple Choice

___ 25. The general formula of a carbohydrate molecule is
    a. $(H_2O)C$
    b. H_2OCC
    c. CH_2O
    d. H_2O

___ 26. Which of the following molecules is *not* a disaccharide?
   a. sucrose
   b. lactose
   c. galactose
   d. maltose

___ 27. Extra sugar molecules in the body are condensed and stored in the liver and muscles as a polymer known as
   a. glycogen
   b. glucose
   c. galactose
   d. glucagon
   e. starch

___ 28. Ketone bodies can be formed by the liver from the hydrolysis (breakdown) of
   a. carbohydrates
   b. proteins
   c. free fatty acids (triglycerides)
   d. nucleic acids
   e. prostaglandins

___ 29. Which of the following molecules forms an integral part of micelles floating in the blood and can also function as a surfactant, decreasing the surface tension of water?
   a. glycogen
   b. water
   c. protein
   d. phospholipid
   e. nucleic acid

___ 30. Which of the following organs does *not* secrete steroid hormones?
   a. liver
   b. ovary
   c. adrenal cortex
   d. testes

B. True or False/Edit

___ 31. Sucrose is a disaccharide of glucose and galactose.
___ 32. Starch is a polysaccharide of glucose, stored in plants.
___ 33. Dehydration synthesis is the use of water to split larger compounds into smaller compounds (digestion).
___ 34. Lipid molecules are characterized by being insoluble in nonpolar solvents, such as water.
___ 35. A fatty acid chain showing a number of double covalent bonds, in which each carbon atom binds with only one hydrogen, is known as a saturated fatty acid chain.
___ 36. Triglycerides are also known as neutral fats because the attached fatty acid groups can no longer release H^+ and function as acids; and therefore, do not alter the acid-base balance.
___ 37. Phospholipids contain both polar and nonpolar sections, which contribute to the hydrophilic and hydrophobic properties, respectively, of these molecules.
___ 38. Cholesterol is the precursor or raw material used by the body for the synthesis of steroid hormones such as testosterone, estrogen, progesterone, and hydrocortisone.
___ 39. Prostaglandins are produced by and are active in almost all organs of the body where they serve a variety of regulatory functions.

III. PROTEINS

Proteins are large molecules composed of amino acid subunits. Since there are twenty different types of amino acids that can be used in constructing a given protein, the variety of protein structures is immense. This variety allows each type of protein to perform very specific functions.

A. Multiple Choice

___ 40. The approximate number of amino acids that form proteins is
   a. eight
   b. twelve
   c. twenty
   d. twenty-three
   e. forty-six

___ 41. In the formation of peptide bonds between two amino acids
   a. condensation or dehydration synthesis occurs
   b. the amino group of one binds with the carboxyl group of the other
   c. a covalent bond is formed between the two amino acids
   d. water is removed from between the two amino acids
   e. All of these occur in the formation of peptide bonds.

___ 42. The helical or spiral structure of a protein best describes its _____ structure.
   a. primary
   b. secondary
   c. tertiary
   d. quaternary

___ 43. Heat irreversibly changes the _____ structure of proteins.
   a. primary
   b. secondary
   c. tertiary
   d. quaternary

___ 44. Hemoglobin and cytochrome molecules are good examples of conjugated (combined) proteins in which the protein is bound to
   a. carbohydrate molecules
   b. lipid molecules
   c. pigment molecules

___ 45. Which of the following is *not* a function of proteins?
   a. add structure or strength to connective tissues
   b. prevent water loss through the skin
   c. catalyze reactions as enzymes
   d. serve as antibodies, preventing infection
   e. serve as cell membrane receptors and carrier molecules
   f. All of these are functions of proteins.

B. True or False/Edit

___ 46. The specific sequence of amino acids is part of the genetic information prescribed by the sequence of nucleic acids.

___ 47. Differences among proteins are due to differences in the functional or R groups of each amino acid.

___ 48. Disulfide (S-S) bonds between neighboring amino acids are strong covalent bonds stabilizing the secondary structure of proteins.

___ 49. Lipoproteins are found in cell membranes and in the plasma or fluid portion of the blood.

___ 50. No other type of molecule in the body serves a wider variety of functions as those served by the proteins.

CHAPTER REVIEW

Please Note: An additional review of chemistry is summarized in **Appendix A** of the laboratory manual entitled, *A Laboratory Guide to Human Physiology, Concepts and Clinical Applications,* by Stuart I. Fox, that accompanies our textbook.

A. Completion
51. _____ spheres are formed when water molecules surround charged particles or _____ which, in turn, attract other water molecules.
52. Molecules that are soluble in water and, therefore, _____ (polar/nonpolar) are said to be **hydro**_____ (philic/phobic); while molecules composed of covalent bonds such as fat molecules are _____ (polar/nonpolar), express few charges, are insoluble in water, and are said to be hydro _____ (philic/phobic).
53. Hydrogen bonding between water molecules is responsible for many of the physical properties of water, including _____ tension and _____ action.
54. An acid is defined as a molecule that can _____ (gain/release) protons (H$^+$) in a solution; thus an acid _____ (raises/lowers) the number of H$^+$ in a solution and _____ (raises/lowers) the pH.
55. Complete this bicarbonate-carbonic acid buffer reaction:
    _____ + H$^+$ ↔ H$_2$CO$_3$
    (bicarbonate)   (_____)   (_____)
56. The three hexose sugars that are structural isomers with the formula C$_6$H$_{12}$O$_6$, are _____, _____, and _____.
57. Animal starch, or _____, is composed of repeating units of _____ molecules and is stored in both the _____ and muscle tissue.
58. Triglycerides are lipids formed _____ by of one molecule of _____ with _____ (#) molecules of _____ acids.
59. The structure of steroid molecules is unique. They feature _____ (#) six-carbon rings joined to one _____ - carbon ring. This structure is seen in the important steroid molecule of the body known as _____, which is the precursor for most steroid hormones in the body. These steroids are primarily synthesized by the _____, _____, and _____ cortex tissues.
60. Proteins are composed of different combinations of _____ (#) individual amino acids, whose amino and _____ groups bind to form _____ bonds; and whose functional or R groups interact to twist the protein into a helix (_____ structure) and then bend and fold onto itself (_____ structure) to form the active protein.
61. Specific regulator proteins found in cell membranes may serve as _____ for other molecules such as hormones, while specific transport molecules are called protein _____.

B. Crossword Puzzle — Chemical Composition of the Body

Across
1. the major buffer molecule of the blood
3. weak bond holding water molecules together
7. molecules containing carbon and hydrogen
9. a glycoprotein secreted from goblet cells
11. common scale of acid-base units
12. element symbol for sodium
13. organic molecule containing carbonyl functional groups
14. element with four valence electrons; forms four bonds
16. functional group found on an alcohol
17. steroids synthesized by the gonads
19. long fatty acid chains with double bonds present
21. what an atom becomes after losing electrons from outermost orbital
24. substance required in hydrolysis reactions
25. water is an example of a _____ solvent
30. solution in which the pH < 7.0
31. also known as "neutral" fat
34. the genetic code macromolecule
35. what results when one or more electrons are gained
36. any charged element or compound

Down
2. bond where electrons are shared equally
4. carbohydrates are composed of carbon, hydrogen, and _____
5. the pigment portion of hemoglobin
6. organic acid functional group
8. bonds in which electrons are shared between two or more atoms
10. fatty acids with no double bonds
11. organic molecule with primary, secondary, and tertiary structure
15. covalent, hydrogen, or ionic _____
18. substance that binds or releases H+ ions in order to stabilize pH
20. nuclear particle most involved in the formation of chemical bonds
22. composed of a nucleus and orbital electron(s)
23. molecule with three six-carbon rings and one five-carbon ring
26. functional group of an amino acid is the R or _____
27. chemical symbol for chlorine
28. solution with pH less than

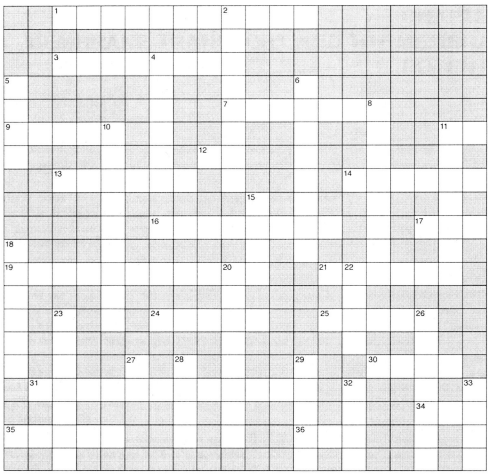

C. Essay

Essay Tutorial

This essay tutorial will answer the first essay question found in the "**Review Activities**" section of each chapter in your *Human Physiology* textbook. Please look for essay question 1. at the end of chapter 2, read it carefully, and let me guide you through one possible answer. Watch for helpful tips and general suggestions on writing the essay or short-answer questions. Learn to spot key words in the questions such as "**Compare**" and "**contrast**" that I have indicated below in bold-face type, and to outline your ideas quickly on a separate piece of paper. This will help you organize your thoughts, express yourself clearly, and result in better test scores. Using similar techniques, try the bonus essay questions that follow on your own. Enjoy!

62. **Compare** and **contrast** nonpolar covalent bonds, polar covalent bonds, and ionic bonds.

Answer. "Compare and contrast" calls for a list of similarities and differences among the three types of bonds, as follows:

Bond	Similarities and Differences
Nonpolar covalent	Share electrons — equally! Results in no +/- charges or "poles." Bond is the strongest.
Polar covalent	Share electrons — equally! Results in + (positive) or - (negative) charges or "poles." O, N, and P are electronegative. Weaker than nonpolar, yet stronger than ionic bonds.
Ionic	Do *not* share electrons! Electrons gained (for example, Cl to Cl⁻) or lost (for example, Na to Na⁺) as NaCl is dissolved in water, Cl⁻ anion; Na⁺ cation. Weakest of three bonds

Note: Although these are "essay" or "short-answer" style questions, in the sciences such as in physiology, answers need not be written in prose or composition-style. Often an answer such as the one above is better organized and displayed more clearly in outline form such as this, or in graphic form, even though the statements may not be complete sentences. Later, your review for exams will be made easier because the information has been condensed and, best of all, it has been assembled and written by you!

63. Since the hydrogen ion (H^+) is, in fact, a proton; what is the molar concentration of H^+ in pure water at 25 C; and explain what changes in H^+ concentration are required both to raise and to lower the pH value of a solution.

64. Describe the carboxyl, hydroxyl, and carbonyl functional groups; include their differences in chemical structure and the corresponding classes of organic molecules they form.

65. Describe dehydration synthesis (or condensation) in the formation of a peptide bond between two neighboring amino acids.

66. List the four main components of a triglyceride molecule; and describe basic differences between saturated and unsaturated fatty acids.

67. Name the lipid class of molecules that forms micelles; and describe the process of micelle formation in water, indicating the direction of the hydrophilic and hydrophobic parts.

68. Describe the primary, secondary, tertiary, and quaternary structures of proteins and how, together, these specific shapes control the specialized activities and functions of these proteins.

Answers — Chapter 2

I. Atoms, Ions, and Chemical Bonds
   A. 1. a, 2. e, 3. a, 4. d, 5. d, 6. a, 7. e, 8. c
   B. 9. F—Organic molecules contain both carbon and hydrogen, 10. T, 11. F—Switch "atomic mass" and "atomic number," 12. F—Replace "cation" with "anion," 13. T, 14. F—Replace "lower" with "raise," 15. T, 16. T, 17. F—Correct: "L-amino acid and D-sugar."
   C. 18. d, 19. f, 20. g, 21. a, 22. c, 23. b, 24. e
   D. See figure 2.10 in the text

Carbonyl	—C=O	
Hydroxyl	—OH	
Sulfhydryl (SH)	—SH	
Amino (NH$_2$)	—NH$_2$	
Carboxyl (COOH)	—C=O, OH	
Phosphate (H$_2$PO$_4$)	—O—P(=O)—OH, OH	

II. Carbohydrates and Lipids
   A. 25. c, 26. c, 27. a, 28. c, 29. d, 30. a
   B. 31. F—Replace "galactose" with "fructose", 32. T, 33. F—Replace "dehydration synthesis" with "hydrolysis," 34. F—Replace "nonpolar" with "polar," 35. F—Replace "a saturated" with "an unsaturated", 36. T, 37. T, 38. T, 39. T

III. Proteins
   A. 40. c, 41. e, 42. b, 43. c, 44. c, 45. f
   B. 46. T, 47. T, 48. F—Replace "secondary" with "tertiary," 49. T, 50. T

Chapter Review
   A. 51. Hydration; ions, 52. polar; philic; nonpolar; phobic, 53. surface; capillary, 54. release; raises; lowers, 55. HCO$_3^-$; (hydrogen ion); (carbonic acid) 56. glucose; fructose; galactose 57. glycogen; glucose; liver 58. condensation; glycerol; three; fatty 59. three; five; cholesterol; testes; overies; adrenal 60. twenty; carboxyl; peptide; secondary; tertiary 61. receptors; carriers

B. Crossword Puzzle

		¹B	I	C	A	R	B	O	²N	A	T	E					
									O								
			³H	Y	D	R	⁴O	G	E	N							
⁵H					X		P				⁶C						
E					Y		⁷O	R	G	A	N	I	⁸C				
⁹M	U	C	U	¹⁰S		G		L			R		O			¹¹P	H
E				A		E		¹²N	A		B		V			R	
			¹³K	E	T	O	N	E		R		O		¹⁴C	A	R	B	O	N
				U					¹⁵B		X		L			T	
				R		¹⁶H	Y	D	R	O	X	Y	L		¹⁷S	E	X
¹⁸B				A					N		L		N			I	
¹⁹U	N	S	A	T	U	R	A	T	²⁰E	D		²¹C	²²A	T	I	O	N
F				E					L				T				
F		²³S		D		²⁴W	A	T	E	R		²⁵P	O	L	A	²⁶R	
E		T							C				M				E	
R		E			²⁷C	²⁸A		T			²⁹H			³⁰B	A	S	E
	³¹T	R	I	G	L	Y	C	E	R	I	D	E		³²M			I		³³N
		O				I		O			L			O			³⁴D	N	A
³⁵A	N	I	O	N		D		N		³⁶I	O	N					U		C
		D								X							E		L

21

CHAPTER 3
CELL STRUCTURE AND GENETIC CONTROL

CHAPTER SCOPE

In this chapter the organic molecules we carefully assembled in chapter 2 will be used to construct a model of a typical **cell**. For now, the cell we build can be any tissue cell — a *neuron, muscle fiber, epithelial* cell or *connective tissue* cell. However, an image of your completed cell should be stored in your memory so that instant recall of its internal structure is available to you during the next three chapters when: cytoplasmic *enzyme* activities are described (chapter 4); cell *respiration and metabolism* in and around the mitochondria are featured (chapter 5); and, detailed descriptions of *cell membrane transport*, including *osmosis and diffusion*, are presented (chapter 6).

Currently the cell **membrane** and the membranes of interior organelles are the focus of intense research efforts. The cell membrane is composed primarily of phospholipids, protein (often with carbohydrates attached), and cholesterol. This active, ever-changing cell boundary appears to be ultimately regulated by the DNA in the nucleus. Within the cell's cytoplasm are the various **organelles**, some with their own surrounding membranes and some without, yet all are suspended in a flexible network of fluid and fibers that make up the **cytoskeleton**. Learning the structure and function of the cell organelles now is important. It will prepare you for understanding why these organelles are found within certain specialized cells and the roles they play as these cells interact with each other and with other tissues of the body.

The genetic information encoded within the molecules of DNA controls the cell's major activities, primarily from the nucleus. The overall purpose of DNA as described here is to: (1) direct the synthesis of RNA, which in turn, directs the synthesis of proteins for use inside the cell and those that will be packaged and secreted outside the cell; (2) prepare the cell for division (**mitosis**); and (3) oversee the formation of sperm and egg gametes (**meiosis**).

I. CELL MEMBRANE AND ASSOCIATED STRUCTURES

The cell is the basic unit of structure and function in the body. Many of the functions of cells are performed by particular subcellular structures known as organelles. The cell membrane allows selective communication between the intracellular and extracellular compartments and aids cellular movements.

A. Multiple Choice

___ 1. The cell membrane is composed primarily of protein and
   a. phospholipids
   b. carbohydrates
   c. nucleic acids
   d. amino acids

___ 2. Which of the following is *not* a function of protein in the cell membrane?
   a. structural support
   b. DNA synthesis
   c. enzymatic control of chemical reactions
   d. receptors for hormones and other regulatory molecules
   e. cellular "markers" or antigens

___ 3. Which of the following organic molecules is *not* commonly found to play an active role in the cell membrane?
   a. carbohydrates
   b. protein
   c. cholesterol
   d. nucleic acids

___ 4. Exocytosis, is best described by the following example of
   a. phagocytosis
   b. pinocytosis
   c. receptor-mediated invagination
   d. secretory vesicle fusion and content release

___ 5. The formation of a food vacuole primarily results from the process of
   a. phagocytosis
   b. pinocytosis
   c. receptor-mediated invagination
   d. exocytosis

B. True or False/Edit

___ 6. The hydrophobic core of cell (plasma) membranes restricts the passage of fat and fat-soluble molecules into and out of the cell.

___ 7. The specialized functions and selective transport properties of the cell (plasma) membrane are believed to be due to its protein content.

___ 8. The flexibility of the cell (plasma) membrane is partly due to the unique ratio between cholesterol and phospholipid molecules present in the membrane.

___ 9. Certain white blood cells (WBCs) and liver cells can help protect the body from invading microorganisms by the process of cellular "eating," or pinocytosis.

___ 10. Both cilia and flagella are composed of microtubule protein pairs arranged in a characteristic "9 + 2" arrangement.

II. CYTOPLASM AND ITS ORGANELLES

Many of the functions of a cell that are performed in the cytoplasmic compartment result from the activity of specific structures called organelles. Among these are the lysosomes, which contain digestive enzymes, and the mitochondria, where most of the cellular energy is produced. Other organelles participate in the synthesis and secretion of cellular products.

A. Multiple Choice

___ 11. Worn-out organelles and phagocytic by-products are characteristically digested within the structure known as a
   a. primary lysosome
   b. secondary lysosome
   c. residual body
   d. secretory vesicle

___ 12. DNA molecules can be found both in the nucleus and in
   a. ribosomes
   b. lysosomes
   c. the Golgi apparatus
   d. mitochondria
   e. the endoplasmic reticulum

___ 13. The organelle that stores calcium ions (Ca^{2+}) in striated (skeletal) muscle cells and is involved in steroid hormone metabolism is the
   a. ribosome
   b. lysosome
   c. Golgi apparatus
   d. mitochondria
   e. endoplasmic reticulum

___ 14. Membranes folded into cristae with matrix material involved in the production of ATP (energy), are characteristics of the organelle known as the
   a. ribosome
   b. lysosome
   c. Golgi apparatus
   d. mitochondria
   e. endoplasmic reticulum

___ 15. Autophagy, a process that destroys worn-out organelles so that they can be continuously replaced, is a function of the
   a. cytoskeleton
   b. lysosome
   c. Golgi apparatus
   d. mitochondria
   e. endoplasmic reticulum

B. True or False/Edit

___ 16. Microtubules and microfilaments are protein fibers that help form the cytoskeleton and provide movement of materials within the cell.

___ 17. Most, if not all, molecules in the cell have a limited life span, and thus must be continuously destroyed and replaced.

___ 18. All of the mitochondria in the cells of an adult were derived from that individual's mother, that is, derived from mitochondria present in her ovum upon fertilization.

___ 19. Smooth endoplasmic reticulum would naturally be abundant in cells that are active in protein synthesis, such as salivary gland cells involved in secretion.

___ 20. The phenomenon of "tolerance" to certain substances, such as drugs, may be accompanied by an increase in the rough endoplasmic reticulum, particularly in liver cells.

___ 21. Mitochondria may be able to reproduce themselves, especially in cells that require greater than normal energy outputs.

C. Label the Figure — The Generalized Cell and the Principal Organelles

It is important to be able to recognize and identify the principal organelles and other important structures of a cell. In figure 3.1 below, write the name of the organelle or structure indicated on the numbered answer line. Then check your work against figure 3.1 in the text and correct any mistakes. How is your spelling? Can you recall the major functions of each organelle and structure?

III. CELL NUCLEUS AND NUCLEIC ACIDS

The genetic code is based on the structure of DNA and is expressed through the structure and function of RNA. DNA and RNA are composed of subunits called nucleotides, and together these molecules are known as nucleic acids. The genetic code is based on the sequences of DNA nucleotides, which serve to direct the synthesis of RNA molecules. It is through the RNA-directed synthesis of proteins that the genetic code is expressed.

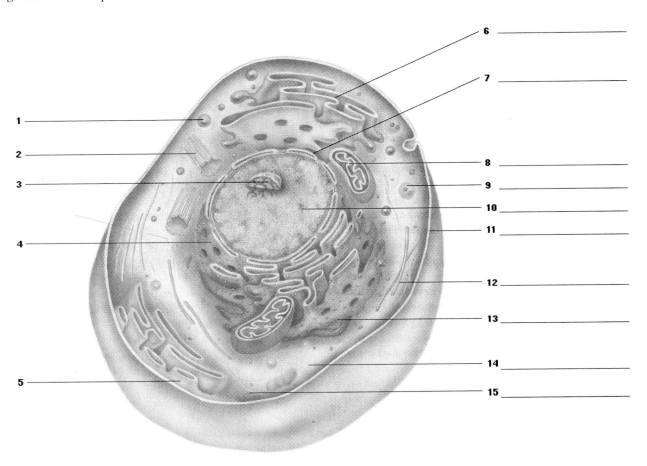

Figure 3.1 The generalized cell and the principal organelles

A. Multiple Choice

___ 22. A five-carbon sugar, a phosphate group, and a nitrogenous base combine to form a larger molecule known as a
   a. protein
   b. nucleic acid
   c. nucleotide
   d. phospholipid
   e. hydrocarbon

___ 23. The nitrogenous base in DNA that is *not* found in RNA is
  a. adenine
  b. guanine
  c. thymine
  d. cytosine
  e. uracil
___ 24. Which of the following is *not* a type of ribonucleic acid (RNA)?
  a. messenger
  b. mitochondrial
  c. transfer
  d. ribosomal
___ 25. Introns (noncoding DNA) and exons (coding DNA) are parts of a gene responsible for directly ordering the synthesis of
  a. pre-mRNA
  b. mRNA
  c. rRNA
  d. tRNA
___ 26. The RNA type that diffuses through nuclear pores to direct the assembly or synthesis of new protein molecules at the ribosomes is
  a. pre-mRNA
  b. mRNA
  c. rRNA
  d. tRNA

B. True or False/Edit
___ 27. Although DNA is the largest molecule in the cell, it has a simpler structure than that of most proteins.
___ 28. The number of purine bases in DNA is equal to the number of pyrimidine bases.
___ 29. Only DNA and mRNA are double-stranded nucleic acids.
___ 30. Positively charged histone proteins spool around negatively charged strands of DNA molecules in the nucleus to form larger chromatin particles called nucleosomes.
___ 31. All three types of RNA are formed from the genetic information contained in the DNA of the nucleus.
___ 32. The synthesis of RNA molecules from DNA is called genetic translation.
___ 33. The genes located within the nucleoli code for the production of messenger RNA (mRNA).
___ 34. Noncoding segments of DNA scattered along a gene that do not participate in transcription of the genetic code are called exons.

IV. PROTEIN SYNTHESIS AND SECRETION

In order for a gene to be expressed, it first must be used as a guide, or template, in the production of a complementary strand of messenger RNA. This mRNA is then itself used as a guide to produce a particular type of protein whose sequence of amino acids is determined by the sequence of base triplets (codons) in the mRNA.

A. Multiple Choice
___ 35. Translation is best defined as the synthesis of
  a. mRNA, tRNA, and rRNA from DNA in the nucleus
  b. pre-mRNA only from DNA in the nucleus
  c. specific proteins from the mRNA base sequence code
  d. new, complementary strands of DNA in the nucleus
___ 36. The RNA type characterized by bending on itself to form a cloverleaf structure that twists further into an upside down "L" shape is called
  a. pre-mRNA
  b. mRNA
  c. rRNA
  d. tRNA
___ 37. Aminoacyl-tRNA synthetase is an enzyme that joins a specific _____ molecule to the end of the tRNA molecule to which it is complementary.
  a. nucleic acid
  b. amino acid
  c. pentose sugar
  d. protein
  e. nucleotide

____ 38. Which of the following is *not* a function of the Golgi apparatus?
   a. preparing proteins for in-cell use
   b. further modification of new proteins (for example, glycoproteins or glycolipids)
   c. organizing proteins by function and destination
   d. packaging the final proteins and shipping them to their destination

B. True or False/Edit

____ 39. The sequence of three bases (a base triplet) in tRNA is called a codon, while the complementary triplet in mRNA is called an anticodon.

____ 40. Proteins that are synthesized for specific functions within a particular cell possess a hydrophobic leader sequence that permits the entry of these proteins into the cisterna of the rough endoplasmic reticulum.

____ 41. The Golgi apparatus and endoplasmic reticulum are responsible for applying the finishing touches on proteins destined for secretion out of the cell.

V. DNA SYNTHESIS AND CELL DIVISION

When a cell is going to divide, each strand of the DNA within its nucleus acts as a template for the formation of a new complementary strand. Organs grow and repair themselves through a type of cell division known as mitosis. The two daughter cells produced by mitosis contain the same genetic information as the parent cell. Gametes contain only half the number of chromosomes as their parent cell and are formed by a type of cell division called meiosis.

A. Multiple Choice

____ 42. The enzyme required to replicate DNA is called
   a. aminoacyl-tRNA synthetase
   b. RNA polymerase
   c. DNA polymerase

____ 43. The phase of the cell cycle during which DNA replicates itself is known as _____ phase.
   a. G_2
   b. G_1
   c. S
   d. M

____ 44. One very important tumor suppressor gene that indirectly blocks the uncontrolled stimulation of cell division common in cancer, is known as
   a. an oncogene
   b. a centrosome
   c. p53
   d. cyclin D

____ 45. The cellular structures composed of protein microtubules that form spindle fibers and pinch off newly formed daughter cells during cell division, best describe the
   a. nucleoli
   b. mitochondria
   c. centrosomes and centrioles
   d. Golgi and endoplasmic reticulum
   e. ribosomes

____ 46. Which of the following share identical base sequences?
   a. two homologous chromosomes
   b. two chromatids
   c. DNA transcribed to mRNA
   d. mRNA translated to tRNA
   e. two X sex chromosomes

____ 47. Which of the following statements about meiosis is *false*?
   a. Each daughter cell is genetically identical to the parent cell.
   b. Final daughter cells are gametes, either four sperm or a single ova.
   c. Each daughter cell contains a total of twenty-three chromosomes.
   d. Each daughter cell receives, at random, either the maternal or the paternal chromosome from each homologous pair.
   e. Crossing-over or mixing of maternal and paternal chromosomes may occur.

B. True or False/Edit

____ 48. DNA is the only type of molecule in the body capable of replicating itself.

____ 49. "Semiconservative" means only one of the two DNA strands is needed to synthesize pre-mRNA during transcription.

____ 50. The nondividing cell is in a part of its life cycle known as interphase, which is further subdivided into G_1, S, and G_2 phases.

___ 51. The nucleus contains twenty-three homologous pairs of autosomal chromosomes, or forty-six chromosomes total.
___ 52. Homologous chromosomes have identical DNA base sequences.
___ 53. Genes that promote the formation of cancer (oncogenes) may cause uncontrolled cell division by activating a specialized group of proteins known as cyclins.
___ 54. Polycythemia is defined as an abnormal increase in the number of circulating red blood cells (RBCs) in the blood, and therefore, is an example of hypertrophy.

CHAPTER REVIEW

A. Matching

___ 55. contains purine and pyrimidine subunits
___ 56. short, stubby DNA of dividing cells
___ 57. formed by the process of endocytosis
___ 58. DNA plus histone protein in nondividing cells
___ 59. has "9 + 2" microtubule pairs (in airways)
___ 60. "powerhouse" organelle of the cell
___ 61. process forming daughter cells called gametes
___ 62. location for RNA synthesis
___ 63. characterized by a fluid-mosaic composition
___ 64. structure responsible for sperm motility
___ 65. forms vesicles for protein secretion
___ 66. right-angle microtubules forming spindles
___ 67. organelle featuring cisternae that process new proteins
___ 68. primary, secondary, or residual bodies
___ 69. process forming two identical daughter cells
___ 70. cell death by shrinking and membrane bubbling
___ 71. proteins known to alter phases of the cell cycle
___ 72. fingerlike projections that aid rapid diffusion

a. cilium
b. cell membrane
c. mitochondrion
d. chromatin
e. flagellum
f. Golgi apparatus
g. endoplasmic reticulum
h. chromosome
i. lysosome
j. nucleus
k. nucleotide
l. meiosis
m. vesicle or vacuole
n. centrioles
o. mitosis
p. microvilli
q. cyclins
r. apoptosis

B. Completion

73. The membranes of cells are dynamic blends of organic molecules, such as _____, _____, and _____, of which the _____ molecules are thought most responsible for _____ transport and other specialized functions of the membrane.

74. "Amoeboid" movements of the cell require cytoplasmic extensions known as _____, which pull the cell along. Other tiny hairlike projections, or _____, from epithelial cells lining the respiratory passages transport sticky _____; while those of the female _____ tract carry the female gamete or _____. Movement is always toward the _____ (inside/outside) of the body. The flagellum is only found on _____ cells, the male gamete.

75. The three methods of endocytosis are _____, _____, and _____-_____ endocytosis. The reverse process, the secretion of proteins and other molecules from secretory vesicles to the _____-cellular (intra/extra) fluid, is known as _____.

76. The organelle that is capable of dividing by itself and that contains DNA derived from the _____ (ovum/sperm) is the _____.

77. Complete the following descriptions of DNA and RNA structure.

Nucleotides:

DNA
(1) _____ sugar
(2) phosphate
(3) base
(a) two purines
adenine
_____
(b) two pyrimidines
_____

RNA
(1) _____ sugar
(2) _____
(3) nitrogenous _____
(a) two purines
_____
(b) two pyrimidines
_____
cytosine

27

In DNA, the base adenine always binds to _____, and the base cytosine always binds to _____. In RNA, the only difference in binding is that adenine binds to _____.

78. Chromatin in a nondividing cell is composed of _____ and postively charged proteins called _____. These proteins spool around negatively charged DNA molecules to form particles known as _____. Histones may act to _____ (stimulate/repress) the expression of genes. The familiar form of DNA is the short, stubby _____, which is seen only when it is _____ (active/inactive) in the _____ (dividing/nondividing) cell. From our parents we inherit genetic information through our _____, which orders the transcription and _____ (synthesis) of only one type of organic molecule: _____.

79. Of the forty-six chromosomes in an adult, _____ (#) are called autosomes and the remaining _____ (#) are the sex chromosomes. In other words, of the twenty-three pairs of chromosomes in an adult, _____ (#) pairs are called autosomes and the remaining _____ (#) pair(s) are the sex chromosomes.

C. Sequencer — Cellular Events

80. In sequence, number the following cellular events as they should occur, starting from the uptake of amino acids into the cytoplasm and ending with the synthesis of a new protein for secretion to the outside of the cell.
Note: Step 1 has been done for you.

___ Newly formed polypeptide (protein) is transported to the Golgi apparatus.
___ Translation occurs as mRNA, tRNA, and rRNA assemble amino acids, forming a growing polypeptide chain with a leader sequence.
___ RNA polymerase unzips the DNA and directs the synthesis of pre-mRNA (transcription).
_1_ Amino acids from blood and extracellular fluid are transported into the cell cytoplasm.
___ The leader sequence is removed during polypeptide synthesis; and, after completion, the new protein floats in the cisternae destined for export.
___ Exocytosis of newly made proteins from the cell membrane.
___ Aminoacyl-tRNA synthetase enzymes locate specific incoming amino acids and bind them to their respective tRNA molecules prior to transcription.
___ Vesicles with new proteins enclosed leave the Golgi apparatus and fuse with the cell membrane.
___ New mRNA diffuses out of the nucleus to the ribosomes attached to the rough endoplasmic reticulum.
___ Newly synthesized proteins are modified and packaged into specialized vesicles.

Now, return to the figure of a cell you labeled in Section II, part C (figure 3.1), and place the numbers from the sequence you completed above where they belong on the figure. This will illustrate the sequence of protein synthesis.

D. Crossword Puzzle — Cell Structure and Genetic Control

Across
1. Gene's "code" sequence of 3 bases
5. Body cells with the highest amount of cholesterol
6. Sequence of 3 bases on messenger (mRNA)
7. The lipid-protein barrier that separates the intracellular from the extracellular
9. Phosphate, sugar, and a nitrogen base
13. Undigested waste in a lysosome is a residual _____
14. Interphase, G_1, S, G_2, and mitosis are parts of the cell's _____
19. The cell with all its component parts is considered a single _____
20. The network of tubules for packaging proteins
21. A dalmatian dog has these
22. Microtubular structure found in all sperm
24. A long, narrow ditch
26. Another name for a tavern
27. The RNA codon for the DNA triplet-AAA
29. Also known as reduction division
30. Membranous sac formed during endocytosis
31. Growth due to an increase in cell number
32. Organelle where mRNA is translated and new proteins are made
35. The process of protein assembly at the ribosome
37. Sex chromosomes designating a female
38. Nonmembranous mass of two rodlike centrioles

Down
1. Small nail; or sailing term
2. Vegetable much like a bean, with pods; soup
3. A type of endocystosis known as "cell eating"
4. Regions of noncoding DNA within a gene
5. DNA replication with one new and one original strand
8. The "A" in DNA or RNA
10. The RNA codon for the DNA triplet-ATC
11. Membrane-bound vesicle with powerful enzymes
12. The process of engulfing by the membrane
15. DNA in a nondividing cell
16. Structure that produces ribosomal RNA for ribosomes
17. The "powerhouse" of the cell
18. Face of the telephone, rotary or push button
22. Another name for triglyceride molecules
23. Rough or smooth _____ reticulum

25. Adenine or guanine
28. The inner fluid portion of mitochondria
29. Month after April
33. Part of a nucleotide is a nitrogen _____

34. The planet Earth has only one _____
36. Genetic defect involving lysosomes, _____-Sachs disease

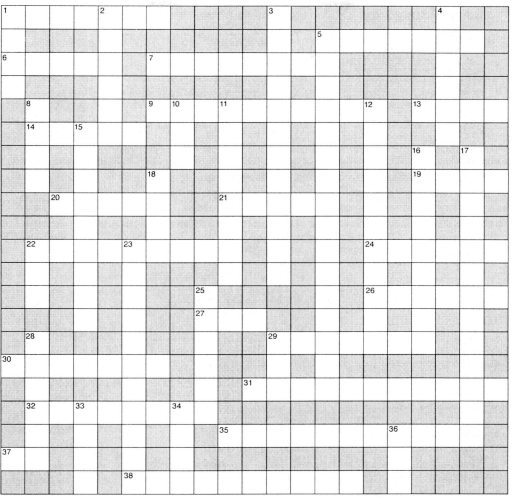

E. Essay

Essay Tutorial

This essay tutorial will answer the first essay question found in the "**Review Activities**" section of your *Human Physiology* textbook. Please look for question 1 at the end of chapter 3, read it carefully, and let me guide you through one possible answer. Watch for key terms in bold-face type, helpful tips and general suggestions on writing the essay or short-answer questions. Enjoy!

81. The cell membrane is an extremely **dynamic** structure. Using **examples**, explain **why** this statement is true.

Answer. The word "dynamic" implies that the membrane is *not* static — that it is energetic, vigorous, and has a tendency to change spontaneously. The "examples" will come from analysis of the membrane composition. The major molecules of membrane structure and specialized function are the proteins —

suspended inside, outside, and throughout the phospholipid bilayer "core" — which are able to move laterally and act in a variety of ways. These actions of proteins include:

1. Structural support or cell shape — including membrane extensions, such as cilia and flagella. With proteins are cholesterol molecules blended into the membrane to alter its flexibility, which is needed by red blood cells to squeeze through capillaries.
2. Cell movements — pseudopod formation during amoeboid movements, such as phagocytosis. Also, all forms of endocytosis (pinocytosis and phagocytosis) and exocytosis are included.
3. Membrane transport — movement of certain molecules across the membrane, a process known as selective permeability.
4. Control of chemical reactions at the membrane by controlling the enzymes (which are proteins) present on the membrane surfaces.
5. Protein receptor molecules for hormones and other regulatory molecules that arrive at the outer membrane surface. Some of these receptors initiate endocytosis and exocytosis (see 2., above).
6. Cellular "markers" or antigens that identify blood and tissue types. Glycoprotein and glycolipids are examples.

OK! How did you do? Now try to answer a few of mine, below.

82. Compare and contrast the structure and function of microtubules in the cell. Include their roles in such structures as cytoskeleton, cilia, flagella, centrioles, and spindle fibers in your answer.

83. Discuss the origin, the three types, and the various functions of lysosomes in the cytoplasm of cells.

84. List and describe the four types of ribonucleic acid (RNA), their structural differences, and the role each plays in protein synthesis.

85. In two columns, list the similarities and differences between mitosis and meiosis.
    Mitosis   Meiosis

Answers — Chapter 3
I. Cell Membrane and Associated Structures
   A. 1. a, 2. b, 3. d, 4. d, 5. a
   B. 6. F—Replace "restricts" with "does not restrict," 7. T, 8. T, 9. F—Replace "pinocytosis" with "phagocytosis," 10. T

II. Cytoplasm and Its Organelles
   A. 11. b, 12. d, 13. e, 14. d, 15. b
   B. 16. T, 17. T, 18. T, 19. F—Replace "smooth" with "rough," 20. F—Replace "rough" with "smooth," 21. T
   C. See figure 3.1 in the text

III. Cell Nucleus and Nucleic Acids
   A. 22. c, 23. c, 24. b, 25. a, 26. b
   B. 27. T, 28. T, 29. F— "mRNA" is single-stranded, 30. T, 31. T, 32. F—Replace "translation" with "transcription," 33. F—Replace "messenger RNA (mRNA)" with "ribosomal RNA (rRNA)," 34. F—Replace "exons" with "introns"

IV. Protein Synthesis and Secretion
   A. 35. c, 36. d, 37. b, 38. a
   B. 39. F—Switch "tRNA" and "mRNA," 40. F—Leader sequences are found only on proteins for export, 41. T

V. DNA Synthesis and Cell Division
   A. 42. c, 43. c, 44. c, 45. c, 46. b, 47. a
   B. 48. T, 49. F—"Semiconservative" means that half of the DNA formed during replication is new; the other half is original, 50. T, 51. F—There are twenty-two pairs of autosomes, or forty-four total, 52. F—Replace "identical" with "different," 53. T, 54. F—Replace "hypertrophy" with "hyperplasia"

VI. Chapter Review
   A. 55. k, 56. h, 57. m, 58. d, 59. a, 60. c, 61. l, 62. j, 63. b, 64. e, 65. f, 66. n, 67. g, 68. i, 69. o, 70. r, 71. q, 72. p
   B. 73. protein; phospholipid; cholesterol; protein; selective, 74. pseudopods; cilia; mucus; genital; ovum; outside; sperm, 75. phagocytosis; pinocytosis; receptor-mediated; extra; exocytosis, 76. ovum; mitochondrion
   77. (1) deoxyribose   (1) ribose
       (2)   (2) phosphate
       (3) nitrogenous   (3) base
           (a) guanine   (a) adenine,
           (b) thymine,   guanine
               cytosine   (b) uracil
                                    cytosine
   thymine; guanine; uracil,
   78. DNA, histones; nucleosome; repress; chromosome, inactive, dividing; DNA, translation, protein. 79. forty-four; two; twenty-two; one
   C. 80. 7, 5, 3, 1, 6, 10, 2, 9, 4, 8

D. Crossword Puzzle

	1 T	R	I	2 P	L	E	T			3 P				4 I	
	A			E						H		5 S	C	H	W	A	N	N
6 C	O	D	O	N		7 M	E	M	B	R	A	N	E		T	
K				T					G		M				R	
	8 A			I		9 N	10 U	C	11 L	E	O	T	I	D	12 E		13 B	O	D	Y
	14 C	15 Y	C	L	E		A		Y		C		C		N		N	
	I	H					G		S		Y		O		D		16 N		17 M
	D	R		18 D			O		T		N		O		19 U	N	I	T
	20 G	O	L	G	I		21 S	P	O	T	S		C		C		T	
		M		A			O		S		E		Y		L		O	
22 F	L	A	23 G	E	L	L	U	M		I		R		24 T	R	E	N	C	H
A		T	N				E		S		V		O		O		H	
T		I	D		25 P				A		26 S	A	L	O	O	N	
	N	O		27 U	U	U		T		I		U		N	
28 M		P		R		29 M	E	I	O	S	I	S		D	
30 V	A	C	U	O	L	E		I		A	V		R	
T		A		N		31 H	Y	P	E	R	P	L	A	S	I	A
32 R	33 I	B	O	S	34 O	M	E						O	
I	A		M		O		35 T	R	A	N	S	L	A	36 T	I	O	N
37 X	X		S	I	O							A	
		E	38 C	E	N	T	R	O	S	O	M	E	Y	

31

CHAPTER 4
ENZYMES AND ENERGY

CHAPTER SCOPE

In the last chapter we learned about the amino acid composition and the structure of proteins. We also studied the process by which proteins are synthesized from information coded in the genes of the chromosomes. Of the body proteins, perhaps the most important group are the **enzymes** — the subject of this chapter. These molecules act as biological catalysts, speeding up chemical reactions in such diverse regions of the body as the stomach and intestine during digestion (chapter 17), in the blood and kidney where the enzyme **carbonic anhydrase** helps maintain *acid-base balance* (chapter 15), and within target cells where various enzymes activate *second messenger systems* in response to visiting hormones (chapter 11). Enzymes also serve as critical facilitators of *cell respiration* and other important metabolic pathways that take place in the cytoplasm and within the mitochondria of all cells to combust fuel molecules and provide energy for the cell's many activities (chapters 5, 18).

As we will see in chapter 5, each step in the breakdown of fuel food molecules and the transfer of energy to **adenosine triphosphate (ATP)** is catalyzed by a specific enzyme. Yet a single defective gene will direct the synthesis of a defective enzyme. Such defective enzymes can cause *inborn errors of metabolism* — which in severe cases may cause nervous system disorders or even death. Because most enzymes are proteins, the delicate tertiary structure of enzymes must be maintained for normal catalysis. Changes in acid-base balance (such as *acidosis* or *alkalosis*) or variations in body temperature (such as *hyperthermia* or *hypothermia*) can disturb this precise architecture and interfere with the ability of enzymes to regulate metabolism.

With a job this vital to life, it is no wonder that enzymes recruit help from other molecules — namely, **coenzymes** and **cofactors**. In this chapter, we will be introduced to two important coenzymes, *NAD* and *FAD*, both derived from water-soluble B vitamins. In similar fashion, these coenzymes function as carriers of hydrogen atoms, shuttling these atoms from place to place along metabolic pathways of the cell. In the next chapter on cell respiration, a third coenzyme (*coenzyme A*) is introduced that will join NAD and FAD in assisting the many metabolic enzymes working to extract and transfer energy from fuel foods to high-energy ATP molecules.

I. ENZYMES AS CATALYSTS

Enzymes are biological catalysts that function to increase the rate of chemical reactions. Most enzymes are proteins, and their catalytic action results from their complex structure. The great diversity of protein structure allows different enzymes to be specialized in their action.

A. Multiple Choice

___ 1. A catalyst is a chemical substance that
    a. increases the rate of a reaction
    b. is not itself changed by the reaction
    c. does not change the nature of the reaction
    d. does not change the final result of the reaction
    e. All of these describe a catalyst.

___ 2. Catalysts make reactions go faster by
    a. increasing the energy level of the reactants
    b. lowering the activation energy
    c. raising the temperature of the reaction
    d. reducing the repulsion between ions within the reactants

___ 3. In enzyme-catalyzed reactions, the reactant molecules are better known as
    a. active sites
    b. substrates

       c. enzyme-substrate complexes
       d. products
____ 4. Enzymes that rearrange atoms within their substrate molecules to form products with the same composition but with a different structure, are called
       a. hydrolases
       b. phosphatases
       c. synthetases
       d. isomerases
____ 5. Different models of the same enzyme (they must have the same active site and catalyze the same reaction) made by different tissues are called
       a. isomers
       b. isomerases
       c. isoenzymes
       d. isomodels

B. True or False/Edit
____ 6. Most proteins are enzymes.
____ 7. Without enzymes all chemical reactions simply will not run.
____ 8. Energy of activation is the amount of energy required for a reaction to proceed.
____ 9. There are enzymes whose names do *not* have the characteristic "-ase" ending, or suffix.
____ 10. Isoenzymes display the same active site and catalyze the same chemical reaction but will differ in composition and structure elsewhere in the molecules.

C. Matching — Enzyme Terms
____ 11. specific binding site for the substrate   a. activation energy
____ 12. another name for substrate molecule   b. isoenzyme
____ 13. formed from enzyme-substrate   c. enzyme
         complex   d. reactant
____ 14. biological catalyst   e. active site
____ 15. enzyme made by different tissues   f. product
____ 16. what is lowered by enzymes

II. CONTROL OF ENZYME ACTIVITY

The rate of an enzyme-catalyzed reaction depends on the concentration of the enzyme, the pH and temperature of the reaction, and on a number of other factors. Genetic control of enzyme concentration, for example, affects the rate of progress along particular metabolic pathways and thus regulates cellular metabolism.

A. Multiple Choice
____ 17. Which of the following does *not* alter enzyme activity?
       a. the temperature and pH of the solution
       b. the concentration of cofactors and coenzymes present
       c. the concentration of oxygen present
       d. the concentration of enzyme and substrate molecules present
____ 18. Pepsin, an enzyme secreted by the stomach lining, would be expected to have an *optimal* pH of
       a. 2
       b. 4
       c. 7.4
       d. 9
       e. 14

____ 19. Which of the following is *least* likely to act as a cofactor?
   a. calcium
   b. magnesium
   c. copper
   d. oxygen
   e. zinc

____ 20. In enzyme-catalyzed reactions, cofactors bind directly to the
   a. enzyme
   b. active site
   c. substrate
   d. Cofactors bind to all of these locations.
   e. Cofactors bind to none of these locations.

____ 21. Coenzymes participate in enzyme-catalyzed reactions by
   a. lowering the activation energy required
   b. transporting hydrogen atoms and small molecules from one enzyme to another
   c. binding to the enzyme, causing conformational changes
   d. providing the pH and temperature optima for the reactions

____ 22. "Saturation" in an enzyme-catalyzed reaction means that the _____ are saturated with _____.
   a. products; enzymes
   b. substrates; products
   c. enzymes; substrates
   d. products; substrates

____ 23. Allosteric inhibition is a mechanism along metabolic pathways by which
   a. inhibition of an earlier step at a branch point along that pathway occurs
   b. structural changes at the active site occurs to interfere with the enzyme
   c. the final product inhibits an earlier enzymatic step (end-product inhibition)
   d. All of these statements describe allosteric inhibition.

____ 24. Inborn errors of metabolism that cause disease result in a (an) _____ (increase/decrease) in the amount of intermediates formed prior to the defective step, and a (an) _____ (increase/decrease) in the number of final products formed along alternate pathways.
   a. increase; increase
   b. increase; decrease
   c. decrease; increase
   d. decrease; decrease

____ 25. The inborn error of metabolism that all newborn babies are tested for and that, once detected, can be controlled by a diet low in one specific amino acid, is known as
   a. albinism
   b. phenylketonuria (PKU)
   c. Gaucher's disease
   d. Tay-Sachs disease
   e. lactose intolerance

B. True or False/Edit

____ 26. Higher temperatures decrease the rate of enzyme activity by altering the tertiary structure of the enzyme.

____ 27. The rate of enzyme activity is decreased by concentrations of hydrogen ion (pH), which are either too high or too low.

____ 28. Alkaline phosphatase is an enzyme with a pH optimum having a lower number than that of acid phosphatase enzymes.

____ 29. Cofactors are derived from water-soluble vitamins.

____ 30. Given a certain number of enzymes, increasing the number of substrate molecules will increase the number of products formed.

____ 31. Reversible reactions are often catalyzed by two different enzymes, one for each direction in the reaction.

___ 32. During metabolism, the product formed by one enzyme can become the substrate for the next enzyme in the pathway.
___ 33. During metabolism, one intermediate can serve as a substrate for two different enzymes, thus ultimately forming two different products.
___ 34. In end-product inhibition, the function of the last product formed is inhibited.

III. BIOENERGETICS

Living organisms require the constant expenditure of energy to maintain their complex structures and processes. Central to life processes are chemical reactions that are coupled, so that the energy released by one reaction is incorporated into the products of another reaction. The transformation of energy in living systems is largely based on reactions that produce and destroy molecules of ATP and on oxidation-reduction reactions.

A. Multiple Choice

___ 35. Which of the following statements about entropy is *false*?
    a. It describes the degree of disorganization of a system.
    b. It is increased as energy is changed to another form.
    c. As it increases the amount of free energy available to do work is reduced.
    d. It is defined by the first law of thermodynamics.
    e. All of these statements regarding entropy are true.

___ 36. Which of the following statements about exergonic reactions is *false*?
    a. They can release energy in the form of heat.
    b. They convert molecules with less free energy to molecules with more free energy.
    c. The combustion of glucose to CO_2 and H_2O is an example.
    d. They convert molecules with less entropy to molecules with more entropy.
    e. All of these statements regarding exergonic reactions are true.

___ 37. Which of the following statements about oxidation-reduction reactions is *false*?
    a. Reducing agents donate electrons to another atom or molecule.
    b. Oxidizing agents accept electrons from another atom or molecule.
    c. An atom or molecule cannot be both an oxidizing and reducing agent.
    d. Oxidation and reduction are always coupled reactions.
    e. All of these statements regarding oxidation-reduction reactions are true.

___ 38. The final electron acceptor in a chain of oxidation-reduction reactions that provides energy for ATP production in the cell is
    a. oxygen
    b. proton (H^+)
    c. electron (e^-)
    d. water
    e. ATP

B. True or False/Edit

___ 39. The first law of thermodynamics states that entropy can be neither created nor destroyed.
___ 40. Only organized or free energy can be used to perform work.
___ 41. Photosynthesis is an example of an endergonic reaction.
___ 42. A calorie is a unit of free energy.
___ 43. Living cells are able to use heat energy to drive most chemical reactions.
___ 44. The breakdown of ATP → ADP + P_i is an exergonic reaction.
___ 45. Oxygen is a very strong oxidizing agent and, thus, a strong electron acceptor in oxidation-reduction reactions.
___ 46. NAD is a coenzyme derived from vitamin B_2.
___ 47. A molecule such as NAD or FAD can be an electron acceptor in one reaction and an electron donor in another.

CHAPTER REVIEW

A. Completion

Assume you have recently consumed a delicious cheeseburger as a source of body fuel. Also, assume that digestion and absorption into the body was successful such that simple sugars (like glucose) from carbohydrates, triglycerides from lipids, and amino acids from proteins are now present in your body cells. Here, the amino acids floating in the cytoplasm are used to make biological catalysts, or 48. _____, as instructed by DNA. The various metal ions assist enzymes by working as 49. _____, while the water-soluble vitamins work primarily as 50. _____. Under optimal conditions of 51. _____ and 52. _____, enzymes can speed up the metabolism of your cheeseburger fuels, releasing 53. _____ from chemical bonds. Therefore, these reactions are 54. _____ (endergonic/exergonic). The combustion of glucose as fuel in the cell results in the formation of 55. _____ and water; while some of the chemical-bond energy is transferred to "high-energy" bonds of 56. _____ or (_____), and the rest of the energy is lost as 57. _____. The formation of this "universal energy carrier" is 58. _____ (endergonic/exergonic), providing the cell with a usable form of energy.

In a similar fashion, triglycerides and amino acids can be combusted in the cell, transferring energy to power the cell's many energy-requiring processes. Complete combustion of these fuels requires that we breathe so that blood can deliver the gas 59. _____, which is the final electron 60. _____ (acceptor/donor) in the cell. In the final step of metabolism, this gas is ultimately 61. _____ (oxidized/reduced) to form 62. _____.

B. Crossword Puzzle — Enzymes and Energy

Across
1. bioenergetics incorporates these first and second laws
3. the cell's "universal energy carrier"
7. reactions that require energy input
10. oxidizing or reducing _____
11. different model of the same enzyme
13. compounds mainly derived from water-soluble vitamins
15. inborn error of phenylalanine (amino acid) metabolism
17. when an atom or molecule gains electrons
18. a new term, or number used to measure the ability of enzymes to convert substrates into products
20. an enzyme acts as a biological _____
21. an enzyme in blood/liver that breaks down hydrogen peroxide
23. a metal ion such as Ca^{2+}, Mg^{2+}, Mn^{2+}, Cu^{2+}, or Zn^{2+}
24. the precise protein structure altered by pH and temperature
26. enzymes work by lowering the energy of _____
28. a unit of heat measurement
30. _____-product inhibition
31. degree of disorganization or less free energy (*hint:* second law of thermodynamics)

Down
2. reactions that release energy
4. enzymes are most affected by pH and _____
5. biological catalyst described in this chapter
6. most metabolic pathways are not linear; rather they are _____
8. loss of electrons from an atom or molecule
9. the first law of thermodynamics conserves _____
12. the pigment missing in the albino due to a defective gene in DNA
14. also known as the *reactant* for enzyme-catalyzed reactions
16. inborn errors of _____

19. a coenzyme derived from vitamin B_2 (riboflavin)
22. energy that is organized and can be used to perform work
25. reversible chemical reactions must obey the law of _____ action
27. a hydrogen-carrying coenzyme derived from niacin
29. the universal suffix for enzymes
32. all enzymes work best at their optimal _____

C. Essay

Essay Tutorial

This essay tutorial will answer the first essay question found in the "**Review Activities**" section of your *Human Physiology* textbook. Please look for question 1. at the end of the chapter 4, read it carefully, and let me guide you through one possible answer. Watch for key terms in bold-face type, helpful tips and general suggestions on writing the essay or short-answer questions. Go ahead try this one, and a few of mine that follow!

63. Explain the relationship between the chemical **structure** and the **function** of an enzyme, and describe how various conditions may alter both the structure and function of an enzyme.

Answer. Most enzymes are proteins. Therefore enzymes exhibit primary, secondary, tertiary, and even quaternary structure. Since enzymes must bind to substrates with the three-dimensional precision of a lock-and-key, any change in the enzyme (the lock) structure can interfere with binding by the substrate (the key).

Inborn errors of metabolism are inherited defects in the gene (DNA) which direct alterations of the enzyme's primary structure (amino acid sequence) and, thus, can cause disease by reducing the activity or the "fit" between the substrate and the enzyme active site. In this way the tertiary structure (bending and folding) of the active site region of the enzyme determines its efficiency. Variation in both pH and temperature from some optimal value can distort or "warp" the delicate active site, reducing the "activity" of the enzyme and decreasing the number of products formed. Finally, the normal function of many enzymes requires the help of coenzymes and/or cofactors obtained from raw material such as vitamins and minerals, respectively. Consequently, a diet deficient in these raw materials can result in less productive enzyme-catalyzed reactions.

64. Describe what is meant by the term "isoenzyme," and include one example of an isoenzyme whose various forms rise abnormally high in the blood, thus aiding in the diagnosis of certain diseases. [*Hint*: see Table 4.2]

65. Describe the variation in the pH experienced by your cheeseburger (from the Completion section) as it travels along the mouth, stomach, and small intestine (pancreas). From each of these locations, name one enzyme, state its optimal pH, and describe a reaction catalyzed by each enzyme. [*Hint*: see Table 4.3]

Note: These last two essay questions were written from information provided by tables — then, would it not make sense to answer each question using a similar table format? Try it!

66. Using phenylketonuria (PKU) as an example, explain how inborn errors of metabolism are inherited and describe how these errors can alter metabolism.

67. Explain the step-by-step processes that occur in the cytoplasm as the chemical-bond energy in glucose is transferred to the "high-energy" bonds of adenosine triphosphate (ATP).

Answers — Chapter 4

I. Enzymes as Catalysts
   A. 1. e, 2. b, 3. b, 4. d, 5. c
   B. 6. F—Most enzymes are proteins, 7. F—Without enzymes reactions *will* run, but much more slowly, 8. T, 9. T, 10. T
   C. 11. e, 12. d, 13. f, 14. c, 15. b, 16. a

II. Control of Enzyme Activity
   A. 17. c, 18. a, 19. d, 20. d, 21. b, 22. c, 23. d, 24. a, 25. b
   B. 26. T, 27. T, 28. F—Replace "lower" with "higher," 29. F—Replace "cofactors" with "coenzymes," 30. T, 31. T, 32. T, 33. T, 34. F—End-product inhibition features inhibition of earlier steps by the last product

III. Bioenergetics
   A. 35. d, 36. b, 37. c, 38. a
   B. 39. F—Replace "entropy" with "energy," 40. T, 41. T, 42. F—Replace "free" with "heat," 43. F—Heat energy is lost from the cell and can't be used, 44. T, 45. T, 46. F—Replace "B_2" with "B_3," 47. T

Chapter Review
   A. 48. enzymes, 49. cofactors, 50. coenzymes, 51. pH, 52. temperature, 53. energy, 54. exergonic, 55. CO_2, 56. adenosine triphosphate; ATP, 57. heat, 58. endergonic, 59. O_2, 60. acceptor, 61. reduced, 62. water

B. Crossword Puzzle

			1.T	2.H	E	R	M	O	D	Y	N	A	M	I	C	S		3.A	4.T	P
				X											5.E			E		
		6.B		7.E	N	D	E	R	G	8.O	N	I	C		N			M		
		R		R						X				9.E		Z		P		
		A	10.A	G	E	N	T			11.I	S	O	E	N	Z	Y	M	E		
		N		O				12.M		D				E		M		R		
	13.C	O	E	N	Z	Y	M	E		A		14.S		R		E		A		
	H		I					L		T		U		G				T		
	E		C					A		I		B		Y			15.P	K	U	
	D	16.M						N		O		S						R		
		17.R	E	D	U	C	T	I	O	N		18.T	U	R	N	O	V	E	R	
	19.F		T					N				R								
20.C	A	T	A	L	Y	S	T		21.C	A	T	A	L	A	S	E				
	D		B						T					22.F						
		23.C	O	F	A	C	T	O	R		24.T	E	R	T	I	A	R	Y		
25.M			L						E											
26.A	C	T	I	V	A	T	I	O	N		27.C	28.A	L	O	R	I	E			
S			S					N		A		S								
S			M			30.E	N	D		31.E	N	T	R	O	P	Y				
														H						

CHAPTER 5
CELL RESPIRATION AND METABOLISM

CHAPTER SCOPE

To place this chapter in perspective, we must realize that all living cells have a continuous need for **energy (ATP)** to perform functions such as membrane transport and generating membrane potentials (chapter 6), transmitting electrical impulses (chapters 7-10), hormone synthesis and secretion (chapter 11), and muscle contraction (chapters 12-14). Ultimately, the energy for these activities comes from the fuel foods we consume, digest, and absorb (digestion: chapter 17); deliver to our cells (circulation: chapters 13 and 14); and combust or metabolize along enzyme-catalyzed pathways. As we learned in the last chapter, much of this energy is lost as heat energy (measured in *calories*) and the remainder is transferred to the synthesis of ATP, which "energizes" cellular functions. We are prepared now to ask questions about cell respiration and to analyze the combustion processes that run continuously in all living cells, thereby maintaining homeostasis.

When we breathe in, where in the body does the *oxygen* go? And, where does the *carbon dioxide* come from that we exhale? And how does this exchange of gases relate to the combustion of fuel food molecules such as **glucose**, **fat** (triglycerides), and **amino acids** and to the subsequent transfer of energy to ATP? Answers to these questions and others regarding **cell respiration** are discussed here.

Also, this chapter illustrates how the metabolic demands for ATP are met by exercising skeletal muscle and other active tissues. A continuous supply of glucose as fuel for ATP synthesis is made available by the carefully regulated cooperation between the *liver* and *muscle* **glycogen** stores. In this way, the concentration of glucose in the blood is maintained homeostatically stable, critical for normal brain and tissue function.

I. GLYCOLYSIS AND THE LACTIC ACID PATHWAY

In cellular respiration, energy is released by the stepwise breakdown of glucose and other molecules, and some of this energy is used to produce ATP. The complete combustion of glucose requires the presence of oxygen and yields thirty ATP per glucose. Some energy can be obtained, however, in the absence of oxygen by the pathway that leads to the production of lactic acid. This process results in the net gain of two ATP per glucose.

A. Multiple Choice

____ 1. Synthesis of large, energy — storage molecules best describes
   a. anabolism
   b. metabolism
   c. catabolism

____ 2. Which of the following molecules is *not* used as a primary source of energy for the cellular synthesis of ATP?
   a. glucose
   b. fatty acids
   c. nucleic acids
   d. amino acids
   e. All of these molecules are used for ATP synthesis.

____ 3. Which of these is *not* a final product of aerobic cell respiration?
   a. carbon dioxide
   b. water
   c. oxygen
   d. energy (ATP)

___ 4. In the respiration of glucose to two molecules of pyruvic acid, four atoms of _____ are removed.
   a. carbon
   b. hydrogen
   c. oxygen
   d. carbon dioxide

___ 5. Which of the following statements about glycolysis is *false*?
   a. It results in the formation of two molecules of pyruvic acid.
   b. It results in the net gain of two ATP molecules.
   c. It can occur with or without oxygen present.
   d. It is exergonic.
   e. All of these statements about glycolysis are correct.

___ 6. As a result of anaerobic respiration, glucose is converted to
   a. pyruvic acid
   b. lactic acid
   c. citric acid
   d. acetyl CoA

___ 7. The organ most responsible for extracting and converting lactic acid to pyruvic acid, and which ultimately reforms and releases free glucose into the bloodstream, is the
   a. liver
   b. brain
   c. cardiac muscle
   d. skeletal muscle
   e. kidney

___ 8. The process in question 7, which describes the conversion of noncarbohydrate molecules into glucose, is known as
   a. glycogenolysis
   b. glycogenesis
   c. gluconeogenesis
   d. glycolysis

___ 9. The Cori cycle is the process by which
   a. liver glycogen is exchanged for muscle glycogen
   b. blood glucose is stored as liver glycogen
   c. muscle lactic acid is stored as muscle glycogen
   d. blood lactic acid is converted to glucose by the liver
   e. liver glucose is converted to lactic acid and released into the bloodstream

B. True or False/Edit

___ 10. Aerobic respiration and ventilation describe two different processes.
___ 11. During aerobic respiration the oxygen we breathe in is converted into carbon dioxide we breathe out.
___ 12. Glycolysis can take place both inside and outside the mitochondrion organelles of the cell.
___ 13. Anaerobic respiration (or lactic acid fermentation) yields a net gain of two ATP molecules.
___ 14. Anaerobic respiration (or lactic acid fermentation) in the cell does not require the presence of oxygen.
___ 15. It is common for certain tissues like skeletal muscle to derive energy (ATP) from anaerobic respiration without permanent injury or damage to the tissue.

II. AEROBIC RESPIRATION

In the aerobic respiration of glucose, pyruvic acid is formed by glycolysis and then converted into acetyl coenzyme A. This begins a cyclic metabolic pathway called the Krebs cycle. As a result of these pathways, a large amount of reduced NAD and FAD (NADH and FADH$_2$) is generated. These reduced coenzymes provide electrons for an energy-generating process that drives the formation of ATP.

A. Multiple Choice

___ 16. In addition to energy (ATP), what is (are) the final product(s) of aerobic respiration?
   a. O_2 and CO_2
   b. CO_2 and H_2O
   c. O_2 and H_2O
   d. CO_2 only

___ 17. Following aerobic respiration, approximately what percent of the chemical bond energy present in a glucose molecule is captured in high-energy bonds of ATP?
   a. 40%
   b. 50%
   c. 60%
   d. 70%
   e. 80%

___ 18. The vitamin from the diet that is converted into coenzyme A and that combines with acetic acid in the mitochondrion is
   a. niacin (B_3)
   b. pantothenic acid
   c. riboflavin (B_2)
   d. pyridoxine (B_6)
   e. vitamin C

___ 19. Which of the following processes does *not* occur during the completion of one circuit around the Krebs cycle?
   a. One GTP molecule is converted to one ATP molecule.
   b. Three NAD molecules are reduced by electrons (H's).
   c. One molecule of oxygen is combined with hydrogen to form water.
   d. One molecule of FAD is reduced by electrons (H's).

___ 20. Which of the following molecules is *not* part of the electron transport chain?
   a. cytochrome
   b. flavoprotein
   c. coenzyme Q
   d. coenzyme A
   e. All of these are part of the electron transport chain.

___ 21. All of the following are formed as a result of the electron transport chain, *except*
   a. carbon dioxide
   b. oxidized NAD
   c. water
   d. ATP
   e. oxidized FAD

___ 22. The **chemiosmotic theory** involves the participation of proton (H^+) pumps that are found within the
   a. nuclear membrane
   b. plasma (cellular) membrane
   c. mitochondrial inner membrane
   d. mitochondrial outer membrane
   e. lysosomal membrane

___ 23. Cyanide is a poison that blocks the electron transfer from cytochrome a_3 to oxygen, therefore *directly* interrupting
   a. glycolysis
   b. Krebs cycle
   c. oxidative phosphorylation
   d. gluconeogenesis

24. The grand total number of ATP molecules generated by the complete aerobic respiration of glucose is
    a. twelve
    b. twenty-four
    c. thirty
    d. thirty-eight
    e. forty-six
25. The breakdown of stored glycogen into individual molecules of glucose-6-phosphate occurs during the process known as
    a. glycolysis
    b. gluconeogenesis
    c. glycogenolysis
    d. glycogenesis
26. The enzyme, found *only* in the liver, that removes phosphate groups and can, thus, release free glucose into the blood, is
    a. glycogen synthetase
    b. glucose-6-phosphatase
    c. glycogen phosphorylase
    d. glucose isomerase
27. Glucose molecules entering skeletal muscle fibers from the blood are "trapped" when quickly converted to
    a. pyruvic acid
    b. glucose-1-phosphate
    c. glucose-6-phosphate
    d. glycogen

B. True or False/Edit

28. In aerobic respiration, the catabolism of a glucose molecule forms pyruvic acid, not lactic acid.
29. The conversion of pyruvic acid to acetyl CoA occurs in the cytoplasm.
30. Glycolysis occurs in the mitochondrion.
31. Iron is the crucial atom within the cytochromes of the mitochondrion that participates in the electron transport chain.
32. Electron transport molecules are fixed within the inner membrane of the mitochondrion and are not part of the matrix.
33. The transfer of energy from the electrons of hydrogen atoms to ATP is an example of an endergonic reaction.
34. The formation of ATP along the electron transport chain, which requires the presence of O_2, is called oxidative phosphorylation.
35. Oxygen is the final electron acceptor of the electron transport chain.
36. The oxygen (O_2) we breathe in is ultimately converted to carbon dioxide (CO_2).
37. In oxidative phosphorylation, each electron pair from $FADH_2$ forms two molecules of ATP, while each electron pair from NADH forms three molecules of ATP.
38. Organic molecules with phosphate groups, such as glucose-6-phosphate, are intracellular "prisoners" and cannot "escape" the cell by crossing the cell membrane.
39. Skeletal muscle can supply the liver with energy in the form of free glucose but the opposite is not true.
40. To maintain a steady supply of ATP, more glucose molecules would have to be burned in tissues that are anaerobic than if the tissues are supplied with oxygen.
41. During exercise, the liver can supply free glucose to many tissues of the body that may have depleted glycogen stores, including the exercising muscles.

III. METABOLISM OF LIPIDS AND PROTEINS

Triglycerides can be hydrolyzed into glycerol and fatty acids. The latter are of particular importance, because they can be converted into numerous molecules of acetyl CoA, that can enter Krebs cycles and generate a large amount of ATP. Amino acids derived from proteins may also be used for energy. This involves deamination (removal of the amine group) and the conversion of the remaining molecule into either pyruvic acid or one of the Krebs cycle molecules.

A. Multiple Choice

___ 42. *Acetyl CoA* is an important metabolic intersection that can lead to the formation of all of the following substances, *except*
   a. CO_2 via Krebs cycle
   b. cholesterol and steroids
   c. ketone bodies
   d. fatty acids and triglycerides
   e. All of these substances are formed from acetyl CoA.

___ 43. The two intermediates of the glucose combustion pathway that directly link glucose metabolism to fat metabolism are
   a. pyruvic acid and phosphoglyceraldehyde
   b. acetyl CoA and pyruvic acid
   c. phosphoglyceraldehyde and acetyl CoA
   d. glucose and pyruvic acid

___ 44. Ranking the following stored energy forms from highest to lowest number of total calories available for the energy needs of the body, the proper sequence is
   1. glycogen (skeletal muscle); 2. glycogen (liver); 3. fat
   a) 1—2—3
   b) 3—2—1
   c) 3—1—2
   d) 2—3—1
   e) 1—3—2

___ 45. In the cytoplasm, the removal of two-carbon acetic acid molecules from the acid end of fatty acids is an important enzymatic process known as
   a. lipogenesis
   b. lipolysis
   c. ß-oxidation
   d. ketosis

___ 46. In the liver, fatty acid metabolism can result in the formation of excess acetyl CoA molecules; this "overflow" pathway ultimately results in the formation of
   a. lactic acid
   b. ketone bodies
   c. cholesterol
   d. bile

___ 47. The formation of nonessential amino acids from essential amino acids and carbohydrates is known as
   a. transamination
   b. ß-oxidation
   c. oxidative deamination
   d. urea cycle
   e. ketosis

48. The vitamin that serves as the required coenzyme for the successful activity of transaminase enzymes is
    a. niacin (B_3)
    b. riboflavin (B_2)
    c. pyridoxine (B_6)
    d. vitamin C
    e. pantothenic acid
49. The enzymatic removal of the amine group from one amino acid, forming ammonia (later converted to urea), and leaving behind a keto acid, is called
    a. ketosis
    b. ß-oxidation
    c. transamination
    d. oxidative deamination
    e. urea cycle
50. The catabolism (breakdown) of this energy source can require the liver to convert toxic ammonia molecules into urea molecules.
    a. carbohydrates
    b. proteins
    c. ketone bodies
    d. fats
51. Which of the following is *not* an energy source that can be found circulating in the bloodstream?
    a. glycogen
    b. glucose
    c. ketone bodies
    d. fatty acids
    e. amino acids
52. The organ with an absolute requirement for blood glucose as its primary energy source is the
    a. brain
    b. heart
    c. skeletal muscle
    d. liver
    e. All of these organs require glucose as its primary energy source.
53. The oxygen debt following strenuous exercise is due, in part, to the *extra* oxygen required for the metabolism of
    a. carbon dioxide
    b. lactic acid
    c. glycogen
    d. fatty acid
    e. None of these require extra oxygen.

B. True or False/Edit

54. Fatty acids are formed by the condensation of many two-carbon acetyl CoA molecules, resulting in the formation of long hydrocarbon chains.
55. Protein accounts for 15% to 20% of the stored calories in the body and is used extensively as an energy source.
56. Lipase enzymes specialize in catalyzing the hydrolysis of triglycerides into glycogen and free fatty acids.
57. Like glucose metabolism, ß-oxidation of fatty acids requires coenzymes NAD and FAD for the transfer of hydrogen atoms and the subsequent release of energy for ATP synthesis.
58. Ketone bodies can be used by many peripheral tissues as an energy source.

___ 59. Growing children excrete less nitrogen than they ingest, therefore they are in a state of *negative* nitrogen balance.
___ 60. Excess amino acids, not used for energy, can be converted to carbohydrate and/or to fat.
___ 61. Of the twenty amino acids required to synthesize protein, about twelve are essential, which means the body must make them.
___ 62. Keto acids can be used in the Krebs cycle as a source of energy, or converted to fat or glucose.

IV. CHAPTER REVIEW

A. Matching — Metabolism Terms

Match the metabolic process on the right with the best descriptive phrase numbered on the left. Write that letter in the space provided.

___ 63. cytochrome oxidation-reduction coupling
___ 64. "hydrogen pumps" explanation for oxidative phosphorylation
___ 65. glycogen to glucose-6-phosphate
___ 66. glucose synthesis from "other" sources
___ 67. one source of reduced NAD and FAD
___ 68. triglyceride to glycerol and fatty acids
___ 69. ATP formation from electron transport
___ 70. fatty acid to acetyl CoA molecules
___ 71. amino acid to keto acid and free amino
___ 72. blood lactic acid converted to glucose (liver)
___ 73. glucose to pyruvic acid (with or without O_2)
___ 74. formation of nonessential amino acids
___ 75. ammonia detoxification in the liver

a. gluconeogenesis
b. oxidative phosphorylation
c. transamination
d. ß-oxidation
e. electron transport system
f. Cori cycle
g. chemiosmotic theory
h. urea cycle
i. glycolysis
j. glycogenolysis
k. Krebs cycle
l. lipolysis
m. oxidative deamination

B. Label the Figure — Cell Metabolic Pathways

The most important metabolic processes are summarized in the text in figure 5.18. Test yourself by attempting to name as many intermediates as possible in figure 5.1 below — then compare your answers with the text figure. As a post-test, erase your work and come back later (before your next exam!) and try it again. Don't expect to name them all the first time — these concepts are difficult.

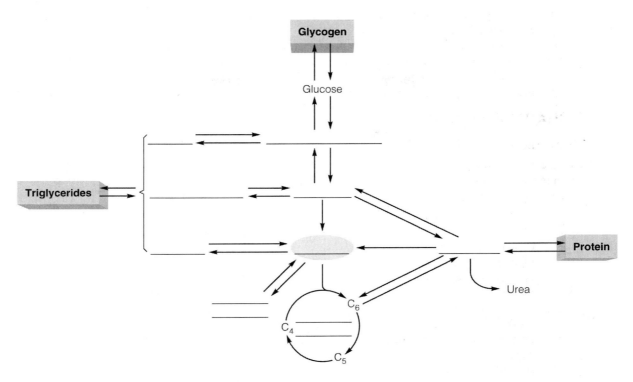

Figure 5.1 Simplified metabolic pathways showing how glycogen, fat (triglycerides), and protein can be interconverted.

C. Matching — Metabolism Compartments

So far in this text we have learned many processes that take place in specific parts of the cell, such as the cytoplasm, plasma membrane, and organelles (ribosomes, mitochondria, among others). These locations can be thought of as "**compartments.**" In this exercise, select the letter of the compartment listed on the right that normally features the process described by the numbered phrases on the left. Write that letter in the space provided.

(*Note*: an answer may be used more than once.)

____ 76. Electron transport chain chemiosmotic "hydrogen pumps"
____ 77. Protein synthesis (translation) of enzymes for metabolism
____ 78. Krebs cycle
____ 79. ß-oxidation of fatty acids to acetyl CoA
____ 80. Blocks transport of phosphorylated molecules
____ 81. Glucose conversion to pyruvic acid molecules
____ 82. Formation of acetyl CoA from pyruvic acid, linking glycolysis to the Krebs cycle
____ 83. Conversion of glycerol to phosphoglyceraldehyde

a. cytoplasm
b. plasma membrane
c. ribosome
d. mitochondrion (membranes)
e. mitochondrion (matrix)

___ 84. Conversion of O_2 gas to water in the electron transport system

___ 85. Formation of CO_2 gas from carboxyl groups

___ 86. Formation of lactic acid from glucose

D. Essay

Essay Tutorial

This essay tutorial will answer the first essay question found in the "**Review Activities**" section of your *Human Physiology* textbook. Please look for question 1 at the end of chapter 5, read it carefully, and let me guide you through one possible answer. Watch for key terms in bold-face type, helpful tips and general suggestions on writing the essay or short-answer questions. Enjoy!

87. **State** the advantages and disadvantages of **anaerobic respiration**.

Note: "**State**" does not necessarily mean to simply "list" or "outline" Rather, it means to describe first the advantages, then the disadvantages, using phrases or complete sentences. Numbering your points may help to organize your answer and assist the reader/instructor in separating each statement. Your discussion then becomes more than just a numbered list. Also notice that by defining the key word "anaerobic" at the start, we help establish a foundation for the rest of the answer. When finished, try a couple of my essay questions that follow, OK?

Answer. Anaerobic respiration refers to the conversion of glucose in the cytoplasm of living cells to pyruvic acid and then to lactic acid, when there exists a temporary absence of oxygen.

Advantages
1. Glycolysis of glucose to pyruvic acid is allowed to continue, despite the fact that fewer ATP (two) are synthesized. This provides cells with a backup or emergency source of ATP.
2. Some peripheral tissues such as skeletal muscles commonly function anaerobically without injury or cell damage for short periods of time.
3. Red blood cells (RBCs) respire anaerobically, thus conserving the hemoglobin-bound O_2 for the tissues.

Disadvantages
1. The potential to make twenty-eight more ATP from glucose is lost.
2. The accumulation of lactic acid in tissues such as skeletal muscle leads to an overall acidosis. By altering the active sites of enzymes, acidosis can interrupt metabolism and lead to the inadequate production of ATP and fatigue.
3. The extra lactic acid produced may place a burden on the liver, that may already be overworked with the Cori Cycle and glycogenesis reactions.
4. Anaerobic respiration is only a temporary backup system for periods of intermittent lack of oxygen and cannot be used as a primary source of energy.

88. You have just consumed a delicious bowl of sugary cereal! In outline form, trace the metabolic pathways taken by the <u>extra</u> glucose molecules as they are converted to triglycerides.

89. So far, you have been introduced to many vitamins that play important roles in metabolism. Briefly, describe the function and physiologic importance of niacin (B₃), riboflavin (B₂), pantothenic acid, and pyridoxine (B₆).

90. We inhale to supply cells with oxygen, and we exhale to exhaust the carbon dioxide by-products of metabolism. In your own words, describe the specific metabolic process in the cell in which O_2 is consumed, as well as the three specific metabolic processes in which CO_2 is produced.

Answers — Chapter 5

I. Glycolysis and the Lactic Acid Pathway
   A. 1. a, 2. c, 3. c, 4. b, 5. e, 6. b, 7. a, 8. c, 9. d
   B. 10. T, 11. F—Replace "carbon dioxide" with "water," 12. F—Glycolysis occurs only in the cytoplasm, 13. T, 14. T, 15. T

II. Aerobic Respiration
   A. 16. b, 17. a, 18. b, 19. c, 20. d, 21. a, 22. c, 23. c, 24. c, 25. c, 26. b, 27. c
   B. 28. T, 29. F—Replace "cytoplasm" with "mitochondrial membrane", 30. F—Replace "mitochondrion" with "cytoplasm", 31. T, 32. T, 33. F—Replace "endergonic" with "exergonic", 34. T, 35. T, 36. F—Replace "carbon dioxide (CO_2)" with "water", 37. T, 38. T, 39. F—Switch "skeletal muscle" and "liver", 40. T, 41. T

III. Metabolism of Lipids and Proteins
   A. 42. e, 43. c, 44. c, 45. c, 46. b, 47. a, 48. c, 49. d, 50. b, 51. a, 52. a, 53. b
   B. 54. T, 55. F—Proteins are not used daily for energy, 56. F—Replace "glycogen" with "glycerol", 57. T, 58. T, 59. F—Replace "negative" with "positive", 60. T, 61. F—There are eight (nine in children [histidine]) essential amino acids which must be included in the adult diet; cells make nonessential amino acids through transamination, 62. T

IV. Chapter Review
   A. 63. e, 64. g, 65. j, 66. a, 67. k, 68. l, 69. b, 70. d, 71. m, 72. f, 73. i, 74. c, 75. h
   B. See figure 5.18 in the text
   C. 76. d, 77. c, 78. e, 79. a, 80. b, 81. a, 82. d, 83. a, 84. d, 85. d and e, 86. a

CHAPTER 6
MEMBRANE TRANSPORT AND THE MEMBRANE POTENTIAL

CHAPTER SCOPE

The important activities that occur at the **plasma membrane** are fully explored in this chapter. To a large extent the protein and phospholipid molecules that make up the composition of the plasma membrane regulate the passage of materials either into or out of the cell's interior. The membrane does have pores through which many substances enter and exit by **simple diffusion**, traveling from higher to lower concentrations. In addition, metabolic gases such as O_2 and CO_2 follow their respective concentration differences (*gradients*) into and out of the cell. Finally, most triglycerides, steroids, and other fat — soluble (nonpolar) molecules may also diffuse across cell membranes based on their solubility in the phospholipid core.

The entry of many nutrients such as simple sugars (for example, glucose) and amino acids (for example, phenylalanine) is not simple, and therefore, requires selective protein "carriers" (**facilitated diffusion**). Other molecules not only require membrane carriers but also require that ATP's metabolic energy be expended in the effort to "pump" these molecules "uphill" in the direction that opposes the concentration gradient (**active transport**). Sodium ions (Na^+) and potassium ions (K^+) are separated from each other by active transport pumps located in the cell membrane. This separation of charged ions results in the *electrical membrane potential*, which in turn, leads to the formation of electrical impulses. Generated in the brain and elsewhere, and conducted throughout the nervous system, these impulses will be described in the next few chapters — running along sensory and motor neurons (chapters 8, 9, and 10) and along muscle fibers (chapter 12).

The movement of water across membranes is a unique form of simple diffusion, flowing from a region of high water concentration to an area of low water concentration (**osmosis**). The concentration of solutions in the body, such as plasma, is regulated by homeostasis and equals approximately 300 milliosmoles (300 mOsm) per liter of water. Nerve receptors (*osmoreceptors*) in the brain monitor body water concentration and, with the cooperation of specific hormones, such as **antidiuretic hormone (ADH)**, regulate the loss of water primarily from the kidney (chapter 16).

I. DIFFUSION AND OSMOSIS

Net diffusion of a molecule or ion through a cell membrane always occurs in the direction of its lower concentration. Nonpolar molecules can penetrate the phospholipid barrier, and small inorganic ions can pass through channels in the membrane. The net diffusion of water through a membrane is known as osmosis.

A. Multiple Choice

____ 1. Which of the following processes is *not* an example of carrier-mediated transport?
   a. facilitated diffusion
   b. osmosis
   c. active transport
   d. All of these processes are carrier-mediated.

____ 2. In general, which of the following substances can *not* pass easily through membranes by the process of simple diffusion?
   a. water
   b. most ions
   c. most lipid-soluble molecules
   d. most proteins or nucleotides
   e. most small organic molecules that are uncharged

___ 3. The energy that "drives" diffusion processes comes from
   a. thermal (heat) energy
   b. metabolic energy
   c. potential energy
   d. kinetic energy
___ 4. The movement of molecules or ions "uphill" from regions of lower to regions of higher concentrations is known as
   a. active transport
   b. facilitated diffusion
   c. osmosis
   d. simple diffusion
   e. None of these descriptions is correct.
___ 5. Which of the following substances can *not* cross the membrane by simple diffusion?
   a. O_2
   b. steroid hormone
   c. CO_2
   d. urea
   e. All of these substances can cross by simple diffusion.
___ 6. The rate of diffusion as measured by the number of diffusing molecules passing through the membrane per unit time is dependent on all of the following factors, *except*
   a. "steepness" of the concentration gradient
   b. simultaneous passage of water molecules
   c. permeability of the membrane to the diffusing substances
   d. surface area of that membrane
___ 7. Molecules that are osmotically active
   a. include plasma proteins such as albumin
   b. cannot readily diffuse across the cell membrane
   c. help regulate the flow of water between the tissues and the blood
   d. do not include water
   e. All of these statements are correct.
___ 8. Osmotic pressure is best defined as the force
   a. generated by the solute gradient across the membrane
   b. exerted by the osmotically active solutes
   c. exerted to oppose the movement of water (osmosis)
   d. generated by the membrane to pump water out of the cell
___ 9. Which of the following statements regarding osmotic pressure is *false*?
   a. Pure water has an osmotic pressure of zero.
   b. A 360 g/L glucose solution has twice the osmotic pressure of a 180 g/L glucose solution.
   c. The greater the solvent concentration, the greater its osmotic pressure.
   d. All of these statements regarding osmotic pressure are true.
___ 10. A 1.0 m glucose solution added to a 2.0 m NaCl solution would form a solution with a total *osmolality* of
   a. 2.0 Osm
   b. 3.0 Osm
   c. 4.0 Osm
   d. 5.0 Osm
___ 11. The milliosmolality of normal human plasma is about
   a. 180 mOsm
   b. 300 mOsm
   c. 0.3 mOsm
   d. 1.86 mOsm
___ 12. Which solution is *not* isotonic to plasma?
   a. 0.3 m glucose
   b. 5% dextrose
   c. 0.15 m NaCl

        d. normal saline
        e. All of these solutions are isotonic to plasma.
____ 13. Red blood cells (RBCs) bled into sea water will _____, since sea water is _____.
        a. crenate; hypotonic
        b. hemolyse; hypotonic
        c. crenate; hypertonic
        d. hemolyse; hypertonic
____ 14. Osmoreceptors, specialized neurons that monitor the osmolality of blood plasma, are located in the
        a. hypothalamus
        b. pituitary
        c. kidney
        d. heart

B. True or False/Edit

____ 15. Simple diffusion may describe the movement of either solute or solvent molecules.
____ 16. Some carrier - mediated processes may occur across the membrane of dead cells.
____ 17. When a concentration difference exists across a membrane, the diffusion of those molecules that are permeable will *strictly* be from the area of higher concentration to the area of lower concentration.
____ 18. Steroid molecules are able to diffuse across cell membranes without carriers because steroids are nonpolar molecules.
____ 19. O_2 and CO_2 gas exchange across the cell membrane occurs by simple diffusion down their respective concentration gradients.
____ 20. Osmosis can be described as water movement in the direction of less dilute to more dilute solutions.
____ 21. The resting neuron membrane is twenty times more permeable to Na^+ ions than to K^+ ions.
____ 22. Microvilli are tiny folds projecting from the apical membranes of epithelial cells found in the intestine and the kidney tubules, that serve to increase the surface area of these membranes for absorption.
____ 23. Osmosis is the net diffusion of water (the solute) across semipermeable membranes.
____ 24. The greater the solute concentration of a solution, the greater its osmotic pressure.
____ 25. One mole of glucose contains the same number of atoms or molecules as one mole of sucrose.
____ 26. One mole of glucose contains the same number of atoms or molecules as one mole of NaCl.
____ 27. Osmolality is determined by the ratio of solute to solvent particles in a solution, not by the chemical nature of the solute molecules.
____ 28. A solution may be isosmotic but not isotonic — as demonstrated when red blood cells are placed in a 0.3 m urea solution.
____ 29. Urea molecules diffuse easily across most cell membranes.
____ 30. Antidiuretic hormone (ADH) acts on the kidney to promote water loss from the body by opposing the reabsorption of water by the nephron.

C. Matching — Transport Process Terms

____ 31. may form tiny ion channels
____ 32. solute transport using thermal energy
____ 33. same osmolality as plasma
____ 34. major role for water in the body
____ 35. role of impermeable solutes in a solution
____ 36. simple diffusion of water
____ 37. concentration difference across cell membranes

a. simple diffusion
b. osmosis
c. gradient
d. solvent
e. solute
f. integral proteins
g. osmotically active
h. isosmotic
i. osmotic pressure

___ 38. a 5% dextrose in water solution
___ 39. molecule that dissolves in a solvent
___ 40. force required only to prevent osmosis
___ 41. solutions such as sea water
___ 42. solutions causing hemolysis
___ 43. hypothalamic neurons regulating plasma osmolality

j. osmoreceptors
k. isotonic
l. hypertonic
m. hypotonic

II. CARRIER — MEDIATED TRANSPORT

Molecules such as glucose are transported across the cell membranes by special protein carriers. Carrier-mediated transport in which the net movement is down a concentration gradient, and which is therefore passive, is called facilitated diffusion. Carrier-mediated transport that occurs against a concentration gradient, and which therefore requires metabolic energy, is called active transport.

A. Multiple Choice

___ 44. Which of the following is *not* a characteristic of membrane carrier proteins?
   a. specificity
   b. competition
   c. denaturation
   d. saturation

___ 45. The transport of glucose molecules from outside the cell, across the membranes, and into most tissue cells (*excluding* the intestine or kidney tubule) occurs by the process of
   a. active transport
   b. simple diffusion
   c. facilitated diffusion
   d. coupled transport

___ 46. Which of the following functions is *not* served by the steep Na^+/K^+ concentration gradient?
   a. It provides energy for the coupled transport of other molecules across the cell membrane.
   b. It keeps Na^+ and water molecules inside the cells.
   c. It can be adjusted by thyroid hormones to help regulate the basal metabolic rate (BMR) of the body.
   d. It serves to produce electrical impulses in nerve and muscle tissue.

___ 47. In the process of secondary active transport called membrane counter-transport (antiport), calcium ion (Ca^{2+})
   a. passively diffuses into the cell as Na^+ is actively moved out of the cell
   b. passively diffuses out of the cell as Na^+ is actively moved out of the cell
   c. is actively moved out of the cell as Na^+ passively diffuses into the cell
   d. is actively moved into the cell as Na^+ passively diffuses out of the cell

B. True or False/Edit

___ 48. Two amino acids can compete for the same carrier protein located in the cell membrane.
___ 49. Secondary active transport (counter-transport) is responsible for keeping the intracellular concentration of calcium (Ca^{2+}) ions very low.
___ 50. Across the cell membrane, both sodium and potassium ions are "pumped" down their concentration gradients.
___ 51. All cells in the body have variable numbers of Na^+/K^+ membrane pumps that are constantly active.

III. THE MEMBRANE POTENTIAL

*The permeability properties of the cell membrane, the presence of nondiffusible negatively charged molecules in the cell, and the action of the Na^+/K^+ pumps, produce an unequal distribution of charges across the membrane. As a result, the inside of the cell is negatively charged compared to the outside. This difference in charge, or potential difference, is known as the **membrane potential**.*

A. Multiple Choice

___ 52. Which of the following substances would *not* be considered a "fixed" anion within the cytoplasm of a cell?
  a. certain steroid molecules
  b. phosphate groups of ATP
  c. certain cellular proteins
  d. certain organic molecules

___ 53. To which of the following cations is the cell membrane most permeable?
  a. sodium
  b. potassium
  c. calcium
  d. iron

___ 54. The cation found in higher concentration inside than outside the cell is
  a. sodium
  b. potassium
  c. calcium
  d. hydrogen

___ 55. The Nernst equation is most often used to estimate the cell's
  a. resting membrane potential
  b. osmotic pressure
  c. threshold potential
  d. equilibrium potential for Na^+ ions or for K^+ ions

___ 56. Using the Nernst equation, the equilibrium potential for Na^+ is
  a. -90 mV
  b. -70 mV
  c. 0 mV
  d. +60 mV

___ 57. A "less negative" membrane potential means
  a. it is "more positive" than the resting potential
  b. it is a number closer to zero mV
  c. the resting membrane potential has moved closer to the sodium equilibrium
  d. All of these statements describe the term "less negative."

B. True or False/Edit

___ 58. "Fixed" anions cannot penetrate the cell membrane.
___ 59. The intracellular Na^+ concentration is lower than the extracellular Na^+ concentration.
___ 60. The equilibrium potential is a theoretical voltage — that is, it does not occur naturally in living cells.
___ 61. A resting membrane potential of -70 mV prevents any diffusion of Na^+ out of the cell.
___ 62. A cell at rest has both Na^+ and K^+ concentrations in perfect equilibrium across the membrane.

CHAPTER REVIEW

A. Completion

63. Passive transport of molecules or ions from regions of high to regions of low concentrations is called _____; and is due to _____ energy rather than metabolic energy.
64. The rate of diffusion depends on: the _____ difference or gradient that exists on two sides of the membrane; the _____ (selectivity) of the cell membrane to the diffusing substance; and is directly proportional to the membrane _____ (for example, microvilli).
65. Lipids such as steroids are _____(polar/nonpolar) molecules and, thus, _____ can/cannot) pass easily through phospholipid layers of the membrane.
66. Osmosis is the simple _____ of _____ molecules from _____ (more/less) dilute solutions to _____ (more/less) dilute solutions.

67. Solute molecules can exert force on the movement of solvent (water). The solute concentration is measured in units called _____, which is directly related to the _____ pressure of a solution.
68. All solutions with the same number of solute particles as plasma are _____, such as _____% NaCl and _____% glucose solutions; and in such solutions, red blood cells (RBCs) _____ (do/do not) gain or lose water.
69. However, increasing the number of solute particles in such solutions results in a _____ - tonic (hyper/iso/hypo) solution in which RBCs would _____ (crenate/hemolyse); while solutions with fewer solutes than plasma are _____ - tonic (hyper/iso/hypo) in which RBCs would _____ (crenate/hemolyse).
70. Water homeostasis is regulated mainly by _____ - receptors located in the _____ of the brain, which control the release of _____ hormone from the _____ pituitary gland; and which directs the kidneys to _____ (lose/reabsorb) body water.
71. Like enzyme proteins, carrier-mediated transport proteins are characterized by _____, _____, and _____. Carrier-mediated transport without the use of energy is _____ and is called _____; whereas carrier-mediated transport requiring metabolic energy is _____ and is called _____.
72. For example, the "uphill" Na^+/K^+ pump maintains the Na^+ concentration high _____ (inside/outside) the cell and K^+ concentration high _____ (inside/outside).
73. Of these two ions, _____ is the more diffusible, and is attracted into the cell by "fixed" _____ (anions/cations).
74. Due to this separation of ions the cell membrane potential at rest is approximately _____ mV, and it is maintained by expending _____ energy in the form of _____.

B. Sequencer

75. Abandoned in the hot desert for long periods of time without water, you have become dehydrated. Your body will sense this water loss and will initiate efforts to correct or compensate for this imbalance (notice this is negative feedback at work!). Read the following list of events and place them in the proper sequence. The last one (8) has been done for you.
    _____ Lower volume of urine is excreted from the body
    _____ Heightened sense of thirst with drinking behavior as the posterior pituitary is stimulated
    _____ Blood volume falls; plasma osmolality (solute/solvent) rises
    _____ Blood volume rises; plasma osmolality (solute/solvent) falls
    _____ Water retention is promoted along the kidney tubules
    __8__ Normal plasma osmolality is restored (homeostasis)
    _____ Osmoreceptors in the hypothalamus are activated
    _____ Antidiuretic hormone (ADH) is released into the bloodstream

C. Crossword Puzzle —Membrane Transport and the Membrane Potential

Across
2. the resting membrane potential is a _____ number, in millivolts
5. as electrolytes dissolve in water they come apart, or
7. when all membrane carriers are saturated, known as the T_m or transport _____
11. the form of transport that includes simple diffusion and osmosis
12. ions may pass through membranes along tiny passageways called _____
14. fingerlike projections or membrane folds; increase the cell surface area for absorption
15. what you receive for solving this puzzle
16. first two letters in the name of the hormone, ADH
19. more than one female egg cell
20. movement of materials "uphill" against concentration gradients is called active _____
21. density of solute molecules per volume of solvent
24. number of Na^+ ions pumped out of the cell as two K^+ ions are pumped into the cell by the Na^+/K^+ pump
25. specific membrane protein made by the cell for transport
29. where a bath can be taken

31. negative ions (such as, proteins)
32. can be abbreviated Osm
33. another name for primary active transport carriers
36. net diffusion of water across a membrane
37. passive carrier-mediated transport
39. boy or girl scout attribute
40. one example of a sugar solute molecule found in this chapter
41. charged particles
42. condition when concentrations of substances across a membrane are no longer different
44. cell membranes are considered to be semi- or _____ permeable
46. what happens to red blood cells when placed in ocean water (hypertonic)
47. hormone lacking in the disease diabetes mellitus
48. a solution with the same osmolality as plasma
51. units used to measure the charge difference across cell membranes
52. organ affected greatly by an excess of K^{+} ions in plasma
53. neurons sensitive to the osmotic pressure and osmolality of plasma

Down
1. genetic material necessary for synthesizing membrane carrier proteins
3. a difference in concentration between two solutions
4. one of three characteristics membrane carriers have in common with enzymes
6. osmotic pressure of pure water
8. example of an osmotically active solute in the plasma
9. change in ice on a hot summer day
10. membrane property — allow some to cross but not others
11. chemical composition of the membrane "core"
13. abbreviation in professional basketball
15. solution with a greater osmotic pressure and osmolality than plasma (for example, sea water)
17. secondary active transport, (for example, glucose uptake from kidney tubule)
18. the body's solvent
22. home for a feathered friend
23. form of energy used to drive the membrane "pumps"
26. the fluid portion of the blood
27. Avogadro's number of molecules; a small furry animal
28. passive movement from an area of high to one of low concentration
30. organ where the hypothalamus and osmoreceptors are located
34. primary intracellular cation
35. what happens to red blood cells when placed in a fresh water lake (hypotonic)
38. artificial removal of waste materials when kidneys fail
43. negative ions trapped within the 600 cell are known as _____
45. diffusion always occurs from higher to _____ concentrations
49. the number of negative charges on a cloride ion
50. worn on a baseball player's head

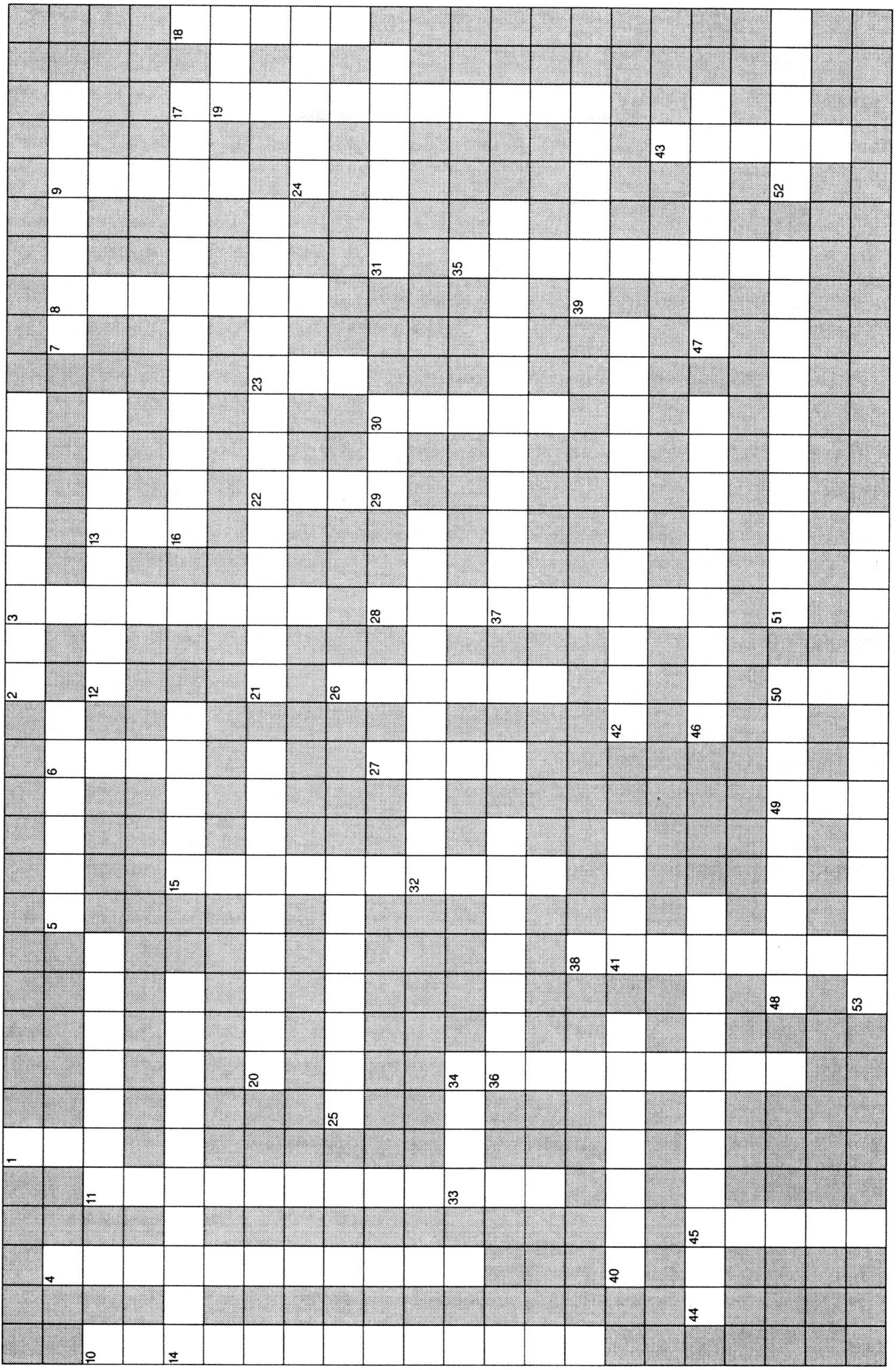

D. Essay

Essay Tutorial

This essay tutorial will answer the first essay question found in the "**Review Activities**" section of your *Human Physiology* textbook. Please look for question 1. at the end of chapter 6, read it carefully, and let me guide you through one possible answer. Watch for key terms in bold-face type, helpful tips and general suggestions on writing the essay or short-answer questions. Enjoy!

76. **Describe** the **conditions** required to produce osmosis, and **explain** why osmosis occurs under these conditions.

Note: This is really two questions in one. First we will describe the conditions producing or causing osmosis, then we will explain why osmosis occurs. Let's begin as we often do by defining the key word in the question — osmosis.

Answer. Osmosis is the net simple diffusion of water molecules (solvent) across a cell membrane that is permeable to water (*note*: not all membranes are permeable to water, such as those in portions of the kidney nephron). The conditions required for osmosis are: (1) the membrane must be relatively impermeable to the solutes on either side; and (2) the concentration of water must be higher on one side of the membrane than on the other. Osmosis now will occur from the side where water concentration is higher (more dilute!) to the side where water concentration is lower (less dilute!). The "impermeable" solutes are unable to cross the membrane and, thus, are said to be *osmotically* active since water will flow in the direction of these solutes in the attempt to "dilute" them. Finally, it is important to observe that when water (which is not compressible) moves throughout the body, the **volume** of that part of the body changes. How did it go? OK, got time for a few more?

77. You are a paramedic at the scene of an accident. You have three glucose (dextrose) solutions in your truck for starting intravenous fluid (IV) treatment — 1%, 5%, and 10% dextrose in water. Which of these solutions is isotonic, which is hypertonic, and which is hypotonic? Describe clearly what would happen if each of these solutions is infused separately.

78. Compare and contrast the terms **osmolality** and **osmotic pressure** — using the terms solute, solvent, and the $\frac{\text{solute}}{\text{solvent}}$ ratio in your explanation.

79. Body water homeostasis is maintained by neuron sensors and hormone effectors participating in a negative feedback loop. Describe this loop, the sensors, the effectors, and the response of the body to too much and too little body water.

80. Describe the interaction between the "fixed anions" and the Na^+/K^+ pump in creating the resting membrane potential. Include the permeability of the membrane to each substance and the role metabolic energy (ATP) plays in forming the membrane potential.

Answers — Chapter 6

I. Diffusion and Osmosis
   A. 1. b, 2. d, 3. a, 4. a, 5. e, 6. b, 7. e, 8. c, 9. c, 10. d, 11. b, 12. e, 13. c, 14. a
   B. 15. T, 16. T, 17. F—Some diffusion will be in the opposite direction, as well, 18. T, 19. T, 20. F—Switch "less" for "more," 21. F—Switch "K^+" and "Na^+," 22. T, 23. F—Replace "solute" with "solvent," 24. T, 25. T, 26. F—One mole of NaCl splits to form two moles of atoms, 27. T, 28. T, 29. T, 30. F—ADH promotes water reabsorption (not loss)
   C. 31. f, 32. a, 33. h, 34. d, 35. g, 36. b, 37. c, 38. k, 39. e, 40. i, 41. l, 42. m, 43. j
II. Carrier-Mediated Transport
   A. 44. c, 45. c, 46. b, 47. c
   B. 48. T, 49. T, 50. F—Replace "down" with "against," 51. T
III. The Membrane Potential
   A. 52. a, 53. b, 54. b, 55. d, 56. d, 57. d
   B. 58. T, 59. T, 60. T, 61. F—Na^+ will diffuse out of the cell due to its steep concentration gradient, 62. F—A cell at rest has both Na^+ and K^+ ions actively separated across the membrane—the basis for the membrane potential

Chapter Review
   A. 63. diffusion; thermal, 64. concentration; permeability; surface area, 65. nonpolar; can, 66. diffusion; water; more; less, 67. osmoles; osmotic, 68. isotonic; 0.9; 5.0; do not, 69. hyper; crenate; hypo; hemolyse, 70. osmo; hypothalamus; ADH; posterior; reabsorb, 71. specificity; competition; saturation; passive; facilitated diffusion; active; active transport, 72. outside; inside, 73. K^+; anions, 74. -70; metabolic; ATP
   B. 75. - 6, 3, 1, 7, 5, 8, 2, 4

C. Crossword Puzzle

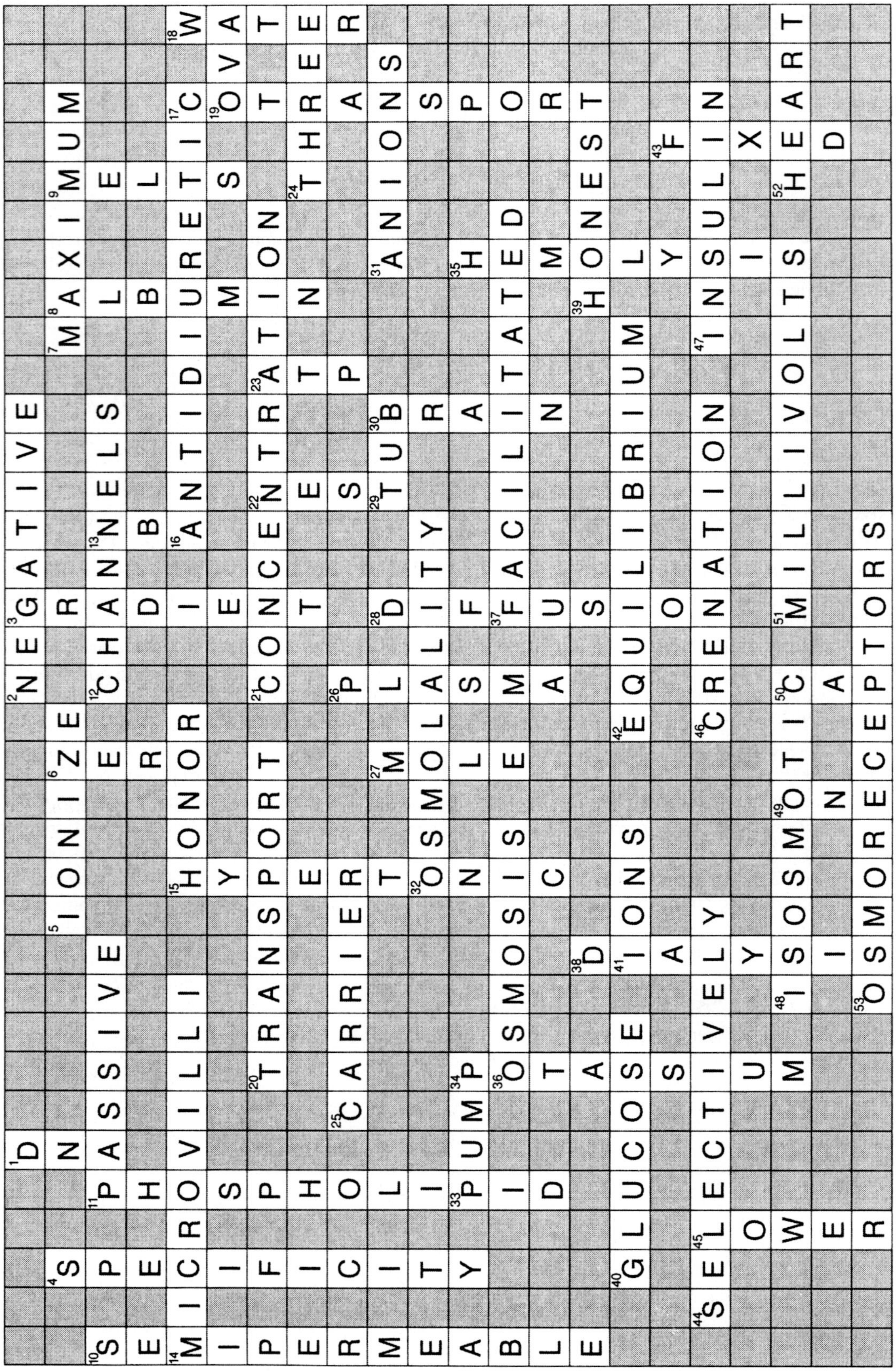

CHAPTER 7
THE NERVOUS SYSTEM: NEURONS AND SYNAPSES

CHAPTER SCOPE

This chapter begins a four-chapter unit (chapters 7 through 10) on the basic structure and function of the nervous system. The electrical potential of a neuron at rest, introduced in the last chapter, now "comes to life" as appropriate stimuli alter the permeability of the cell membrane to ions. The synchronized opening and closing of Na^+ and K^+ gates result in the movement of electrical charges that generates a nerve impulse or **action potential**.

Action potentials reach the end of each neuron where these electrical signals are either transmitted directly to the next cell in the sequence via *gap junctions*, or are responsible for activating the release of specialized **neurotransmitter** chemicals. Released from vesicles into the synaptic space, these neurotransmitters diffuse a short distance, binding to specialized receptors integrated in the membrane of the next effector cell in the conduction pathway, and promoting the formation of new action potentials. Effector cells, such as another neuron, a muscle fiber (chapters 12, 13), or a gland cell (chapters 11, 20), will then respond.

The action of specific neurotransmitters, especially *acetylcholine* (ACh), is also described in this chapter. Others, such as the **catecholamines** (*dopamine*, *norepinephrine*, and *epinephrine*) and a growing number of less well-known neurochemicals (*amino acids*, *polypeptides*, and *nitric oxide*) are particularly active in the CNS. It is important to have a solid understanding of the nervous system's structure and function presented in these four chapters for a successful (and enjoyable) comprehension of the organ system chapters that follow. The nervous system forms the basic communication network linking all tissues of the body to the brain and to each other. As will be featured in chapter 11, the nervous system's fast electrical signals (action potentials) are supplemented by slower-responding chemical messengers (*hormones*). Both systems cooperate effectively in the maintenance of overall body homeostasis.

I. NEURONS AND SUPPORTING CELLS

The nervous system is composed of neurons, which produce and conduct electrochemical impulses, and supporting cells, which assist the functions of neurons. Neurons are classified according to structure and function; the various types of supporting cells perform specialized functions.

A. Multiple Choice

    1. Which of the following is *not* a function of neurons?
        a. respond to physical and chemical stimuli
        b. conduct electrical impulses
        c. release specific chemical regulators
        d. All of these are neuron functions.

    2. Nissl bodies of the perikaryon are composed of
        a. mitochondria
        b. rough endoplasmic reticulum
        c. Golgi apparatus
        d. lysosomes

    3. A grouping of cell bodies located within the CNS is known as a
        a. tract
        b. nerve
        c. nucleus
        d. ganglion

    4. Involuntary effectors (glands, smooth or cardiac muscle) are innervated (stimulated) by
        a. autonomic nerves
        b. efferent nerves

       c. motor nerves
       d. All of these nerves innervate involuntary effectors.
___ 5. The most common type of neuron (motor neuron, for example) is
       a. bipolar
       b. multipolar
       c. pseudounipolar
___ 6. Myelin sheaths around axons within the CNS are formed by
       a. Schwann cells
       b. microglia
       c. astrocytes
       d. oligodendrocytes
___ 7. The most abundant supporting cell in the CNS, which forms perivascular feet associated with the blood-brain barrier, is the
       a. astrocyte
       b. oligodendrocyte
       c. satellite cell
       d. microglia

B. True or False/Edit

___ 8. The nervous system is composed of two principal types of cells — neurons and supporting cells (neuroglia or glial cells).
___ 9. Neurons cannot divide by mitosis, although some neurons can regenerate severed portions or sprout new branches under some conditions.
___ 10. In the brain, neurons outnumber glial cells five to one.
___ 11. Orthograde (forward flow) and retrograde (reverse flow) transport in neurons is characteristic of rapid axonal transport.
___ 12. Association neurons (interneurons) are located entirely within the central nervous system (CNS).
___ 13. All axons in the CNS, but not in the peripheral nervous system (PNS), are surrounded by the sheaths of Schwann.
___ 14. The only dendrites that have myelin sheaths are those of the sensory neurons located within the PNS.
___ 15. Spaces (pores) are found between endothelial cells lining the capillaries of the brain, and thus form the blood-brain barrier.

C. Label the Figure — Neuron Structure

Study figure 7.1 and notice the differences in structure between sensory and motor neurons. Then correctly label each neuron type using the term "sensory" or "motor." Complete the exercise by labeling the various parts of each neuron in the space provided. (When finished, check your work with figure 7.1 in your textbook.)

II. ELECTRICAL ACTIVITY IN AXONS

The permeability of the axon membrane to Na^+ and K^+ is regulated by gates, which open in response to stimulation. Net diffusion of these ions occurs in two stages: first Na^+ moves into the axon, then K^+ moves out. This flow of ions, and the changes in the membrane potential that result, constitute an event called an action potential or a nerve impulse.

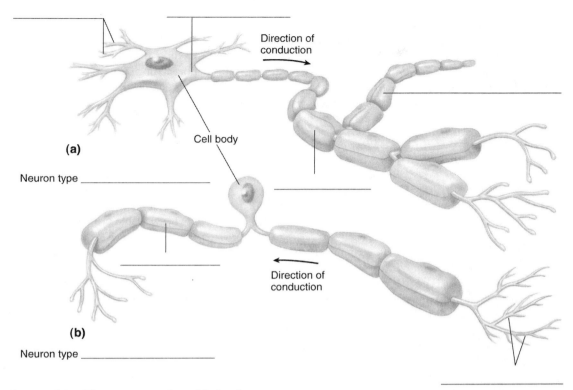

Figure 7.1 The structure of two kinds of neurons.

A. Multiple Choice

___ 16. The term "voltage regulated" means that the membrane
   a. gates open and close with changes in the membrane potential
   b. potential is controlled by the Na$^+$/K$^+$ pumps
   c. will not respond unless electrically stimulated
   d. potential can only be seen with an oscilloscope

___ 17. Arrange these action potential events in proper sequence:
   1. Membrane depolarization begins. 2. K$^+$ gates begin to open. 3. K$^+$ gates begin to close. 4. Na$^+$ gates begin to open. 5. Na$^+$ gates begin to close. 6. membrane repolarization begins
   a. 1, 2, 4, 3, 5, 6
   b. 2, 6, 3, 4, 1, 5
   c. 4, 6, 2, 1, 5, 3
   d. 1, 4, 2, 5, 6, 3

___ 18. Which statement about the action potential or nerve impulse is *false*?
   a. Only a relatively small number of Na$^+$ and K$^+$ ions actually diffuse across the membrane.
   b. Each action potential includes both positive and negative feedback loops.
   c. The Na$^+$/K$^+$ pumps are directly involved in creating the action potential.
   d. During the action potential, Na$^+$ and K$^+$ total concentrations are not significantly changed.
   e. Repolarization requires the outward diffusion of K$^+$ ions.

___ 19. When a stimulus of greater strength is applied to a neuron
   a. identical action potentials are produced more frequently (more are produced per minute)
   b. the total amplitude (height) of each action potential increases also
   c. the neuron fires a steady barrage of action potentials for a longer duration of time

___ 20. Action potentials conducted without *decrement* means conducted without
   a. decreasing its velocity
   b. altering the threshold potential

  c. decreasing its amplitude
  d. altering the Na$^+$ or K$^+$ concentrations in the neuron
___ 21. Which of the following statements about the conduction velocity of action potentials along myelinated axons when compared to that along unmyelinated axons, is *false*?
  a. Conduction velocity in the myelinated axon is very fast, approaching 225 miles per hour.
  b. Cable properties within the myelinated axon increase the conduction velocity.
  c. Nodes of Ranvier increase the conduction velocity.
  d. Saltatory conduction increases the conduction velocity.

B. True or False/Edit

___ 22. Within a collection of axons (or nerves), a low-intensity stimulus will only activate those few fibers with low thresholds, whereas high-intensity stimuli can activate fibers with higher thresholds.

___ 23. Compared to metal wires, the axon is a very poor electrical conductor.

___ 24. High-speed conduction of neural impulses is made possible due to the cable properties of the axon.

___ 25. The action potential generated at the end of the axon looks different from that formed at the axon nearest the cell body.

___ 26. Action potentials conducted along thicker, unmyelinated fibers are conducted faster than those along thin, unmyelinated fibers; and are *substantially* faster if the axon is myelinated.

___ 27. Thick myelinated fibers would be expected to mediate (to come in the middle of or to control) slow responses in the viscera (to and from internal organs and smooth muscle).

___ 28. Saltatory conduction of action potentials is made possible by the interruptions in the myelin sheath along axons, known as nodes of Ranvier.

III. THE SYNAPSE

Axons end close to, or in some cases at the point of contact with, another cell. Once action potentials reach the end of an axon, they directly or indirectly stimulate (or inhibit) the other cell. In specialized cases, action potentials can directly pass from one cell to another. In most cases, however, the action potentials stop at the axon ending where they stimulate the release of a chemical neurotransmitter that affects the next cell.

A. Multiple Choice

___ 29. The only synapse that has bidirectional conduction is
  a. axodendritic
  b. axosomatic
  c. axoaxonic
  d. dendrodentritic
  e. All are one-directional only.

___ 30. Electrical synapses (for example, smooth and cardiac muscle fibers) are characterized by having two adjoining cells that
  a. are about equal in size
  b. have contact areas with low electrical resistance
  c. have gap junctions present between them
  d. All of these characterize electrical synapses.
  e. None of these characterize electrical synapses.

___ 31. As the intensity of the stimulus in a presynaptic neuron increases, the number of vesicles undergoing exocytosis _____, and the number of released neurotransmitter molecules _____.
  a. increases; increases
  b. increases; decreases
  c. decreases; increases
  d. decreases; decreases

____ 32. The ion that must flow into the presynaptic neuron ending to activate the release of neurotransmitter chemicals from synaptic vesicles is
   a. sodium
   b. potassium
   c. calcium
   d. iron
   e. hydrogen

____ 33. Which of the following events is *not* involved in the release of neurotransmitter chemicals from the presynaptic terminal boutons?
   a. opening of voltage-regulated calcium channels
   b. turning off the Na$^+$/K$^+$ membrane pumps
   c. activation of intracellular enzymes known as protein kinases
   d. exocytosis of membrane-bound vesicles
   e. phosphorylation of synapsin proteins in the membrane of the synaptic vesicles.

B. True or False/Edit

____ 34. Myoneural and neuromuscular junctions mean the same thing - that is, they refer to a neuron-to-muscle synapse.

____ 35. Synaptic transmission is electrical rather than chemical.

____ 36. Gap junctions are characteristic features of smooth and cardiac muscle cells (fibers), brain neurons, and even many embryonic tissues.

____ 37. The synaptic cleft refers to the swollen ending of the presynaptic axon terminal.

____ 38. Voltage-regulated channels are found in the postsynaptic membrane and open in response to depolarization.

____ 39. Depolarization of the postsynaptic membrane results in an EPSP, whereas hyperpolarization of the postsynaptic membrane results in an IPSP.

IV. ACETYLCHOLINE AS A NEUROTRANSMITTER

When acetylcholine (ACh) binds to its receptor, it directly or indirectly causes the opening of chemically regulated gates. In most cases, this produces a depolarization called an excitatory postsynaptic potential, or EPSP. In some cases, however, ACh causes a hyperpolarization known as an inhibitory postsynaptic potential, or IPSP.

A. Multiple Choice

____ 40. *Acetylcholine* (ACh) is a neurotransmitter released from all these neurons *except*
   a. specific CNS neuron endings
   b. somatic motor neurons at the neuromuscular junction
   c. specific autonomic neuron endings
   d. All of these neurons release ACh.

____ 41. Which of the following is *not* a property of chemically regulated gated channels?
   a. They respond best to membrane potential changes.
   b. They are located on the postsynaptic membrane.
   c. They can allow Na$^+$ and K$^+$ diffusion simultaneously through opened ion channels.
   d. They are activated by neurotransmitters binding to specific receptor molecules.

____ 42. Which of the following statements describes *nicotinic* receptors (as opposed to muscarinic ACh receptors)?
   a. These receptors are formed from only a single subunit.
   b. These receptors activate G-proteins located in the cell membrane.
   c. These receptors do not contain an ion channel.
   d. Once opened, for example, can permit the outward diffusion of K$^+$ and hyperpolarization.
   e. Once opened, for example, can permit the inward diffusion of Na$^+$ and depolarization.

____ 43. Acetylcholinesterase (AChE) is an enzyme located on or immediately outside the
   a. presynaptic membrane
   b. postsynaptic membrane

        c. axon terminal cytoplasm
        d. vesicles released by exocytosis

___ 44. The drug curare reduces the size of end plate potentials on the membrane of muscle fibers by
        a. competing with ACh for attachment to the receptor proteins
        b. blocking the release of ACh from presynaptic vesicles
        c. enhancing the breakdown of ACh by the enzyme, AChE
        d. blocking the flow of Na^+ through open ion channels

___ 45. *Myasthenia gravis* is a muscle weakness disease caused by
        a. antibodies blocking and destroying ACh receptors
        b. blocking the release of ACh from presynaptic vesicles
        c. enhancing the breakdown of ACh by AChE
        d. blocking the flow of Na^+ through open ion channels

___ 46. The first voltage-regulated gates encountered along the neuron membrane, which initiate the formation of action potentials, are located on the
        a. dendrite
        b. cell body
        c. axon hillock portion of the axon
        d. axon terminal
        e. postsynaptic membrane

B. True or False/Edit

___ 47. The effects of acetylcholine (ACh) can be either excitatory or inhibitory.
___ 48. ACh is transported into the postsynaptic cell cytoplasm, where it produces its effects.
___ 49. Neurotransmitters operating chemically regulated gates, do *not* directly result in action potentials, but rather initially produce EPSPs and IPSPs.
___ 50. Acetylcholinesterase (AChE) is an enzyme that inactivates ACh, thus serves to uncouple the electrochemical conduction of the nerve impulse.
___ 51. The bond between ACh and its receptor protein is exceptionally strong.
___ 52. Unlike action potentials, excitatory postsynaptic potentials (EPSPs) can summate and have no refractory period.
___ 53. Curare , a drug first used on poison darts by South American Indians, interrupts neuromuscular transmission and results in a spastic form of paralysis.
___ 54. EPSPs become action potentials at the initial segment portion of the axon.
___ 55. Somatic motor neurons always make synapses with skeletal muscle fibers, releasing ACh molecules that bind to nicotinic receptors on the motor end plate and result in end plate potentials.
___ 56. Alzheimer's disease is thought to be caused by a loss of CNS neurons that release the neurotransmitter, serotonin.

V. MONOAMINES AS NEUROTRANSMITTERS

There are a variety of chemicals in the CNS that function as neurotransmitters. Among these are the family of monoamines that include dopamine, norepinephrine, and serotonin. Although these molecules are in the same chemical family and have similar mechanisms of action, they are used by different neurons for different functions.

A. Multiple Choice

___ 57. All of the following regulatory molecules are in the chemical family known as monoamines, *except:*
        a. acetylcholine
        b. epinephrine
        c. dopamine
        d. serotonin
        e. norepinephrine

___ 58. Which of the following is *not* used to inhibit the stimulatory effects of monoamines released from presynaptic vesicles?
   a. reuptake (pump) into the presynaptic neuron ending
   b. enzyme degradation(breakdown) by monoamine oxidase (MAO) enzymes
   c. receptor blockade and inhibition by specific receptor antibodies
   d. enzyme degradation by catecholamine-O-methyltransferase (COMT) enzymes
   e. All of these inhibit the effects of released monamines.

___ 59. Adenylate cyclase is an important enzyme that
   a. inhibits cAMP by converting it into inactive metabolites
   b. phosphorylates other proteins to open postsynaptic membrane channels
   c. converts ATP to cAMP and pyrophosphate in the postsynaptic cell cytoplasm
   d. catalyzes the conversion of ADP and phosphate to active ATP

___ 60. Cocaine stimulates the synapses of specific neurons that release dopamine, by
   a. inhibiting enzyme inactivation of dopamine
   b. blocking dopamine reuptake into the presynaptic axon
   c. mimicking the effects of dopamine on the postsynaptic cell
   d. facilitating the release of dopamine from the presynaptic cell terminal

___ 61. *Parkinson's disease* is caused by loss of neurons that secrete the neurotransmitter
   a. acetylcholine (ACh)
   b. norepinephrine
   c. serotonin
   d. GABA
   e. dopamine

___ 62. Amphetamines are drugs that cause general arousal in behavior by stimulating specific pathways that use _____ as a neurotransmitter
   a. ACh
   b. norepinephrine
   c. serotonin
   d. GABA
   e. dopamine

B. True or False/Edit

___ 63. Serotonin is derived from the amino acid, tryptophan.
___ 64. Norepinephrine is also known as adrenalin, a hormone secreted by the adrenal cortex.
___ 65. Epinephrine is both a hormone and a neurotransmitter molecule.
___ 66. Dopamine is only a neurotransmitter molecule and not a hormone.
___ 67. Drugs that inhibit MAO (and COMT) ultimately promote the effects of monoamine neurotransmitter action.
___ 68. Instead of opening ionic channels directly in the postsynaptic membrane, monoamine neurotransmitters act through a second messenger molecule, such as cyclic adenosine monophosphate (cAMP).
___ 69. Schizophrenia may be caused, in part, by overactivity of the specific dopaminergic pathways.
___ 70. Sympathetic neurons of the PNS use norepinephrine as a neurotransmitter at their terminal synapse with smooth muscles, cardiac muscle, and glands.

VI. OTHER NEUROTRANSMITTERS

There are a surprisingly large number of different molecules that appear to function as neurotransmitters. These include some amino acids and their derivatives, many polypeptides, and even the gas nitric oxide.

A. Multiple Choice

___ 71. Which of the following neurotransmitters is *inhibitory*?
   a. glycine
   b. aspartic acid

c. norepinephrine
d. glutamic acid

___ 72. The most prevalent brain neurotransmitter is
   a. ACh
   b. norepinephrine
   c. serotonin
   d. GABA
   e. dopamine

___ 73. The neurotransmitter that appears to be involved in such clinical problems as Huntington's chorea, status epilepticus (seizures), and severe alterations in mood and emotions, is
   a. ACh
   b. norepinephrine
   c. serotonin
   d. GABA
   e. dopamine

___ 74. The brain neurotransmitters that may have opioid (pain relieving) properties is
   a. enkaphalin peptides
   b. dynorphin polypeptides
   c. ß-endorphins
   d. All of these are endogenous opiods.
   e. None of these are endogenous opiods.

___ 75. Which of the following statements about nitric oxide (NO) is *false*?
   a. NO acts locally to relax the smooth muscles of blood vessel walls, resulting in vessel dilation.
   b. NO is occasionally used by dentists as an analgesic (painkiller).
   c. NO acts as a neurotransmitter of certain neurons in both the PNS and the CNS; and in the immune system, helps to kill bacteria.
   d. NO stimulates the production of cyclic guanosine monophosphate (cGMP), that can act as a second messenger in the cytoplasm.
   e. NO appears to be involved in such processes as erection of the penis, dilation of respiratory passageways, and learning and memory.

B. True or False/Edit

___ 76. Certain amino acids neurotransmitters excite effectors by forming EPSPs, and others inhibit CNS neurons by producing IPSPs.

___ 77. Both GABA (gamma-aminobutyric acid) and glycine are excitatory CNS neurotransmitters.

___ 78. Inhibitory neurotransmitters may cause inhibition by hyperpolarizing the postsynaptic membranes of their target cells.

___ 79. Synaptic plasticity means that neurons may release either classical neurotransmitters or polypeptides known as neuromodulators; and that synapses are formed and reformed continuously even in the mature brain.

___ 80. Naloxone is a drug that mimics (imitates) the analgesic action of the endogenous opioids produced naturally by the brain.

___ 81. Through its action on the smooth muscle of blood vessels, nitric oxide (NO) gas can be used to treat pulmonary hypertension.

VII. SYNAPTIC INTEGRATION

The summation of a number of EPSPs may be needed to produce a depolarization of sufficient magnitude to stimulate the postsynaptic cell. The net effect of EPSPs on the postsynaptic neuron is reduced by hyperpolarization (IPSPs), which is produced by inhibitory neurotransmitters. The activity of neurons within the central nervous system is thus the net result of both excitatory and inhibitory effects.

A. Multiple Choice

___ 82. EPSPs produced by many different presynaptic fibers converging on a single postsynaptic neuron, causing summation on the postsynaptic dendrites and cell body, best describes
    a. synaptic plasticity
    b. temporal summation
    c. synaptic inhibition
    d. spatial summation

___ 83. Inhibitory postsynaptic potentials (IPSPs)
    a. result in hyperpolarization of the postsynaptic membrane
    b. may be caused by opening postsynaptic K^+ gates
    c. may be caused by opening postsynaptic Cl^- gates
    d. lower the membrane potential; more negative than resting
    e. All of these statements regarding IPSPs are correct.

___ 84. Which of the following is *not* characteristic of the term, *presynaptic inhibition*?
    a. The axon of the first neuron synapses with the axon (rather than the dendrite) of the second neuron.
    b. It can result from the opening Cl^- gates, producing hyperpolarization and forming IPSPs.
    c. The first neuron is partially depolarized by the neurotransmitter from the second neuron.
    d. Lesser amounts of neurotransmitter is released by the first neuron due to fewer action potentials arriving at the axon terminal.
    e. All of these are characteristic of presynaptic inhibition.

B. True or False/Edit

___ 85. Temporal summation of EPSPs in the postsynaptic neuron is caused by the combined effect of successive waves of transmitter released from presynaptic neurons.

___ 86. Long term potentiation (LTP) refers to the enhancement of synaptic transmission that may involve nitric oxide and may represent a mechanism of neural "learning" or memory.

___ 87. Most postsynaptic neuron responses are determined by the algebraic balance between hundreds or thousands of incoming EPSPs and IPSPs.

CHAPTER REVIEW

A. Matching — Neuron Terms

___ 88. membrane potential returns toward resting
___ 89. as stimulus strength increases more neurons fire
___ 90. another name for "spike" potential
___ 91. upward oscilloscope deflection (hypopolarization)
___ 92. action potential amplitude never varies
___ 93. downward oscilloscope deflection below resting
___ 94. time of depolarization (Na^+ gates open)
___ 95. time of depolarization (K^+ gates open)
___ 96. transmission of electric charge through the cytoplasm of neurons

a. depolarization
b. hyperpolarization
c. repolarization
d. all-or-none
e. action potential
f. cable property
g. recruitment
h. absolute refractory period
i. relative refractory period

B. Completion

97. The nervous system is divided into two parts — the central nervous system and the _____ nervous system. The CNS includes the _____ and _____ _____, featuring collections

of cell bodies called _____ and bundles of axons called _____. The PNS collections of cell bodies are _____ and axons are _____. 98. Neurons contain _____ which receive stimuli, whereas the _____ conducts impulses away from the _____. 99. Sensory or _____ neurons are _____ in structure, conducting impulses _____ (toward/away from) the CNS — whereas a _____ or efferent neuron is _____ in structure and conducts impulses _____ (toward/away from) the CNS. There are _____ (#) different categories of neuroglial cells. (Do you remember *why* each is significant? See *table 7.3* in the text.) 100. A depolarizing stimulus opens _____-regulated Na⁺ and K⁺ gates, causing the all-or-none _____ potential — which is separated from the next by a period of time called a _____ period. This time period is first _____, during which the neuron will never respond, and then _____, during which supramaximal stimuli are required. Stronger stimuli increase the _____ of action potentials. 101. Electrical synapses called _____ junctions are found in _____ muscle, _____ muscle, and sometimes in the brain. 102. By the process of _____, chemical synapses release vesicles containing _____ molecules, which open _____ regulated gates. The resulting depolarizations are _____, meaning they can be added, or _____ as EPSPs at the initial segment of the axon _____, reach threshold, and fire action potentials. 103. CNS neurotransmitters that have short-term and long-term effects include the catecholamines _____ and _____ that ultimately form second messengers called _____. Two known inhibitory neurotransmitters in the CNS are _____ and _____. They _____-polarize (de/re/hyper) the postsynaptic membrane forming IPSPs by opening chemically regulated gates to _____ or _____ ions. 104. Neuron inhibition can be pre- or postsynaptic, preventing the formation of _____ potentials, whereas EPSPs are excitatory and are often summated both _____ and _____, thus facilitating the formation of nerve impulses.

C. Sequencer — The Action Potential

105. In sequence, number the following events that take place along the membrane of an activated neuron axon leading to the formation and completion of an action potential. If this is fuzzy to you, see the second section in your text chapter that describes the electrical activity in axons. *Note*: The last event (8) has been marked for you.

　____ K⁺ gates begin to open while Na⁺ gates begin to close
　____ Outward diffusion of K⁺ may result in an overshoot in the membrane potential below -60 mV (hyperpolarization)
　____ Na⁺ diffuses through open gates into the axon, further depolarizing the axon (example of positive feedback!), as the membrane potential rapidly approaches +40 mV
　____ Neuron membrane at rest (-65 mV), voltage-regulated gates are closed
　____ Na⁺ gates open, the membrane potential reaches its threshold potential level
　__8__ Refractory periods along the axon membrane prevent subsequent action potentials from running together.
　____ Depolarizing stimulus begins to open voltage-regulated Na⁺ gates (followed later by K⁺ gates opening)
　____ Membrane potential at around +40 mV sharply reverses its direction and returns toward resting (repolarization)

D. Essay

Essay Tutorial

This essay tutorial will answer the first essay question found in the "**Review Activities**" section of your *Human Physiology* textbook. Please look for *Essay Question* 1. at the end of chapter 7, read it carefully, and let me guide you through one possible answer. Watch for key terms in bold-face type, helpful tips and general suggestions on writing the essay or short-answer questions. Enjoy!

106. Compare the **characteristics** of **action** potentials with those of **synaptic** potentials.

Answer. Study table 7.5 in the text, and note that the three column headings are similar to the boldfaced key terms in the question. As an example of graded synaptic potentials, the text has chosen to feature excitatory postsynaptic potentials (EPSPs). Read this table carefully. Notice that this *EPSPs* column could just as easily have been written to describe inhibitory postsynaptic potentials (IPSPs). Could you do this? Try it, by making the appropriate changes in the wording already present in the table. Good luck.

Now, try the following essay questions — and remember, tables are acceptable formats for answering physiology essay questions.

107. During the formation of an action potential (nerve impulse), the membrane potential *never* reaches the Na$^+$ equilibrium potential at +60 mV. Use the flow of Na$^+$ and K$^+$ through gates in the living neuron to explain why this does not happen.

108. Distinguish between the absolute and relative refractory periods of an axon. Include the role of ion gates and the physiologic significance of these periods *in vivo* (in the body).

109. Describe those features of the action potential that represent both positive and negative feedback loops.

110. Compare voltage-regulated gates with chemically-regulated gates on the neuron membrane. Include differences in their location and their function.

Answers — Chapter 7

I. Neurons and Supporting Cells
   A. 1. d, 2. b, 3. c, 4. d, 5. b, 6. d, 7. a
   B. 8. T, 9. T, 10. F—Switch "neurons" with "glial cells," 11. T, 12. T, 13. F—Switch "CNS" with "PNS," 14. T, 15. F—Brain endothelial cells have no spaces but do form a blood — brain barrier
   C. Label the Figure — Neuron Structure; See figure 7.1 in the text

II. Electrical Activity in Axons
   A. 16. a, 17. d, 18. c, 19. a, 20. c, 21. b
   B. 22. T, 23. T, 24. F—Cable properties in unmyelinated axons result in very slow conduction of impulses, 25. F—All action potentials look the same—"all or none," 26. T, 27. F—Replace "thick myelinated" with "thin unmyelinated", 28. T

III. The Synapse
   A. 29. d, 30. d, 31. a, 32. c, 33. b
   B. 34. T, 35. F—Switch "electrical" for "chemical," 36. T, 37. F—Replace "synaptic cleft" with "terminal boutons," 38. F—Replace "postsynaptic membrane" with "axon," 39. T

IV. Acetylcholine as a Neurotransmitter
   A. 40. d, 41. a, 42. e, 43. b, 44. a, 45. a, 46. c
   B. 47. T, 48. F—ACh cannot cross the membrane, so it binds and opens ion channel gates for Na^+ and K^+, 49. T, 50. T, 51. F—Replace "strong" with "weak," 52. T, 53. F—Replace "spastic" with "flaccid," 54. T, 55. T, 56. F—Replace "serotonin" with "Ach"

V. Monoamines and Neurotransmitters
   A. 57. a, 58. c, 59. c, 60. b, 61. e, 62.e
   B. 63. T, 64. F—Delete "Nor" to make "Epinephrine," and replace "cortex" with "medulla," 65. F—Epinephrine is only a hormone, 66. T, 67. T, 68. T, 69. T, 70. T

VI. Other Neurotransmitters
   A. 71. a, 72. d, 73. d, 74. d, 75. b
   B. 76. T, 77. F—Replace "excitatory" with "inhibitory," 78. T, 79. T, 80. F—Replace "mimics (imitates)" with "blocks," 81. T

VII. Synaptic Integration
   A. 82. d, 83. e, 84. b
   B. 85. T, 86. T, 87. T

Chapter Review
   A. 88. c, 89. g, 90. e, 91. a, 92. d, 93. b, 94. h, 95. i, 96. f
   B. 97. peripheral; brain, spinal cord, nuclei, tracts; ganglia, nerves, 98. dendrites, axon, cell body, 99. afferent, pseudounipolar, to, motor, multipolar, from; six, 100. voltage, action, refractory; absolute, relative; frequency, 101. gap, smooth, cardiac, 102. exocytosis, neurotransmitter, chemically; graded, summated, hillock, 103. dopamine, norepinephrine, cAMP; glycine, GABA; hyper, K^+, Cl^-, 104. action, temporally; spatially
   C. 105. 5, 7, 4, 1, 3, 8, 2, 6

CHAPTER 8
THE CENTRAL NERVOUS SYSTEM

CHAPTER SCOPE

The *brain* and *spinal cord* are structural and functional nervous tissue of the body that together compose the **central nervous system** (CNS). The action potentials (nerve impulses) that come into the brain via sensory (*afferent*) neurons and exit via motor (*efferent*) neurons are interconnected by numerous *association* neurons. Within specific portions of the brain these action potentials are interpreted, giving us the ability to speak, express emotion, be motivated, move muscles, and remember things.

The deeper structures of the brain, such as the **thalamus, hypothalamus,** and **medulla oblongata,** are critical interpretive and relay centers for information traveling into and out of the brain. In addition, this more primitive area of the brain provides an essential link to the complex endocrine system. Triggered by nerve impulses, endocrine glands release many hormones that ultimately control many of the body's homeostatic processes, especially those of the *viscera* (internal tissues).

The spinal cord can be subdivided into ascending (sensory) and descending (motor) *tracts* (axon bundles). The spinal cord houses the pathways for the motor neurons originating in the **motor cortex** (*precentral gyrus*), that controls voluntary muscle contractions. This route directs nerve impulses down through important brain regions such as the **basal nuclei** (or *basal ganglia*) and the **cerebellum**, where rough, voluntary commands are modulated into smooth, coordinated contractions. Selected spinal cord tracts (and cranial nerves) also carry sensory action potentials in the opposite direction. Many of these ascending pathways ultimately arrive at the **sensory cortex** (*postcentral gyrus*) for interpretation of the various senses. The sensory system will be described in more detail in the next chapter. Of further interest is the *simple reflex arc*, a pathway of both sensory and motor neurons joined at the spinal cord, that is an integral part of all voluntary muscle movements.

I. STRUCTURAL ORGANIZATION OF THE BRAIN

The brain is composed of an enormous number of association neurons, with accompanying neuroglia, arranged in regions and subdivisions. These neurons receive sensory information, direct the activity of motor neurons, and perform such higher brain functions as learning and memory.

A. Multiple Choice

____ 1. The embryonic tissue layer that eventually forms the epidermis of the skin and the nervous system is the
   a. ectoderm
   b. mesoderm
   c. endoderm

____ 2. The telencephalon and diencephalon are subdivisions of the
   a. prosencephalon
   b. mesencephalon
   c. rhombencephalon

____ 3. Neuron cell bodies and dendrites deep within the brain form gray aggregations or gray matter known as
   a. the cortex
   b. ventricles
   c. the cerebrum
   d. nuclei

B. True or False/Edit

___ 4. Eventually, the neural tube will become the central nervous system in the growing embryo.

___ 5. The hindbrain, or mesencephalon, eventually divides into the metencephalon and myelencephalon brain regions.

___ 6. The hollow center of the neural tube eventually forms the ventricle cavities of the brain and central canal of the spinal cord.

___ 7. The adult brain receives about 20% of the total blood flow from the heart each minute.

II. CEREBRUM

The cerebrum, consisting of five paired lobes within two convoluted hemispheres, contains gray matter in its cortex and in deeper cerebral nuclei. Most of what are considered to be the higher functions of the brain are performed by the cerebrum.

A. Multiple Choice

___ 8. The largest portion of the brain (80% of its mass) is the
   a. cerebellum
   b. cerebrum
   c. hypothalamus
   d. basal ganglia
   e. None of these is the largest portion of the brain.

___ 9. Which of the following is *not* a lobe of the cerebral cortex?
   a. occipital
   b. parietal
   c. insula
   d. cerebellar
   e. temporal

___ 10. Which of the following does *not* send somatesthetic sensory information to the cerebral cortex sensory area located in the postcentral gyrus?
   a. skin (cutaneous)
   b. muscle fibers
   c. tendons
   d. joints
   e. All of these regions are somatesthetic sensory areas.

___ 11. Somatesthetic sensory information is interpreted in the
   a. cerebellum
   b. precentral gyrus
   c. basal ganglia
   d. postcentral gyrus
   e. occipital cortex

___ 12. The size of the sensory and motor maps on the cerebral cortex are determined by the
   a. size of the area represented in square meters
   b. precise location of the area represented in the body
   c. highest density of receptors or greatest number of effectors in the area represented
   d. time of development during embryonic growth

___ 13. The lobe interpreting sensory information from the cochlea, and for processing both auditory and visual information, is the
   a. frontal
   b. parietal
   c. temporal
   d. occipital
   e. insula

___ 14. Which of the following new techniques for visualizing the brain utilizes complex manipulation of x-ray absorption data obtained from tissues of different densities?

        a. computer tomography (CT)
        b. positron-emission tomography (PET)
        c. magnetic resonance imaging (MRI)
___ 15. Which of the following new techniques for visualizing the brain creates excellent images by detecting emitted radio wave signals released from stimulated protons aligned in the tissues?
        a. computer tomography (CT)
        b. positron-emission tomography (PET)
        c. magnetic resonance imaging (MRI)
___ 16. The EEG pattern recorded from the parietal and occipital regions that is characteristic in awake yet relaxed persons is
        a. alpha
        b. beta
        c. theta
        d. delta
___ 17. The basal nuclei (or basal ganglia) are masses of gray matter that function primarily in the
        a. perception of auditory and visual stimuli
        b. control of voluntary movements
        c. relay of sensory and motor information
        d. synthesis and release of important regulatory hormones
___ 18. The study of speech and language disorders (aphasias) have contributed greatly to our understanding of the brain, particularly that region known as
        a. basal ganglia
        b. cerebellum
        c. Broca's and Wernicke's areas
        d. limbic system
___ 19. That brain region formerly known as the "smell brain" but now known as a center for basic emotional drives is the
        a. hypothalamus
        b. pituitary
        c. limbic system
        d. basal ganglia
        e. Broca's and Wernicke's areas
___ 20. Which of the following processes is *not* thought to be regulated by the hypothalamus and limbic system?
        a. absolute fear
        b. language interpretation
        c. feeding and satiety
        d. sexual drive and sexual behavior
        e. aggression (rage)
___ 21. That portion of the brain thought to be involved primarily in the consolidation of short-term into long-term memory, is the
        a. cerebral cortex
        b. hypothalamus
        c. limbic system
        d. hippocampus
        e. basal ganglia

B. True or False/Edit
___ 22. The elevated folds of the cerebral surface are sulci, and the depressed grooves are called gyri.
___ 23. The precentral gyrus is located in the frontal lobe and is involved in control of motor neuron activity.
___ 24. The fingers and face have a higher density of sensory receptors and more muscles for innervation, and so, have a correspondingly larger representation on the sensory and motor regions of the cerebral cortex, respectively.

___ 25. The parietal lobe is the primary area for vision and for the coordination of eye movements.
___ 26. The upper caudate nucleus and the lower lentiform nucleus make up the corpus striatum, a prominent portion of the basal nuclei (ganglia).
___ 27. Each cerebral hemisphere ultimately receives information from both sides of the body as they intercommunicate via the corpus callosum tracts.
___ 28. *Cerebral lateralization* refers to the specialty of function delegated to one hemisphere or the other, while *cerebral dominance* is related to the concept of handedness (right or left).
___ 29. The left hemisphere is more adept than the right hemisphere at visuospatial tasks, such as reading maps or finding the way around an unfamiliar house.
___ 30. People with *Broca's aphasia* produce incomprehensible speech that has been described as a "word salad".
___ 31. The *Papez circuit* refers to the closed pathways that interconnect the limbic system, the thalamus, and the hypothalamus for processing information regarding emotion.
___ 32. Long-term memory may involve relatively permanent changes in the neurons and synapses involved, such as the synthesis of new proteins.

C. Label the Figure — Lobes and Important Regions of the Left Cerebral Cortex

The cerebral cortex is characterized by numerous folds and grooves called **convolutions**. The elevated folds of the convolutions are called *gyri*, and the depressed grooves are the *sulci (fissures)*. Each cerebral hemisphere is subdivided by deep sulci, or fissures, into five lobes, four of which are visible from the surface. Study figure 8.1 below and label the four lobes and the two sulci (the lateral sulcus and the central sulcus). Next, on the lines of the figure that point to the various cortical brain regions, write the important general function attributed to that area of the brain. Then, compare your answers with those in figure 8.6 in your text. Pay particular attention to the sensory and motor areas that located adjacent to the central sulcus. Study hard!

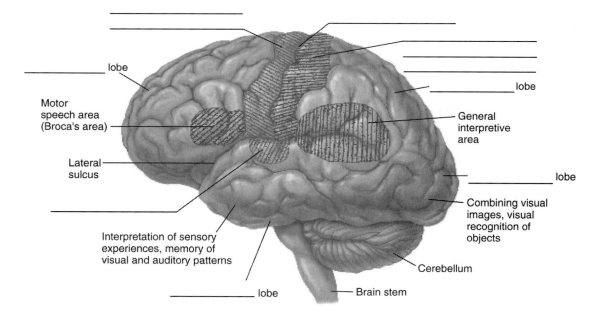

Figure 8.1

The lobes of the left cerebral hemisphere showing the principle motor and sensory areas of the cerebral cortex.

III. DIENCEPHALON

The diencephalon is the part of the forebrain that contains such important structures as the thalamus, hypothalamus, and pituitary gland. The hypothalamus performs numerous vital functions, most of which relate directly or indirectly to the regulation of visceral activities by way of other brain regions and the autonomic nervous system.

A. Multiple Choice

___ 33. That portion of the brain acting primarily as a relay center through which all sensory information (except smell) passes on the way to the cerebrum, is the
   a. thalamus
   b. hypothalamus
   c. hippocampus
   d. limbic system
   e. basal nuclei (ganglia)

___ 34. Melatonin is a hormone secreted by the
   a. thalamus
   b. hypothalamus
   c. pituitary gland
   d. pineal gland
   e. None of these brain regions secrete melatonin.

___ 35. The *choroid plexus* located in each of the cerebral ventricles is primarily responsible for
   a. relaying sensory information to the cortex
   b. altering motor control over voluntary muscle action
   c. synthesizing neurotransmitters for cranial nerves
   d. secreting cerebrospinal fluid (CSF)

___ 36. Which of the following vital physiologic functions is *not* centered in the hypothalamus?
   a. hunger
   b. thirst
   c. control over heart rate and blood pressure
   d. control over body temperature ("thermostat")
   e. control over pituitary gland secretion of hormones

___ 37. A "somatic response" refers to a response by the
   a. whole body
   b. sensory system only
   c. skeletal (voluntary) muscles only (for example, shivering)
   d. visceral glands of the autonomic (involuntary) nervous system only
   e. skin and connective tissues (muscle and bone)

B. True or False/Edit

___ 38. The only sensation that is *not* relayed through the thalamus en route to the cerebrum for interpretation is the sense of taste.
___ 39. The hormone melatonin may play a role in the hormonal control of reproduction.
___ 40. With regard to hunger, the hypothalamus has opposing "feeding" and "satiety" (fullness) centers that are located in the lateral and medial regions, respectively.
___ 41. The supraoptic and paraventricular nuclei are specialized neurons located in the hypothalamus where the important hormones *vasopressin (ADH)* and *oxytocin* are made.
___ 42. The anterior pituitary is known as the *neuro*hypophysis, while the posterior pituitary is known as the *adeno*hypophysis.
___ 43. The *hypothalamo-hypophyseal tract* connects the hypothalamus to the posterior pituitary gland.

IV. MIDBRAIN AND HINDBRAIN

The midbrain and hindbrain contain many important relay centers for sensory and motor pathways, and are particularly important in the control of skeletal movements by the brain. The medulla oblongata, a vital region of the hindbrain, contains centers for the control of breathing and cardiovascular function.

A. Multiple Choice

___ 44. That portion of the brain housing the "four bodies" known as the corpora quadrigemina is the
   a. midbrain
   b. hindbrain
   c. diencephalon
   d. prosencephalon
   e. erebellum

___ 45. The *apneustic* center and *pneumotaxic* center that work together to influence respiratory movements, are located in the
   a. hypothalamus
   b. cerebellum
   c. midbrain
   d. pons
   e. medulla oblongata

___ 46. Damage to the cerebellum, the second largest structure in the brain, usually results in
   a. long-term and short-term memory loss
   b. loss of visual and auditory reflexes
   c. loss of respiratory and cardiovascular control
   d. ataxia or lack of muscular coordination

___ 47. Which of the following is *not* a vital center within the medulla oblongata portion of the myelencephalon?
   a. vasomotor center (diameter of blood vessels)
   b. center for rage and aggression (deep emotion)
   c. parasympathetic inhibitory control of the heart rate
   d. respiratory center (with the pons) for control of breathing
   e. All of these are vital centers in the medulla oblongata.

___ 48. That portion of the brain most responsible for the general arousal of the cerebral cortex when a variety of sensory sources are activated, is the
   a. cerebellum
   b. hypothalamus
   c. limbic system
   d. medulla oblongata
   e. reticular activating system (RAS)

B. True or False/Edit

___ 49. The *superior colliculi* of the corpora quadrigemina portion of the midbrain are involved in visual reflexes, while the *inferior colliculi* are involved in auditory reflexes.

___ 50. The *mesencephalon* is also known as the hindbrain and contains the cerebral peduncles, red nucleus, and the substantia nigra.

___ 51. The *metencephalon* is composed of the pons and the cerebrum.

___ 52. The *pons* contains several nuclei (cell bodies of neurons) associated with the control and interpretation of specific cranial nerves.

___ 53. The *cerebellum* receives sensory information from proprioceptors and, through relays with other nuclei, coordinates muscle movements.

___ 54. The *pyramids* of the medulla are characterized by crossing-over or decussation of nerve fiber tracts to the contralateral (opposite) side of the medulla.

___ 55. Falling asleep and loss of consciousness due to anesthesia perhaps both involve suppression of the *reticular activating system* (RAS).

V. SPINAL CORD TRACTS

Sensory information from receptors throughout most of the body is relayed to the brain by means of ascending tracts of fibers that conduct impulses up the spinal cord. When the brain directs motor activities, these directions are in the form of nerve impulses that travel down the spinal cord in descending tracts of fibers.

A. Multiple Choice

___ 56. The term "funiculi" refers to
  a. specific clusters of motor and sensory nuclei (cell bodies) in the spinal cord
  b. spinal cord ascending and descending columns of axons (myelinated, white matter)
  c. regions of gray matter crossovers (decussations) in the spinal cord
  d. autonomic vital centers located in the spinal cord

___ 57. Which of the following descending tracts is *not* extrapyramidal?
  a. reticulospinal
  b. corticospinal
  c. rubrospinal
  d. vestibulospinal
  e. All of these tracts are extrapyramidal.

B. True or False/Edit

___ 58. Unlike the brain, the spinal cord white matter is located in a central "H" pattern, with gray matter found on the outside.

___ 59. The spinothalamic and corticospinal tracts are both descending tracts in the spinal cord.

___ 60. All descending motor tracts from the brain eventually cross over and, thus, innervate muscles on the contralateral side of the body.

___ 61. The two major groups of descending tracts from the brain are the corticospinal (pyramidal) and extrapyramidal tracts.

___ 62. The positive Babinski sign, or reflex (upward movement of the toes) indicates damage to the extrapyramidal motor pathway.

VI. CRANIAL AND SPINAL NERVES

The central nervous system communicates with the body by means of nerves that exit the CNS from the brain (cranial nerves) and spinal cord (spinal nerves). These nerves, together with aggregations of cell bodies located outside the CNS, constitute the peripheral nervous system.

A. Multiple Choice

___ 63. How many pairs of **cranial** nerves exit the brain?
  a. twelve
  b. eighteen
  c. twenty-four
  d. thirty-eight
  e. forty-six

___ 64. How many pairs of **spinal** nerves exit the spinal cord?
  a. twelve
  b. twenty-four
  c. thirty-one
  d. forty-six
  e. fifty-two

___ 65. The dorsal root ganglion region of the spinal cord contains the
  a. axons of motor (efferent) and sensory (afferent) spinal neurons
  b. cell bodies of motor and sensory spinal neurons
  c. cell bodies of sensory spinal neurons only
  d. axons of sensory spinal neurons only
  e. cell bodies of motor spinal neurons only

___ 66. The ventral root portion of the spinal cord is composed of
  a. axons of sensory (afferent) spinal neurons
  b. nuclei (cell bodies) of sensory spinal neurons
  c. axons of motor (efferent) spinal neurons
  d. nuclei (cell bodies) of motor spinal neurons

B. True or False/Edit

___ 67. Most cranial nerves are classified as mixed nerves because they contain both sensory and motor fibers.
___ 68. All spinal nerves are classified as mixed nerves.
___ 69. The cell bodies of all somatic motor neurons are located in the dorsal root ganglia.
___ 70. A reflex arc occurs when some sensory stimulus produces an unconscious (that is, the brain is not directly involved) motor response.

CHAPTER REVIEW

A. Completion

71. The embryonic brain develops into: a forebrain made up of the _____ and the _____; the midbrain which is the _____; and the hindbrain, which contains the _____ and the _____.

72. Cerebrospinal fluid (CSF) is secreted by capillaries called _____, which are found in brain cavities called _____. The large neuron tract that connects the two hemispheres is the _____ _____, which links the _____ (left/right) hemisphere, which is normally dominant in language and analytical ability, with the _____ (left/right) hemisphere, which is normally strong in pattern and face recognition, music, and song creativity.

73. The cerebral cortex and basal ganglia are _____ (gray/white) matter due to collections of cell bodies, whereas the _____ (gray/white) matter is primarily _____. Damage to the _____ (left/right) cerebral cortex produces speech disabilities called _____, involving two specific areas. The area involved in speech comprehension is _____'s area, whereas _____'s area is required for the act of speaking.

74. The two brain regions most associated with emotion are the _____ _____ and the _____. The two forms of memory are _____-_____ and _____-_____, which appear to involve various brain areas in a very complex way.

75. In the diencephalon the important sensory relay center is the _____; the epithalamus contains a _____ for CSF production and the _____ gland synthesizing the hormone _____. The diencephalon includes the hypothalamus and pituitary gland.

76. The hypothalamus houses centers for control of _____, _____, _____, and emotions. It also has *direct* neuron contact with the _____ (anterior/posterior) pituitary and *indirect* contact via _____ with the _____ (anterior/posterior) pituitary gland.

77. Visual reflexes are coordinated in the _____ _____ of the corpora _____, whereas auditory reflexes involve the _____ _____.

78. The pons has two centers for breathing control called the _____ and _____ centers. A few _____ nerves have cell bodies originating in the pons. The medulla oblongata _____ also regulates _____ and controls cardiovascular functions as well.

79. Sensory information travels up _____ tracts, while the two motor tracts are _____. These motor tracts are the _____ or corticospinal tracts—which are nonstop neurons, crossing over or _____ in the medulla oblongata controlling fine muscle movement — and the _____ tracts — composed of many indirect connections among various brain regions and the muscles.

80. There are _____ (#) pairs of cranial nerves which are either _____ (sensory or motor) only or mixed. All _____ (#) pairs of spinal nerves are _____, with cell bodies of sensory neurons in the _____ ganglion, and motor neurons exiting the spinal cord along the _____ root. Sensory, association, and motor neurons may all interact in the subconscious pathway known as the _____.

B. Crossword Puzzle — The Central Nervous System

Across
1. part of the diencephalon—control over the pituitary gland
5. cerebral gray matter
6. descending (motor) tracts may be _____-pyramidal or pyramidal
9. mesencephalon region
10. this system may be a center for various emotions
11. metencephalon region for control and coordination of skeletal muscle movements
12. fluid produced by the choroid plexus of the ventricles
13. area required for mechanical performance of speech
16. afferent neurons of the reflex arc, for example
18. the telencephalon and diencephalon
20. function common to the limbic system and hypothalamus
21. a word for internal tissue functions—controlled by the hypothalamus
24. language disability
25. dorsal or ventral _____
26. important relay center for sensory information
27. a visceral function of the hypothalamus (seek water!)
28. in most people one or the other of these is dominant
29. sensory and motor neurons are part of the _____ arc

Down
2. gland controlled mainly by the hypothalamus
3. hormones from the hypothalamus control the _____ pituitary
4. area of the cortex involved in speech comprehension
5. cerebral hemispheres are joined by the corpus _____
6. test used to measure electrical activity in the brain
7. that part of the neuron that makes brain matter "gray" is the cell _____
8. the metencephalon and the myelencephalon combined
9. important function of the medial temporal lobes, especially the hippocampus
12. consists of two hemispheres
14. important function of the left cerebral cortex—Wernicke's and Broca's areas
15. fluid-filled brain cavities
17. a visceral function controlled by the hypothalamus
19. the thalamus is an important _____ center for sensory information
22. twelve pair of _____ nerves
23. metencephalon source of cranial nerves V through VIII

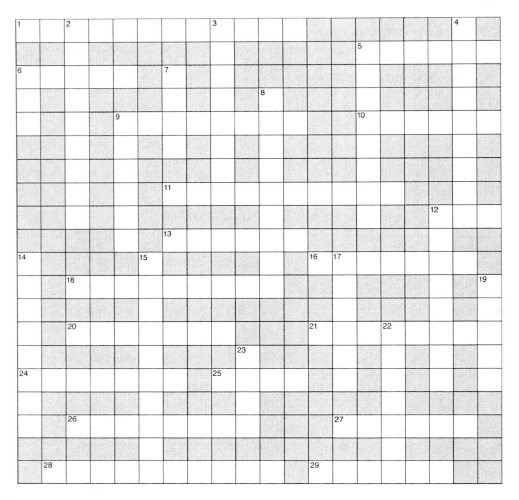

C. Essay

Essay Tutorial

This essay tutorial will answer the first essay question found in the "**Review Activities**" section of your *Human Physiology* textbook. Please look for *Essay Question* 1. at the end of chapter 8, read it carefully, and let me guide you through one possible answer. Watch for key terms in bold-face type, helpful tips and general suggestions on writing the essay or short-answer questions. Enjoy!

81. Define the term **decussation** and explain its significance in terms of the **pyramidal** motor system.

Answer: First, define the term decussation as the crossover of neuron fibers from one side of the brain or spinal cord to the other. The pyramidal tracts are exclusively descending and originate primarily from the motor (precentral gyrus) cortex, traveling nonstop to the spinal cord. Along the way, however, these neurons decussate in the medulla oblongata, forming visible triangular patterns on the dorsal surface of the medulla—hence the name pyramids. The major significance of this crossing-over means that the right cerebral hemisphere controls the muscles of the left half of the body, while the left hemisphere controls muscles of the right side of the body.

[You see, some "essay" answers can be short and sweet. However, always reread the question to be sure that all parts of the question have been answered. Too many of my students have needlessly lost important points with incomplete answers. Have you? For extra practice, try a couple more, OK?]

82. What does *EEG* stand for? Explain the neuron events that are responsible for the erratic cycles recorded on the EEG.

83. Describe the location of the *cerebellum*, its size, and explain how it functions in the indirect control over the coordination of voluntary muscle movements.

84. Describe the location of *Wernicke's* and *Broca's areas* in the cerebral cortex, and explain the evidence from neurosurgery and from damage to these areas which led to our current understanding of how speech is formed and interpreted.

85. A pesky mosquito lands on your left arm! Trace the action potentials that originate in your motor cortex (precentral gyrus) along the pyramidal tracts to the muscles of the opposite arm to swat the insect. *Note*: Keep track of left and right.

Answers — Chapter 8

I. Structural Organization of the Brain
   A. 1. a, 2. a, 3. d
   B. 4. T, 5. F—Replace "mesencephalon" with "rhombencephalon," 6. T, 7. T

II. Cerebrum
   A. 8. b, 9. d, 10. e, 11. d, 12. c, 13. c, 14. a, 15. c, 16. a, 17. b, 18. c, 19. c, 20. b, 21. d
   B. 22. F—Switch "sulci" and "gyri" 23. T, 24. T, 25. F—Replace "parietal" with "occipital," 26. T, 27. T, 28. T, 29. F—Switch "left" and "right," 30. F—

Replace "Broca's" with "Wernicke's," 31. T, 32. T
C. Label the Figure — Lobes and Important Regions of the Left Cerebral Cortex. See figure 8.6 in the text.
III. Diencephalon
   A. 33. a, 34. d, 35. d, 36. c, 37. c
   B. 38. F—Replace "taste" with "smell," 39. T, 40. T, 41. T, 42. F—Switch "anterior" and "posterior," 43. T
IV. Midbrain and Hindbrain
   A. 44. a, 45. d, 46. d, 47. b, 48. e
   B. 49. T, 50. F—Replace "hindbrain" with "midbrain," 51. F—Replace "cerebrum" with "cerebellum," 52. T, 53. T, 54. T, 55. T
V. Spinal Cord Tracts
   A. 56. b, 57. b
   B. 58. F—Switch "white" and "gray," 59. F—"Spinothalamic" tracts are ascending, 60. T, 61. T, 62. F—Replace "extrapyramidal" with "pyramidal"
VI. Cranial and Spinal Nerves
   A. 63. a, 64. c, 65. c, 66. c
   B. 67. T, 68. T, 69. F—Cell bodies of somatic motor neurons are located in the spinal cord, 70. T

Chapter Review
   A. 71. telencephalon, diencephalon, mesencephalon, metencephalon, myelencephalon, 72. choroid plexi, ventricles; corpus callosum, left, right, 73. gray, white, axons; left, aphasias; Wernicke, Broca, 74. limbic system, hypothalamus; short-term, long-term, 75. thalamus, choroid plexus, pineal, melatonin, 76. hunger, thirst, temperature; posterior, hormones, anterior, 77. superior colliculi, quadrigemina, inferior colliculi, 78. apneustic, pneumotaxic; cranial; oblongata, breathing, 79. ascending, descending; pyramidal, decussating; extrapyramidal, 80. twelve, sensory; thirty-one, mixed, dorsal root, ventral; reflex arc

B. Crossword Puzzle

	¹H	²Y	P	O	T	H	A	L	³A	M	U	S					⁴W	
		I					N					⁵C	O	R	T	E	X	
⁶E	X	T	R	A		⁷B		T				A				R	
E		U				O		E		⁸H		L				N	
G		I		⁹M	I	D	B	R	A	I	N		¹⁰L	I	M	B	I	C
		T		E		Y		I		N			O			C	
		A		M				O		D			S			K	
		R		O		¹¹C	E	R	E	B	E	L	L	U	M		E	
		Y		R				R					M			¹²C	S	F
				Y		¹³B	R	O	C	A	S					E	
¹⁴L				¹⁵V				I		¹⁶S	¹⁷E	N	S	O	R	Y	
A		¹⁸F	O	R	E	B	R	A	I	N		A				E		¹⁹R
N				N						T			B			E
G		²⁰E	M	O	T	I	O	N			²¹V	I	S	²²C	E	R	A	L
U				R			²³P			N		R	U	A
²⁴A	P	H	A	S	I	A	²⁵R	O	O	T		G		A		M		Y
G				C			N					N	
E		²⁶T	H	A	L	A	M	U	S		²⁷T	H	I	R	S	T
				E								A	
	²⁸H	E	M	I	S	P	H	E	R	E	²⁹R	E	F	L	E	X

85

CHAPTER 9
THE AUTONOMIC NERVOUS SYSTEM

CHAPTER SCOPE

This is the third chapter of the four-chapter unit on the nervous system and is entirely devoted to the subconscious or involuntary control over *smooth muscle, cardiac muscle,* or *glands*. Neurons of the autonomic nervous system are always **motor** (efferent) and are classified as either **sympathetic** or **parasympathetic**. There are a variety of neurotransmitters released by autonomic neurons. The action of these neurons is largely dependent upon the neurotransmitter chemical that is released from the presynaptic axon terminal and upon which specific type of receptor type that is waiting on the postsynaptic membrane to receive these neurotransmitters.

There are two major types of autonomic neuron receptors — those that are **adrenergic**, receiving norepinephrine, epinephrine, and related neurotransmitter substances; and those that are **cholinergic**, receiving acetylcholine (ACh). Interestingly, because the receptor types can vary from neuron to neuron, the same neurotransmitter may cause the *response* of one neuron to differ from that of another neuron. Sometimes *antagonistic*, sometimes *complementary*, and sometimes *cooperative*, typical autonomic neuron responses are described in this chapter. Since these neurons are all motor, many of their action potentials originate, and are controlled by higher brain centers such as the **hypothalamus, limbic system, cerebellum**, and **cerebrum**.

If we take time in this chapter to understand well the structure and function of the **autonomic nervous system (ANS)**, the effort will be quickly rewarded in a better understanding of the chapters that follow — endocrine (chapter 11), cardiovascular (chapters 13, 14), respiratory (chapter 15), renal (chapter 16), and reproduction (chapter 20).

I. NEURAL CONTROL OF INVOLUNTARY EFFECTORS

The autonomic nervous system helps to regulate the activities of cardiac muscle, smooth muscle, and glands. In this regulation, impulses are conducted from the CNS by an axon that synapses with a second autonomic neuron. It is the axon of this second neuron in the pathway that innervates the involuntary effectors.

A. Multiple Choice

____ 1. Which of the following is *not* an effector (target) of autonomic nervous system (ANS) motor neurons?
    a. cardiac muscle
    b. exocrine glands
    c. skeletal muscle
    d. endocrine glands
    e. smooth muscle

____ 2. Somatic motor neurons have cell bodies located _____ the CNS that send axons to _____; usually under _____ control.
    a. outside; skeletal muscle; involuntary
    b. inside; the viscera; voluntary
    c. outside; the viscera; involuntary
    d. inside; skeletal muscle; voluntary
    e. outside; the viscera; voluntary

____ 3. Which of the following statements does *not* describe *denervation hypersensitivity*?
    a. autonomic target tissues become more sensitive than normal to stimulating agents
    b. muscle effectors enter a state of flaccid paralysis and atrophy
    c. can result from severing (cutting) autonomic motor neurons

d. an example is restoring the secretion of acid from the stomach following vagotomy (severing the vagus nerve)

B. True or False/Edit

____ 4. Autonomic motor nerves innervate organs whose functions are *not* usually under voluntary control.

____ 5. The word *viscera* refers to the organs located within the body cavities.

____ 6. Unlike somatic motor neurons, autonomic motor neurons always involve two neurons in the efferent pathway.

____ 7. A *ganglion* is defined as a collection of cell bodies inside the CNS (brain and spinal cord).

____ 8. Ganglia are an integral part of the somatic motor pathway.

____ 9. Cardiac muscle (the heart) and many smooth muscles can contract rhythmically even in the absence of autonomic nerve stimulation.

____ 10. Unlike somatic motor neurons that always cause stimulation of skeletal muscle effectors, some autonomic nerves release neurotransmitter substances that inhibit the activity of their effectors.

II. DIVISIONS OF THE AUTONOMIC NERVOUS SYSTEM

Preganglionic neurons of the sympathetic division of the autonomic system originate in the thoracic and lumbar levels of the spinal cord and send axons to sympathetic ganglia, which parallel the spinal cord. Preganglionic neurons of the parasympathetic division, by contrast, originate in the brain and in the sacral level of the spinal cord, and send axons to ganglia located in or near the effector organs.

A. Multiple Choice

____ 11. Which statement regarding autonomic sympathetic neurons is *false*?
   a. They are usually activated as a single unit (mass activation).
   b. They emerge from the brain and sacral regions.
   c. They form white and grey rami communicantes fibers.
   d. They may have ganglia located along the spinal cord.

____ 12. Which of the following ganglia is *not* a collateral (prevertebral) ganglion?
   a. celiac
   b. superior mesenteric
   c. inferior mesenteric
   d. cervical

____ 13. Which system is *not* served by postganglionic fibers that arise from the *collateral* (prevertebral) ganglia?
   a. respiratory
   b. digestive
   c. urinary
   d. reproductive
   e. All of these systems are served by these postganglionic fibers.

____ 14. Which of the following statements about parasympathetic neurons is *false*?
   a. Like sympathetics, they travel within spinal nerves.
   b. They synapse in terminal ganglia, either next to or within the organs innervated.
   c. They originate in the brain or sacral spinal cord regions (the craniosacral division).
   d. Postganglionic fibers are usually shorter than those of sympathetic neurons.
   e. They send preganglionic fibers to the visceral organs, such as the heart, lungs, esophagus, intestine, among others.

B. True or False/Edit

____ 15. Both sympathetic and parasympathetic neurons have preganglionic cell bodies located inside the CNS and postganglionic cell bodies located outside the CNS.

____ 16. Preganglionic sympathetic neurons are myelinated, and thus, called *white* rami communicantes, while postganglionic sympathetic fibers are unmyelinated, and therefore, known as the *gray* rami communicantes.

___ 17. The convergence of impulses from the spinal cord to the ganglia and the divergence of impulses within the ganglia usually result in the mass activation of almost all postganglionic fibers as a unit.
___ 18. The cortex of the adrenal gland is a modified sympathetic ganglion.
___ 19. Neurons whose cell bodies originate in the medulla oblongata and whose axons serve as cranial nerves, would be classified as parasympathetic.
___ 20. Sympathetic neurons show great divergence from preganglionic to postganglionic fibers, whereas parasympathetic neurons diverge only a little.

III. FUNCTIONS OF THE AUTONOMIC NERVOUS SYSTEM

The sympathetic division activates the body to "fight or flight," largely through the release of norepinephrine from postganglionic fibers and the secretion of epinephrine from the adrenal medulla. The parasympathetic division often produces antagonistic effects through the release of acetylcholine from its postganglionic fibers. The actions of both divisions of the autonomic nervous system must be balanced in order to maintain homeostasis.

A. Multiple Choice

___ 21. Which neuron does *not* release acetylcholine (ACh) as a neurotransmitter?
   a. preganglionic sympathetic fibers
   b. postganglionic sympathetic fibers
   c. preganglionic parasympathetic fibers
   d. postganglionic parasympathetic fibers

___ 22. *Catecholamines* are substances derived from the amino acid, tyrosine, and include all of the following *except*
   a. acetylcholine (ACh)
   b. epinephrine
   c. dopamine
   d. norepinephrine

___ 23. Which of the following is *not* a ß-adrenergic response?
   a. slowing down (relaxation) of the digestive tract muscular motility, such as peristalsis
   b. opening of the airways or bronchioles in the lung
   c. increasing the force and rate of the heart beat
   d. dilating the smooth muscle of the skin and splanchnic blood vessels
   e. relaxing the smooth muscle wall of the urinary bladder

___ 24. The drug that aids the suffering of asthmatics by serving as a $ß_2$ agonist to dilate the airways of the lung, is
   a. terbutaline
   b. atenolol
   c. phenylephrine
   d. clonidine

___ 25. Which statement about *muscarinic* receptors is *false*?
   a. They are not found in autonomic ganglia or at the neuromuscular junctions of skeletal muscle fibers.
   b. They are stimulated by extracts from poisonous mushrooms.
   c. They are subtypes of adrenergic receptors.
   d. They are not affected by the drug, curare, which specifically blocks nicotinic receptors.
   e. They can be found on the target organs of specific postganglionic parasympathetic fibers.

___ 26. Which of the following molecules is *not* a proposed neurotransmitter of the select group of "nonadrenergic noncholinergic" postganglionic autonomic axons?
   a. adenosine triphosphate (ATP)
   b. gamma aminobutyric acid (GABA)
   c. vasoactive intestinal peptide (VIP)
   d. nitric oxide (NO)
   e. All of these are candidate neurotransmitters.

___ 27. The separate effects of sympathetic and parasympathetic innervation of the pacemaker region of the heart can best be described as
   a. antagonistic
   b. complementary
   c. cooperative (synergistic)

___ 28. The effects of sympathetic and parasympathetic innervation on the urinary and reproductive systems are
   a. antagonistic
   b. complementary
   c. cooperative (synergistic)

___ 29. The effects of sympathetic and parasympathetic stimulation on the salivary gland secretion are
   a. antagonistic
   b. complementary
   c. cooperative (synergistic)

___ 30. Which of the following target tissues is (are) innervated *only* by the sympathetic neurons?
   a. adrenal medulla
   b. arrector pili muscle
   c. sweat glands
   d. most blood vessels
   e. All of these are only innervated by sympathetics.

___ 31. That brain region that most *directly* controls the activity of the autonomic nervous system, is the
   a. medulla oblongata
   b. pituitary gland
   c. cerebellum
   d. hypothalamus
   e. basal ganglia

___ 32. Which system does *not* have its control center in the *medulla*?
   a. cardiovascular system
   b. pulmonary system
   c. urinary system
   d. reproductive system
   e. immune system

___ 33. The *hypothalamus* does *not* contain the control center for the homeostatic regulation of
   a. body temperature
   b. various emotional states
   c. hunger
   d. breathing
   e. thirst

B. True or False/Edit

___ 34. Sympathetic and parasympathetic neurons usually release different neurotransmitters from their respective postganglionic neuron axons.

___ 35. Those sympathetic postganglionic neurons activating blood vessels in skeletal muscle and in sweat glands are unique in their release of acetylcholine (ACh) instead of norepinephrine (NE).

___ 36. Adrenergic stimulation by epinephrine, usually secreted by the adrenal medulla, and by norepinephrine, secreted from sympathetic nerve endings, can produce both excitatory and inhibitory effects.

___ 37. The two subtypes of alpha receptors produce their effects by stimulating increases in the production of the second messenger, cyclic AMP (cAMP), within the target cell cytoplasm.

___ 38. The response of a target cell when norepinephrine binds to I_1 receptors results in a rise in intracellular calcium (Ca^{2+}) concentration that serves as a "second messenger" molecule.

___ 39. Stimulation of alpha-adrenergic receptors located on smooth muscle fibers in the walls of blood vessels almost always results in contraction and vasoconstriction.

___ 40. The activation of somatic motor neurons or preganglionic autonomic neurons results in cholinergic effects that can be both excitatory and inhibitory.
___ 41. Both nicotinic and muscarinic receptors bind with and respond to the neurotransmitter, acetylcholine (ACh).
___ 42. Parasympathetic neuron stimulation of the pacemaker region of the heart increases the heart rate.
___ 43. In the digestive system, activation of parasympathetic neurons increases intestinal movements and intestinal secretions.
___ 44. Increased sympathetic neuron activity causes blood vessels to constrict, whereas vasodilation results from a decrease in sympathetic nerve activity.
___ 45. Cooling of the body can be accomplished by sweat glands in the trunk that secrete both a watery sweat that evaporates and a chemical, bradykinin, that dilates surface blood vessels to help radiate heat.
___ 46. The vagus nerve is a mixed nerve, containing both sensory and motor neuron fibers.
___ 47. Thermoregulation, the regulation of heat gain or loss by the body, is accomplished without the direct involvement of the parasympathetic nervous system.
___ 48. Blushing, pallor, fainting, breaking out in a cold sweat, a racing heartbeat, and "butterflies in the stomach", are only some of the many visceral reactions that accompany emotional activation of the hypothalamus.

C. Label the Figure — Autonomic Nervous System Neurotransmitters

Neurons of the autonomic nervous system are motor (efferent) and release the neurotransmitters acetylcholine (ACh) and norepinephrine (NE). Those synapses with receptors for acetylcholine are called *cholinergic* and those with receptors for norepinephrine are called *adrenergic*. Study figure 9.1 and locate the nine blank spaces at the autonomic synapses. Write either *ACh* or *NE* in the spaces provided. When finished, check your work with figure 9.8 in the text.

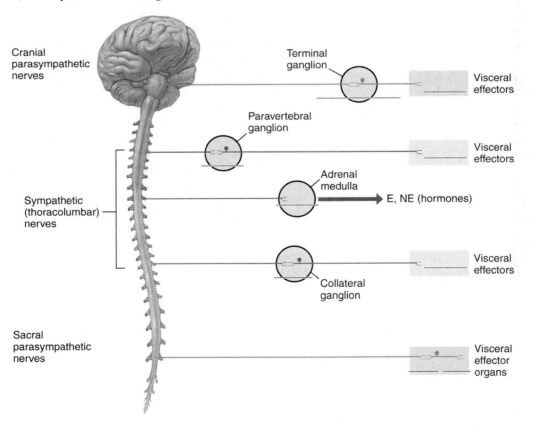

CHAPTER REVIEW

A. Completion

49. Autonomic neuron axons are always motor or _____, originating in the _____ or _____ as preganglionic neurons. Postganglionic neurons originate from collections of _____ outside the CNS, known as _____.
50. The three target or _____ cells at the end of autonomic neurons are _____ _____, _____ _____, and _____.
51. Severing or cutting autonomic neurons results in an increase in responsiveness at the target cell. This characteristic of autonomic neurons is called _____. Preganglionic sympathetic neurons emerge from the _____ and _____ levels of the spinal cord, whereas preganglionic parasympathetic fibers originate in the _____ and _____ levels of the spinal cord.
52. Cell bodies of postganglionic sympathetic neurons are located in ganglia called the sympathetic or _____ ganglia; the _____ ganglia (which include the celiac and mesenteric) innervate organs of the digestive, _____, and _____ systems. Modified sympathetic ganglion cells are located directly in the medulla of the _____ gland.
53. Many cranial nerves are _____ (pre-/post-) ganglionic _____ (sympathetic/parasympathetic) neurons with _____ (long/short) postganglionic neurons because the ganglia are located close to or _____ the target cells.
54. "Fight or flight" results from the release of the neurotransmitter _____ from postganglionic _____ (sympathetic/parasympathetic) neurons—effects called _____.
55. All preganglionic fibers and all postganglionic fibers that are _____ (sympathetic/parasympathetic) release only the neurotransmitter _____, and their effects are called _____. Beware — sympathetic fibers that innervate _____ _____ and those that innervate _____ in skeletal muscles are cholinergic!
56. Norepinephrine binds to two groups of receptor proteins, known as _____ and _____, with two subtypes for each (1 and 2), which produce _____ (adrenergic/cholinergic) effects in various organs of the body.
57. In organs stimulated by both sympathetic and parasympathetic neurons (_____ innervation), the actions between these two types of neurons will be _____, _____, or _____.
58. The two most important regions of the brain directly responsible for the control of autonomic nervous system activity are the _____ _____ and the _____.

B. Crossword Puzzle—The Autonomic Nervous System

Across
1. Autonomic nervous system action on salivary glands
3. One origin for preganglionic neurons of the sympathetic division
6. Related to the female gonad
7. Key economic indicator
8. Change in the autonomic effector that may occur when disconnected from its innervation
11. Most common (85%) catecholamine released from the adrenal medulla during sympathetic stimulation
13. Specialized receptors on the postsynaptic membrane that recognize ACh
16. Long cranial nerve (X)
19. Alcohol form of a steroid molecule
20. Double chain of sympathetic ganglia outside the spinal cord
22. Autonomic effectors include smooth muscle, cardiac muscle, and _____
23. Division of the autonomic nervous system including spinal nerves that exit the brain and lower spinal cord (lumbar)
26. Emergency distress signal
27. If not the beginning
28. Subconscious or involuntary division of the nervous system
30. Spinal cord origin of preganglionic sympathetic neurons
32. Adrenergic effects include heart stimulation and _____ of the bronchi
33. Actions taken involving the law
34. One type of muscle innervated by autonomic neurons
35. Autonomic neurons originating from ganglia located outside the central nervous system (CNS)

37. Drug that inhibits the effects of parasympathetic nerve stimulation (anticholinergic)
38. Cats love to play with balls of this material (not yarn)
39. Drug that acts as a beta-blocker on both the heart and the bronchioles of the lung
41. Preganglionic neurons of the parasympathetic division of the autonomic nervous system (ANS) originate here
42. Specialized receptors on the postsynaptic membrane that recognize catecholamines (for example, epinephrine)
43. Common time piece

Down

2. Adrenergic receptor proteins are grouped as either _____ or beta
4. Autonomic nerves can have either excitatory or _____ effects on their target organs
5. Action of the autonomic nervous system on the regulation of the reproductive and urinary systems
7. Collections of neuron cell bodies located outside the CNS
9. Word vital to all "real" shoppers
10. Autonomic portion of the adrenal glands—activated during "fight-or-flight"
12. Nucleic acid used in the synthesis of proteins
13. Deoxyribonucleic acid (DNA) is commonly called the genetic _____
14. Any chemical synthesized by and released from presynaptic neurons
15. Autonomic neurons originating from the brain or spinal cord
17. "Fight-or-flight" division of the autonomic nervous system
18. Adrenergic effects include heart stimulation and blood vessel _____
21. Drug that promotes cholinergic effects of parasympathetic nerve stimulation
24. Smallest unit of matter
25. Action of the autonomic nervous system on the heart and pupils
29. Include the celiac, superior, and inferior mesenteric ganglia
31. Area of the brain stem most in control of autonomic system activity is the medulla _____
36. Excessive secretion of growth hormone (GH) can result in a pituitary _____
40. Fishing outing requires a rod 'n' _____

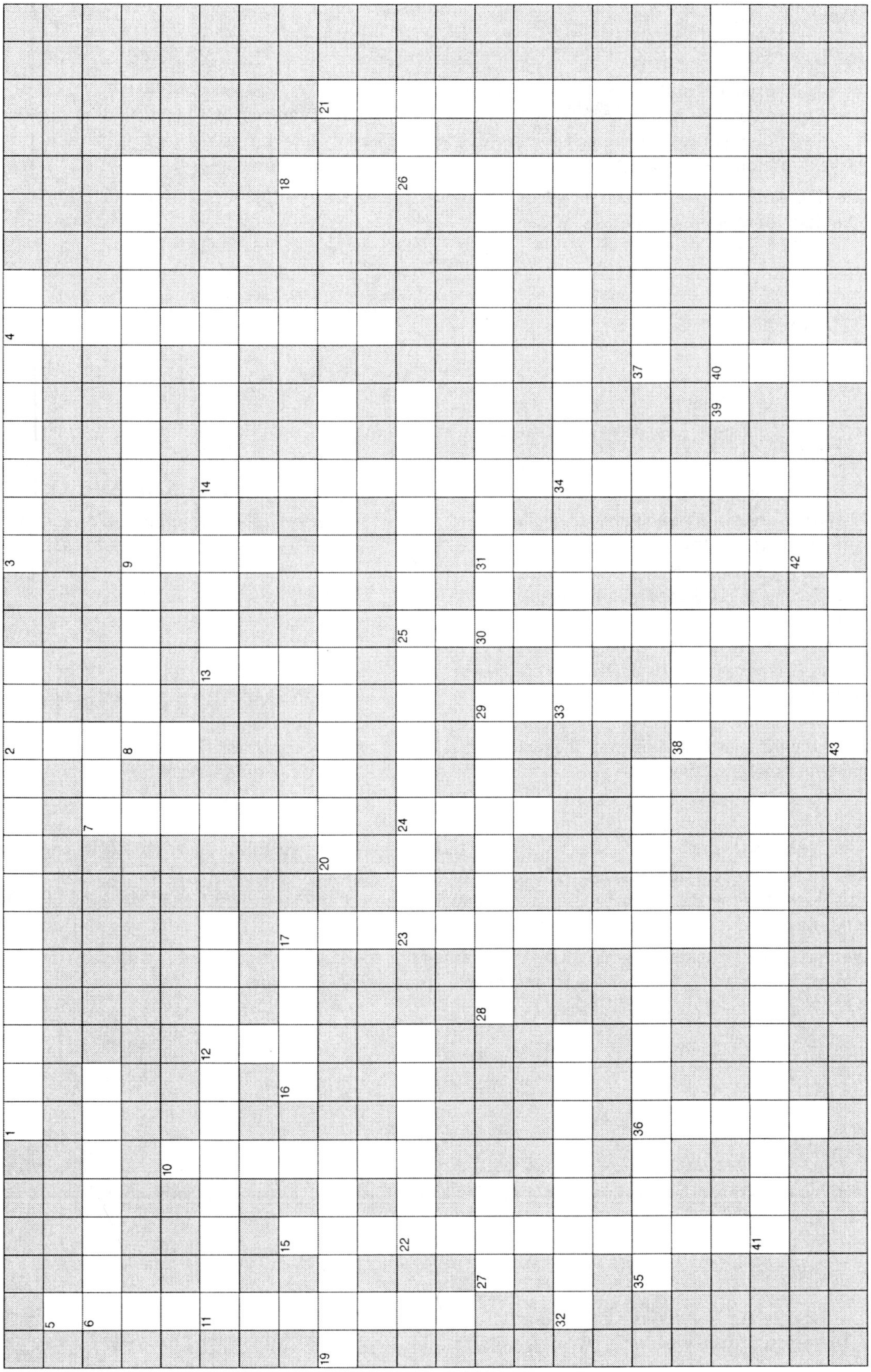
1
2
3
4
5
6
7
8
9
10
11
12
13
14
15
16
17
18
19
20
21
22
23
24
25
26
27
28
29
30
31
32
33
34
35
36
37
38
39
40
41
42
43

C. Essay

Essay Tutorial

This essay tutorial will answer the first essay question found in the "**Review Activities**" section of your *Human Physiology* textbook. Please look for *Essay Question* 1. at the end of chapter 9, read it carefully, and let me guide you through one possible answer. Watch for key terms in bold-face type, helpful tips and general suggestions on writing the essay or short-answer questions. Enjoy!

59. Compare the sympathetic and parasympathetic systems in terms of the **location** of their **ganglia** and the **distribution** of their **nerves.**

Answer. This question can easily be answered by creating a numbered outline within a "mini-table" such as that which follows:

Sympathetic	Parasympathetic
1. Ganglia — double (left and right) chain close to and parallel to the vertebrae (*paravertebral*); or farther out from the spinal cord in *collateral* ganglia (celiac, superior, and inferior mesenteric ganglia); and the direct "hotline" to the *adrenal medulla*.	1. Terminal ganglia are located on or close to the target cells.
2. Nerve distribution — preganglionic nerves exit the thoracic and lumbar areas of the spinal cord with branches from the head down to the lower abdomen.	2. Preganglionic nerve exits the brain or sacral region of the spinal cord. Many cranial nerves such as III, VII, IX, and X (vagus nerve); may innervate the same or different cells.

Do you notice how organized your answers can be? Students who spend the time and effort constructing tables like this one will be rewarded with quick "table-at-a-glance" learning tools before exam time — and professors will enjoy the easier grading as a bonus! Keep up the good work! Now try a couple more if time permits.

60. Explain how sympathetic innervation of the adrenal medulla follows a "hotline" pathway from the brain, directing the "fight-or-flight" response to emergency situations.

61. Define the terms **adrenergic** and **cholinergic**; and describe the anatomical distribution of these autonomic effects.

62. Name the two most important areas of the brain controlling autonomic activity (involuntary); and describe the various physiologic systems that are controlled by these two regions.

Answers — Chapter 9

I. Neural Control of Involuntary Effectors
   A. 1. , 2. , 3.
   B. 4. , 5. , 6. , 7. —Replace "inside" with "outside," 8. F—Replace "somatic" with "autonomic," 9. T, 10. T
II. Divisions of the Autonomic Nervous System
   A. 11. b, 12. d, 13. a, 14. a
   B. 15. T, 16. T, 17. F—Switch "convergence" with "divergence," 18. F—Replace "cortex" with "medulla," 19. T, 20. T
III. Functions of the Autonomic Nervous System
   A. 21. b, 22. a, 23. d, 24. a, 25. c, 26. b, 27. a, 28. c, 29. b, 30. e, 31. a, 32. e, 33. d
   B. 34. T, 35. T, 36. T, 37. F—Replace "alpha" with "beta," 38. T, 39. T, 40. F—They are excitatory only, 41. T, 42. F—Replace "increases" with "decreases," 43. T, 44. T, 45. T, 46. T, 47. T, 48. F—Replace "hypothalamus" with "limbic system"
   C. Autonomic Nervous System Neurotransmitters; See figure 9.8 in the text.

Chapter Review
   A. 49. efferent, brain, spinal cord; cell bodies, ganglia, 50. effector, smooth muscle, cardiac muscle, glands, 51. denervation hypersensitivity; thoracic, lumbar, brain, sacral, 52. paravertebral, collateral, urinary, reproductive; adrenal, 53. pre-, parasympathetic, short, within, 54. norepinephrine (NE), sympathetic, adrenergic, 55. parasympathetic, ACh, cholinergic; sweat glands, blood vessels, 56. alpha, beta, adrenergic, 57. dual, antagonistic, complementary, cooperative, 58. medulla oblongata, hypothalamus

B. Crossword Puzzle

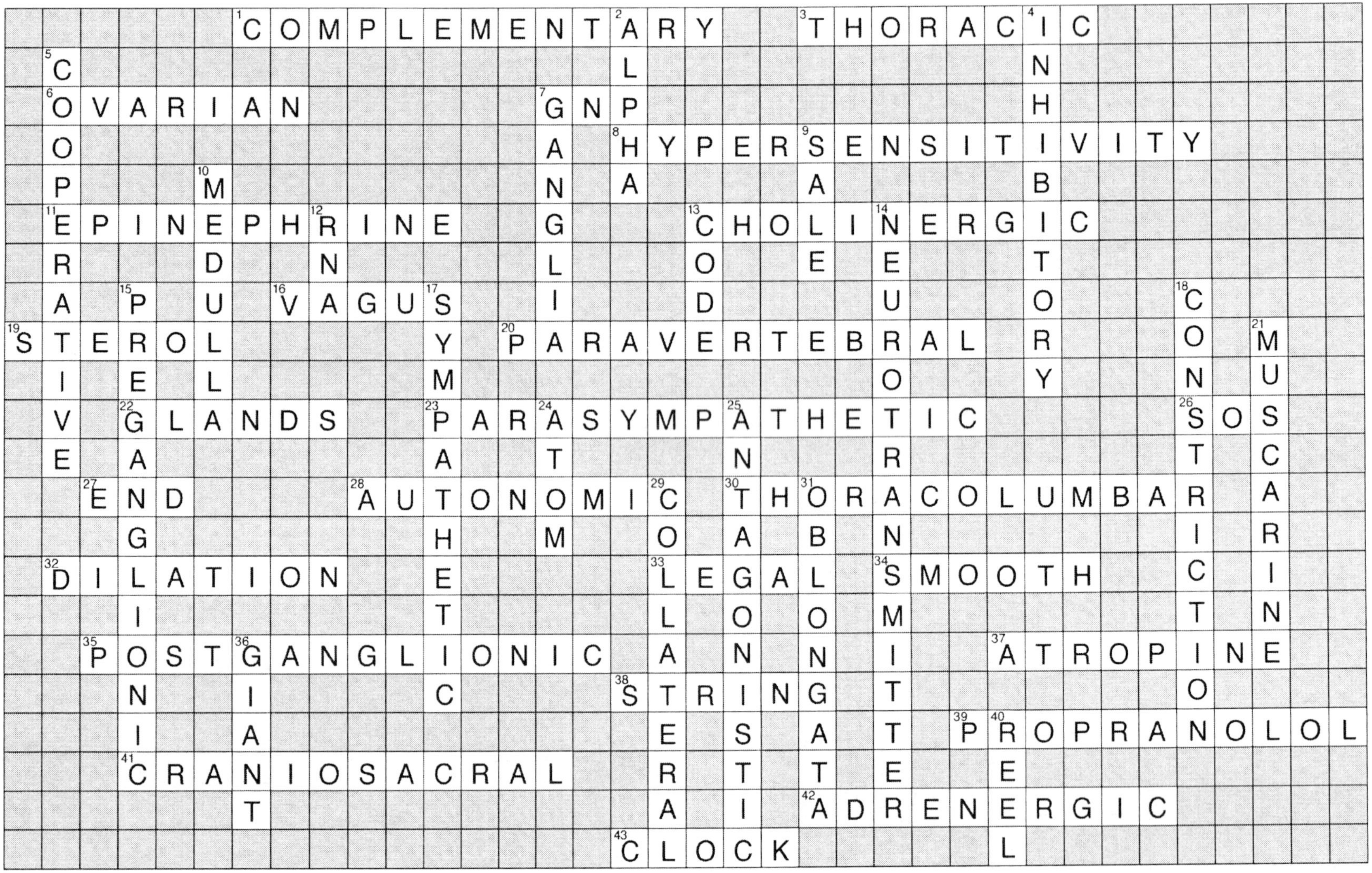

CHAPTER 10
SENSORY PHYSIOLOGY

CHAPTER SCOPE

Earlier (chapter 8), we explored the brain and spinal cord, pointing out important regions such as the **sensory cortex** (postcentral gyrus), the **auditory cortex** (temporal) the **visual cortex** (occipital) and the deeper, specialized nuclei for interpretation of **taste** and **smell**. This chapter examines characteristics of the many specialized structures known as *sensory receptors* that allow us to perceive a variety of disturbances in our environment. When appropriately stimulated, these receptors generate electrical impulses or action potentials that are directed to the brain for interpretation.

Sensory receptors in the skin (**cutaneous**) such as those sensitive to changes in temperature, pressure, touch, and pain provide us with our most familiar contact with the surrounding world. The specialized sensory receptors for taste (*gustation*), smell (*olfaction*), and sensation of balance (*vestibular equilibrium*) are not as familiar to us, yet they use many of the same principles that apply to the cutaneous receptors. In addition, the ear and the eye as unique receptors for **hearing** and **vision** are clearly presented. Each of these receptors generate nerve impulses that the brain interprets, incorporates with other input, and then responds to appropriately.

I. CHARACTERISTICS OF SENSORY RECEPTORS

Each type of sensory receptor responds to a particular modality of environmental stimulus by causing the production of action potentials in a sensory neuron. These impulses are conducted to parts of the brain that provide the proper interpretation of sensory perception when that particular neural pathway is activated.

A. Multiple Choice

    1. Which of the following is *not* a chemoreceptor?
       a. taste bud
       b. olfactory epithelium
       c. hot and cold receptors
       d. aortic and carotid bodies
       e. All of these are chemoreceptors.

    2. Which of the following is *not* a mechanoreceptor?
       a. touch receptor
       b. pain receptor
       c. pressure receptor
       d. inner ear hair cell (for hearing)
       e. vestibular hair cell (for balance)

    3. Which of the following is *not* a proprioceptor?
       a. muscle spindle
       b. Golgi tendon organ
       c. touch and pressure receptors
       d. joint receptors

    4. Which of the following is *not* a cutaneous receptor?
       a. touch receptor
       b. joint receptor
       c. pain receptor
       d. temperature receptor
       e. All of these are cutaneous receptors.

    5. Which of the following sensations does *not* adapt quickly, if at all, to constant stimuli?
       a. temperature
       b. touch

       c. pain
       d. odor
       e. All of these sensations adapt quickly.
   ___ 6. Which of the following does *not* apply to the *law of specific nerve energies*?
       a. Stimulation of a sensory nerve fiber produces only one sensation, such as touch, cold, pain, and so on.
       b. Each sensory neuron responds to its own normal, or adequate, stimulus with a characteristic sensation.
       c. Sensory neurons may respond to "injury currents" as readily as they do to "normal" stimuli.
       d. Paradoxical cold is an example of the law of specific nerve energies.
       e. All of these apply.
   ___ 7. The pacinian corpuscle is a cutaneous receptor for
       a. heat
       b. cold
       c. touch
       d. pressure
       e. pain
   ___ 8. The difference between a strong stimulus (for example, *hot*) and a weak stimulus (for example, *warm*) is that the strong stimulus
       a. produces a greater number of action potentials per unit of time (frequency)
       b. produces action potentials having greater strength (amplitude)
       c. routes action potentials to more sensitive brain areas
       d. produces action potentials that last a longer period of time (duration)

B. True or False/Edit

___ 9. The term "modality" refers to the quality of sensation, such as sound, light, pressure, and so on.
___ 10. Sensory receptors are actually specialized neurons or dendrites of such neurons that may be free or encapsulated within nonneural structures.
___ 11. Nociceptors provide us with a sense of body position.
___ 12. Receptors that produce a relatively constant rate of firing as long as the stimulus is maintained are known as *phasic* receptors.
___ 13. Receptor potentials are the same as generator potentials since they are formed in sensory nerve endings (receptors) and serve to generate action potentials.
___ 14. All generator potentials reach threshold and fire action potentials from the periphery toward the brain.

II. CUTANEOUS SENSATIONS

There are several different types of sensory receptors in the skin, each of which is specialized to be maximally sensitive to one modality of sensation. A receptor will be activated when a given area of the skin is stimulated; this is the receptive field of that receptor. A process known as lateral inhibition helps to sharpen the perceived location of the stimulus on the skin.

A. Multiple Choice

___ 15. The *medial lemniscus* is a sensory fiber tract of second-order neurons relaying cutaneous information to the
       a. thalamus
       b. medulla oblongata
       c. spinal cord
       d. cerebral cortex
       e. None of these regions receives information from the medial lemniscus.
___ 16. Somatesthetic action potentials are perceived by the
       a. thalamus
       b. medulla oblongata
       c. spinal cord
       d. cerebral cortex (postcentral gyrus)

___ 17. The tip of the index finger is very sensitive because
    a. the size of each receptive field is very small
    b. the density of its touch receptors is very high
    c. its representative area on the cortex is very large
    d. All of these help explain this fingertip sensitivity.

___ 18. Which statement about lateral inhibition is *false*?
    a. It occurs via inhibitory interneurons in the central nervous system (CNS).
    b. Weaker, neighboring input is inhibited from reaching the brain.
    c. It is characteristic only of receptors in the skin (cutaneous).
    d. It results in a sharpening of sensation with perception that is more well-defined than the original stimulus that was applied.

B. True or False/Edit

___ 19. Somatesthetic sensors include sensations from cutaneous receptors and proprioceptors.

___ 20. Somatesthetic information is projected to the postcentral gyrus of the ipsilateral cerebral hemisphere for interpretation.

___ 21. The larger area of the cortex devoted to the interpretation of face and hand sensation is due to the higher density of sensory receptors in the face and hands.

___ 22. The two-point threshold test is used to measure the minimum distance on the skin between neighboring receptive fields for touch.

III. TASTE AND OLFACTION

The receptors for taste and olfaction respond to molecules that are dissolved in fluid, and are thus classified as chemoreceptors. Although there are only four basic modalities of taste, they combine in various ways and are influenced by sensations of olfaction, thus permitting a wide variety of different sensory experiences.

A. Multiple Choice

___ 23. Which of the following is *not* characteristic of taste buds?
    a. They have microvilli at their apical (top) opening to the surface.
    b. They are characterized as interoceptors.
    c. They respond to chemicals dissolved in saliva.
    d. Along the tongue, they are innervated by two different cranial nerves.
    e. Although taste bud cells are not neurons, they are able to depolarize and release chemical transmitters when stimulated.

___ 24. Which is *not* one of the four basic taste modalities?
    a. bitter
    b. metallic
    c. salty
    d. sour
    e. sweet

___ 25. Which is *not* a characteristic of olfactory sensation?
    a. Olfactory receptors can be classified as chemoreceptors and exteroceptors.
    b. Olfactory receptors are bipolar neurons that are unique, dividing by mitosis to replace themselves every month or two.
    c. Olfactory information (smell) is perceived in the limbic system region of the cerebral cortex.
    d. Smells can affect both memory and emotion.
    e. All of these are characteristic of olfactory sensation.

B. True or False/Edit

___ 26. Chemoreceptors can be characterized as interoceptors or exteroceptors based on the source of the chemical stimuli.

___ 27. Both salt and sour tastes are mediated by receptors that are coupled to G-proteins that, in turn, activate second-messenger systems within the cytoplasm of the receptor cell.

___ 28. Although taste can be neatly grouped into four modalities, smell is not as easily classified into specific groups of odors.

___ 29. Despite the recent discovery of a large family of genes (thousands in number) that code for olfactory receptor proteins, the fact that humans can distinguish up to 10,000 different odors continues to be unexplained.

___ 30. Before taste buds and olfactory receptors can respond, the stimulating chemicals must first be dissolved in a fluid medium.

IV. VESTIBULAR APPARATUS AND EQUILIBRIUM

The sense of equilibrium is provided by structures in the inner ear, collectively known as the vestibular apparatus. Movements of the head cause fluid within these structures to bend extensions of sensory hair cells, and this mechanical bending results in the production of action potentials.

A. Multiple Choice

___ 31. Which of the following is *not* part of the vestibular apparatus?
   a. cochlea
   b. otolith organs
   c. utricle
   d. saccule
   e. semicircular canals

___ 32. Information about *linear* acceleration is sensed by
   a. the utricle only
   b. the saccule only
   c. the semicircular canals
   d. both the utricle and saccule

___ 33. The receptors for the sense of equilibrium are modified epithelial cells called
   a. chemoreceptors
   b. proprioceptors
   c. stereocilia
   d. hair cells
   e. kinocilia

___ 34. Arrange the following events in proper sequence.
   1. Hair cell membrane is depressed; hair cells depolarize.
   2. Stereocilia are bent in the direction of the kinocilium.
   3. Newly generated action potentials race along the eighth cranial nerve.
   4. The body (and head) move or accelerate linearly.
   5. Hair cells release synaptic transmitter substances.
      a. 2, 5, 4, 1, 3
      b. 4, 3, 2, 1, 5
      c. 4, 2, 1, 5, 3
      d. 2, 3, 1, 5, 4

___ 35. The *otolith* membrane is an important part of the
   a. utricle and saccule
   b. vestibular apparatus
   c. semicircular canals
   d. cochlea

___ 36. Hair cells, ampulla, and cupula are located in the
   a. utricle and saccule
   b. vestibular apparatus
   c. semicircular canals
   d. cochlea

___ 37. Angular or rotational acceleration is sensed by
   a. the utricle only
   b. the saccule only

      c. the semicircular canals
      d. both the utricle and saccule

B. True or False/Edit

____ 38. The sense of equilibrium can be described as the orientation of the body with respect to the pull of gravity.

____ 39. The sensory receptors of the vestibular apparatus and cochlea are located within a tubular "membranous labyrinth" filled with fluid, called perilymph.

____ 40. Perilymph is similar in ionic composition to cerebrospinal fluid (CSF).

____ 41. Rotational or angular acceleration is sensed by the semicircular canals.

____ 42. Hyperpolarization of hair cell membranes reduces the quantity of synaptic transmitter released that, in turn, reduces the frequency (impulses per minute) of action potentials.

____ 43. The *utricle* is most sensitive to vertical acceleration, while the *saccule* is most sensitive to horizontal acceleration.

____ 44. Vestibular nystagmus refers to involuntary oscillations of the eyes, which may occur after a spinning person is stopped abruptly; and is also a symptom of Meniere's disease.

____ 45. The duct of Hensen is a tiny hole that permits the continuous flow of endolymph from the vestibular apparatus to the cochlea.

V. THE EARS AND HEARING

Sound causes vibrations of the tympanic membrane. These vibrations, in turn, produce movements of the middle ear ossicles, which press against a membrane called the oval window in the cochlea. The movements of the oval window produce pressure waves within the fluid of the cochlea, which in turn cause movements of a membrane called the basilar membrane. Sensory hair cells are located on the basilar membrane, and the movements of this membrane in response to sound result in the bending of the hair cell processes. This stimulates action potentials in sensory fibers, which are transmitted to the brain and interpreted as sound.

A. Multiple Choice

____ 46. The *pitch* of a sound is directly related to the _____ of sound waves and is measured in units called _____.
      a. amplitude; hertz
      b. frequency; hertz
      c. amplitude; decibels
      d. frequency; decibels

____ 47. Which of the following is *not* part of the functional unit of the cochlea known as the *organ of Corti*?
      a. Reissner's membrane
      b. basilar membrane
      c. tectorial membrane
      d. inner and outer hair cells with sensory fibers

____ 48. The louder the sound intensity entering the ear, the greater the
      a. amplitude of action potentials formed by sensory hair cells
      b. frequency of action potentials formed by sensory hair cells
      c. displacement of the basilar membrane
      d. Both a and c are correct.
      e. Both b and c are correct.

____ 49. Which of the following is *not* part of the neural pathway leading to the interpretation of sound by the brain?
      a. the sensory hair cells of the organ of Corti
      b. the inferior colliculus of the midbrain (corpora quadrigemina)
      c. the vestibulocochlear (eighth cranial) nerve
      d. the thalamus (medial geniculate)
      e. All of these are part of the neural pathway for sound.

___ 50. Which of the following is *not* true of *conduction* deafness?
   a. It impairs hearing at all sound frequencies.
   b. It results when the transmission of sound waves from the air through the middle ear to the oval window is impaired.
   c. It may be caused by otitis media or otosclerosis.
   d. It is the cause of age-related hearing deficits known as presbycusis.
   e. All of these are true regarding conduction deafness.

B. True or False/Edit

___ 51. The intensity or loudness of a sound is directly related to the amplitude of the sound waves, and it is measured in units known as decibels.
___ 52. The auditory (eustachian) tube is a normally collapsed passageway leading from the inner ear to the nasopharynx.
___ 53. Damage to the tympanic membrane or middle ear ossicles, such as that caused by otitis media or otosclerosis, results in conduction deafness.
___ 54. The cochlear duct conducts pressure waves created by sound, and contains endolymph that bathes the sensory hair cells of the organ of Corti.
___ 55. The greater the displacement of the basilar membrane and the bending of the stereocilia, the greater the frequency of action potentials produced which will be perceived as a louder sound.
___ 56. High pitched sounds produce peak displacement closer to the base of the basilar membrane, while lower pitched sounds cause peak displacement further toward the apex.
___ 57. Nerve or sensory deafness can be caused by otitis media.

VI. THE EYES AND VISION

Light from an observed object is focused by the cornea and lens onto the photoreceptive retina at the back of the eye. The focus is maintained on the retina at different distances between a visual object and the eyes by variations in the curvature of the lens.

A. Multiple Choice

___ 58. The structures of the eye that transmit and refract light are the
   a. lens and cornea
   b. lens and choroid
   c. cornea and iris
   d. cornea and choroid
   e. lens and sclera
___ 59. The structure of the eye that is darkly pigmented to absorb light within the eyeball, and thereby prevent reflection, is the
   a. cornea
   b. sclera
   c. choroid
   d. ciliary body
   e. retina
___ 60. Which of the following statements about the autonomic nerve control over smooth muscles of the pupil is *true*?
   a. Parasympathetic stimulation of circular muscles causes the iris to dilate.
   b. Parasympathetic stimulation of radial muscles causes the iris to constrict.
   c. Sympathetic stimulation of the radial muscles causes the iris to constrict.
   d. Sympathetic stimulation of the radial muscles causes the iris to dilate.
___ 61. *Glaucoma* is best described as a condition in which the
   a. lens and cornea may become cloudy or translucent, making it difficult for light to be transmitted
   b. retina may become detached, resulting in blindness
   c. canal of Schlemm is blocked, causing the intraocular pressure to rise
   d. normal pigments of the retina are not synthesized, so that light reflection interferes with vision

___ 62. The portion of the eye with the greatest *refractive index* (where light is refracted most) is the
  a. cornea
  b. aqueous humor
  c. lens
  d. vitreous body
  e. retina
___ 63. Which statement about visual field halves and the retina halves is correct?
  a. The left visual field focuses on the left half-retina.
  b. The left visual field focuses on the right half-retina.
  c. The nasal half-retina of the right eye receives the same image as the temporal half-retina of the left eye.
  d. The nasal half-retina of the right eye receives the same image as the nasal half-retina of the left eye.
  e. Both b and c are correct.
___ 64. *Accommodation*, the ability of the eyes to keep the image focused on the retina as distance is changed, results from contraction of the
  a. circular muscles
  b. ciliary muscles
  c. radial muscles
  d. pupil
___ 65. Which of the following about *myopia* is *false*?
  a. It is also known as nearsightedness.
  b. It may result from an eyeball that is too short.
  c. It is corrected by glasses with concave lenses.
  d. The blurry image is focused in front of the retina.
___ 66. A cylindrical lens is prescribed to correct for
  a. astigmatism
  b. myopia
  c. hyperopia
  d. presbyopia
  e. Cylindrical lenses are not used for correction.

B. True or False/Edit

___ 67. Light of longer wavelengths (infrared) or shorter wavelengths (ultraviolet) than the visible light spectrum, cannot be seen by the human eye.
___ 68. The anterior and posterior chambers are filled with a fluid called the vitreous body.
___ 69. At the optic disc region of the eyeball neurons exit only, whereas blood vessels both enter and exit from the optic disc.
___ 70. Both the visual field and the retina of each eye are divided into halves because light entering the eye is bent (refracted).
___ 71. An image will be seen in perfect focus only when the light waves from an object are bent (refracted) to a point on the retina itself.
___ 72. As an object moves away from you, the ciliary muscle relaxes, placing tension on the zonular fibers that pull the lens flatter or less convex to keep the image in focus.
___ 73. Myopia is also known as farsightedness.
___ 74. Astigmatism can be an abnormal curvature of either the cornea or the lens or both.

C. Label the Figure — Anatomy of the Eye

Identify each structure indicated by the lines in figure 10.1, the internal anatomy of the eyeball. As you write each term in the space provided, verbally (to your study partner) state the function of each structure. Check your anatomy recall with figure 10.27 in your text, and check your physiology with chapter 10.

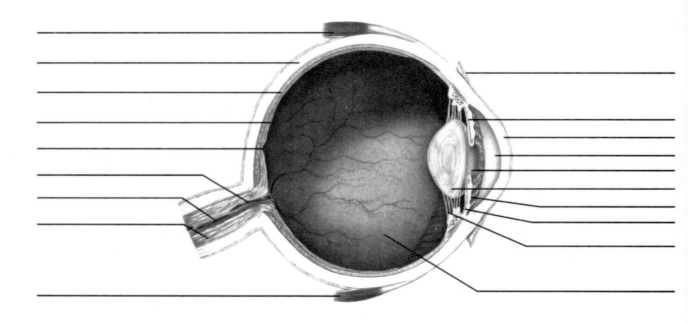

Figure 10.1 The internal anatomy of the eyeball.

VII. THE RETINA

There are two types of photoreceptor neurons: rods and cones. Both receptor cell types contain pigment molecules that undergo dissociation in response to light, and it is this photochemical reaction that eventually results in the production of action potentials in the optic nerve. Rods provide black-and-white vision under conditions of low light intensities, whereas cones provide sharp color vision when light intensities are greater.

A. Multiple Choice

___ 75. The neurons in the retina whose axons gather to form the optic nerve tract are called
    a. bipolar cells
    b. ganglion cells
    c. horizontal cells
    d. amacrine cells
    e. photoreceptor cells

___ 76. The only neurons of the light-activated retina responsible for directly generating the all-or-none action potentials that are conveyed out the optic nerve are the
    a. photoreceptor cells only
    b. bipolar cells and horizontal cells
    c. ganglion cells and amacrine cells
    d. horizontal cells only

___ 77. As opposed to rods, the cones
    a. are less sensitive in low light conditions
    b. provide color vision
    c. provide greater visual acuity (sharpness of detail)
    d. are more responsive in the daylight
    e. All of these correctly describe cones.

___ 78. Which color (wavelength of light) is *not* designated as one of the three types of cones?
    a. blue
    b. red

c. yellow
d. green

___ 79. The pitted portion of the retina upon which the image of the objects we look at falls, and which contains almost all cones for greatest visual acuity, is called the
   a. ganglion cell layer
   b. optic disc
   c. fovea centralis
   d. pigmented epithelium
   e. choroid layer

___ 80. Most (70% to 80%) of the ganglion cell axons from the retina exit the eye as the optic nerve and pass immediately to the
   a. superior colliculus of the midbrain (optic tectum)
   b. lateral geniculate bodies of the thalamus
   c. striate cortex of the occipital lobe
   d. Brodmann areas 17, 18, and 19 of the occipital lobe

B. True or False/Edit

___ 81. Light must pass through several neuron cell layers before striking the photoreceptors (rods and cones).

___ 82. Ganglion cells of the retina synapse with, and are interconnected laterally to, amacrine cells.

___ 83. Cones contain a purple pigment known as *rhodopsin*, that is partially derived from vitamin A obtained from food in the diet.

___ 84. During the *bleaching reaction*, there is a gradual increase in photoreceptor sensitivity, which reaches a maximum at about twenty minutes.

___ 85. The *dark current* is the continuous leakage of Na^+ through special Na^+ channels, diffusing into the photoreceptor cells.

___ 86. Light appears to hyperpolarize (inhibit) the rod and cone photoreceptors, causing the release of lower amounts of inhibitory neurotransmitter chemicals, and ultimately resulting in stimulation of the bipolar cells.

___ 87. The convergence of photoreceptors onto ganglion cells in the fovea centralis region of the retina is lower for the cones (1:1) than for the rods.

___ 88. The axons from the retina that pass through the superior colliculus of the midbrain (optic tectum) is needed to activate motor pathways and answer the visual question "What is it?"

___ 89. Smooth pursuit movements and saccadic eye movements are two types of eye movements coordinated by the lateral geniculate bodies of the thalamus.

___ 90. The superior colliculus (tectal system) is involved in contraction of the ciliary muscles of the iris during both accommodation and the pupillary reflex.

VIII. NEURAL PROCESSING OF VISUAL INFORMATION

Electrical activity in ganglion cells of the retina, and in neurons of the lateral geniculate nucleus and cerebral cortex, is evoked in response to light on the retina. The way in which each neuron type responds to light at a particular point on the retina provides information about the way the brain interprets visual information.

A. Multiple Choice

___ 91. Which of the following types of neurons is *not* a cortical neuron found in the striate cortex region of the occipital lobe (Brodmann's areas 17, 18, and 19)?
   a. simple
   b. circular
   c. complex
   d. hypercomplex
   e. rectangular

___ 92. Neurons of the visual (occipital) cortex respond to all of the following forms of stimuli *except*
   a. slits or bars of light
   b. straight lines with a specific orientation and direction

c. particular lengths, corners or edges
d. circles with on and off centers with surrounds

B. True or False/Edit

___ 93. Ganglion cells with on-center receptive fields are stimulated by light at the center of their visual fields, whereas those inhibited by light at the center and stimulated by light in the surround have off-center fields.

___ 94. Lateral geniculate neuron receptive fields, like ganglion cell receptive fields of the retina, are circular with an antagonistic center and surround areas.

CHAPTER REVIEW

A. Match 'n' Spell — Sensory Physiology

Match the lettered items on the right to the numbered statements on the left - then write out the word (or phrase) in the center space provided. Be sure to spell the terms correctly!

___ 95. measurement of sound wave frequency _____	a.	receptor
___ 96. maintaining near and distant focus on the retina _____	b.	decibel
___ 97. oscillatory movements of the eyes _____	c.	hertz
___ 98. receptor for pain sensation _____	d.	proprioceptor
___ 99. each receptor has lowest threshold to one modality _____	e.	chemoreceptor
___ 100. dendritic nerve endings, specialized neurons, or specialized epithelial cells _____	f.	mechanoreceptor
	g.	tonic receptor
___ 101. muscle, tendon, or joint receptor _____	h.	phasic receptor
___ 102. receptor firing continuously when stimulated _____	i.	nocioreceptor
___ 103. test for the density of touch receptors _____	j.	thermoreceptor
___ 104. cutaneous receptor for heat and cold _____	k.	law of specific nerve energies
___ 105. receptor that adapts to constant stimulation _____		
___ 106. the somatesthetic cortex of the cerebrum _____	l.	two-point threshold
___ 107. touch and pressure receptors, for example _____	m.	postcentral gyrus
___ 108. unit of sound intensity _____	n.	utricle and saccule
___ 109. sensory structure of the semicircular canals _____	o.	cupula
___ 110. connects the scala vestibuli to the scala tympani _____	p.	nystagmus
___ 111. responsible for linear acceleration _____	q.	helicotrema
___ 112. sensory structures for perception of sound _____	r.	semicircular canals
___ 113. abnormal curvature of the lens or cornea _____	s.	organ of Corti
___ 114. responsible for angular/rotational acceleration _____	t.	kinocilium
___ 115. primary pathway for visual reflexes (colliculus) _____	u.	myopia
___ 116. unique projection from vestibular hair cells _____	v.	geniculostriate
___ 117. eyeball is too short—farsighted _____	w.	hyperopia
___ 118. main pathway for action potentials from the retina _____	x.	tectal pathway
___ 119. eyeball is too long—nearsighted _____	y.	astigmatism
___ 120. carotid body, osmo-, smell, or taste receptor _____	z.	accommodation

B. Essay

Essay Tutorial

This essay tutorial will answer the first essay question found in the "**Review Activities**" section of your *Human Physiology* textbook. Please look for *Essay Question* 1. at the end of chapter 10, read it carefully, and let me guide you through one possible answer. Watch for key terms in bold-face type, helpful tips and general suggestions on writing the essay or short-answer questions. Enjoy!

121. **Define** the term *lateral inhibition* and give examples of its **effects** in **three** sensory systems.

Answer. As the question is asking, the first step in the answer is to define *lateral inhibition* — the central nervous system phenomenon by which sensory information is "sharpened" by inhibition of incoming neighboring (lateral) field information from the periphery of that region which is maximally stimulated. Three sensory systems utilizing lateral inhibition are the senses of touch (cutaneous), hearing, and vision. In the skin, a single touch is felt when a blunt object touches the skin because the surrounding fields have been "laterally inhibited" at the level of the central nervous system. Similarly, in the discrimination of different pitches of sounds with similar frequencies, neural activity is "laterally inhibited" so that the hair cells along the basilar membrane which are maximally displaced by sound waves are selected for interpretation by the auditory cortex of the brain while hair cells with neural activity from the surrounding regions are suppressed. Lateral inhibition is also at work in the processing of visual information at the level of the ganglion cells in the retina. Here, the receptive fields of each ganglion cell resembles a "bull's eye" with a central core area and an outer surround area that oppose one another, that is, are antagonistic. Those ganglion cells that have **on-center fields** are excited by light at the center of their visual fields while the surround is suppressed (or inhibited laterally). Those ganglion cells that have **off-center fields** are inhibited by light in the center and stimulated by light in the surround. Due to the distribution of these two types of ganglion cell fields along the retinal surface, incoming light excites some and inhibits some of these fields — which translates later at the occipital (striate) cortex as sharper visual acuity.

Note: Don't be frustrated if your answer doesn't resemble this one. These answers are intended to be as all-encompassing as possible using various concepts from the text. Try some more!

122. Congratulations! You are the "middle C" note entering the ear canal from a nearby piano. Carefully trace your pathway through the rest of the ear until your vibrations die at the round window. Now, describe *how* and *where* your vibrations formed action potentials in the cochlea.

123. Describe the location and response of the olfactory receptors to odors. Now trace their unique pathway to the brain for interpretation. How is smell different from other senses?

124. Distinguish between *tonic* and *phasic* receptors, including examples of each.

125. Explain the two-point touch threshold test and its possible application to acupressure and acupuncture treatment.

Answers — Chapter 10

I. Characteristics of Sensory Receptors
  A. 1. c, 2. b, 3. c, 4. b, 5. c, 6. e, 7. d, 8. a
  B. 9. T, 10. T, 11. F—Replace "nociceptor" with "proprioceptor," 12. F—Replace "phasic" with "tonic," 13. T, 14. F—Generator potentials are graded, and thus may be subthreshold

II. Cutaneous Sensations
  A. 15. a, 16. d, 17. d, 18. c
  B. 19. T, 20. F—Replace "ipsilateral" with "contralateral," 21. T, 22. T

III. Taste and Olfaction
  A. 23. b, 24. b, 25. e
  B. 26. T, 27. F—Replace "salt and sour" with "sweet and bitter," 28. T, 29. T, 30. T

IV. Vestibular Apparatus and Equilibrium
  A. 31. a, 32. d, 33. d, 34. c, 35. a, 36. c, 37. c
  B. 38. T, 39. F—Replace "perilymph" with "endolymph," 40. T, 41. T, 42. T, 43. F—Switch "vertical" and "horizontal," 44. T, 45. T

V. The Ears and Hearing
  A. 46. b, 47. a, 48. e, 49. e, 50. d
  B. 51. T, 52. F—Replace "inner" with "middle," 53. T, 54. T, 55. T, 56. T, 57. F—Otitis media causes conduction deafness

VI. The Eyes and Vision
  A. 58. a, 59. c, 60. d, 61. c, 62. a, 63. e, 64. b, 65. b, 66. a
  B. 67. T, 68. F—Replace "vitreous body" with "aqueous humor," 69. T, 70. T, 71. T, 72. T, 73. F Replace "Myopia" with "Hyperopia," 74. T
  C. See figure 10.27 in the text.

VII. The Retina
  A. 75. b, 76. c, 77. e, 78. c, 79. c, 80. b
  B. 81. T, 82. T, 83. F—Replace "Cones" with "Rods," 84. F—Replace "The bleaching reaction" with "Dark adaptation," 85. T, 86. T, 87. T, 88. F—Replace "What" with "Where," 89. F—Replace "lateral geniculate bodies of the thalamus" with "superior colliculus", 90. T

VIII. Neural Processing of Visual Information
  A. 91. b, 92. d
  B. 93. T, 94. T

Chapter Review
  A. 95. c, 96. z, 97. p, 98. i, 99. k, 100. a, 101. d, 102. g, 103. l, 104. j, 105. h, 106. m, 107. f, 108. b, 109. o, 110. q, 111. n, 112. s, 113. y, 114. r, 115. x, 116. t, 117. w, 118. v, 119. u, 120. e

CHAPTER 11
ENDOCRINE GLANDS: SECRETION AND ACTION OF HORMONES

CHAPTER SCOPE

Now that we have explored the nervous system and its complex electrical communication network, it is time to study the chemical communication network. This discussion will feature the important role of chemical messengers, or **hormones,** in the regulation of whole body homeostasis. Tissues that secrete hormones are derived from *glandular epithelium,* eventually developing into endocrine glands that are located in various places throughout the body. In this chapter, hormones are classified based on their chemical composition. The variety of mechanisms by which hormones activate their target cells are then described.

Steroid hormones and *thyroid gland* hormones can diffuse *through* the target cell membranes to exert their effects on receptors located in the cytoplasm. In contrast, *protein* hormones and other related polar hormones cannot penetrate the cell membrane. Most of these protein and polar hormones, consequently, must activate **second messenger** systems that, in turn, will operate within the cytoplasm of the target cells. **Cyclic AMP, cyclic GMP, Ca^{2+}** ions, and **tyrosine kinase** are described in their roles as second messengers for such hormones and other "first" messengers such as neurotransmitters that arrive at, but are not permitted direct entrance into the target cells. Not surprisingly, the production of these hormones is regulated by complex negative feedback mechanisms.

This chapter includes a guided tour of many endocrine glands in the body, describing the hormones, target organs, and the primary hormonal effects. Many of these glands and hormones will be studied in more detail later in the book. Interestingly, this list will include adipose tissue as an endocrine gland, secreting the hormone, leptin whose primary target is the hypothalamus where appetite is suppressed. Starting with the **pituitary gland** and its complex interaction with the hypothalamus, the text moves on to the **adrenal gland** (*cortex* and *medulla*) and hormonal effects on the cardiovascular system (chapters 13 and 14); the **thyroid, parathyroid, pancreas, pineal,** and **thymus** glands and their effects on metabolism (chapter 18); the **gastrointestinal tract** (chapter 17); and then **gonads** and the **placenta** (chapter 20).

The final discussion is an introduction to the chemical nature and physiological roles of locally important **autocrine** and **paracrine** regulators, such as *prostaglandins* and *growth factors*. In summary, a variety of hormones, together with autocrine, and paracrine chemicals are essential messengers made by the body tissues in the continuous effort to maintain constant internal body processes (homeostasis).

I. ENDOCRINE GLANDS AND HORMONES

Hormones are regulatory molecules secreted into the blood by endocrine glands. Chemical categories of hormones include steroids, amines, polypeptides, and glycoproteins. Interactions occur between the various hormones to produce effects that may be synergistic, permissive, or antagonistic.

A. Multiple Choice

____ 1. All hormones can be grouped into the following general chemical categories, *except*
   a. catecholamines (epinephrine and norepinephrine)
   b. polypeptides and glycoproteins
   c. nucleic acids
   d. steroids

____ 2. The steroid hormones
   a. are derived from cholesterol
   b. are lipid molecules
   c. are not water-soluble

       d. include the sex hormones and corticosteroids
       e. All of these describe steroid hormones.
___ 3. The hormones that contain the element *iodine* are
       a. triiodothyronine (T_3) and tetraiodothyronine (T_4)
       b. catecholamines (epinephrine and norepinephrine)
       c. sex steroids
       d. corticosteroids
       e. glycoproteins
___ 4. Which of the following properties is *not* required for a particular chemical, such as a neurotransmitter or hormone to function as a physiological regulator in the body?
       a. target cells with specific receptor proteins to which that chemical must bind
       b. the chemical must open specific ion channels for the rapid diffusion of ions to occur
       c. the chemical-receptor combination must cause a specific sequence of changes in the target cells
       d. there must be a mechanism for quickly turning off the action of the chemical
___ 5. Polypeptide hormones called *prohormones*
       a. are often derived from prehormones
       b. include proinsulin from the endocrine beta cells of the pancreas
       c. are usually less active "parent" or precursor molecules
       d. are usually longer-chained molecules than those of the active hormone
       e. All of these statements about prohormones are correct.
___ 6. Which of the following statements does *not* describe the *synergistic* effects of hormones?
       a. two or more hormones working together to produce a particular result
       b. effects that may be additive or complementary
       c. enhancing the activity of a second hormone at a target cell
       d. the action of epinephrine and norepinephrine on the heart rate
       e. the action of FSH and testosterone on spermatogenesis during puberty
___ 7. The interaction between which of the following hormone pairs is *not* an example of the *permissive* effect of a first hormone for a second hormone?
       a. estrogen for prolactin on the mammary glands
       b. parathyroid hormone (PTH) for vitamin D_3 on blood Ca^{2+} levels
       c. estrogen for progesterone on the uterus
       d. glucocorticoids for catecholamine actions
       e. All of these hormone pairs display permissive effects.
___ 8. The half-life period of most hormones ranges from
       a. seconds to minutes
       b. minutes to hours;
       c. hours to days
       d. days to weeks
       e. weeks to months
___ 9. Pulsatile (noncontinuous) secretion of hormones
       a. describes how many polypeptide and glycoprotein hormones are released
       b. is needed to prevent desensitization of target cells
       c. includes the release of GnRH and LH as examples
       d. All of these statements describe pulsatile secretion.

B. True or False/Edit

___ 10. A list of endocrine glands should include the heart, liver, hypothalamus, kidneys, and adipose tissue.

___ 11. Although these hormones are *not* steroids, T_3 and T_4 are small and nonpolar; and thus can be taken orally without being inactivated by enzymes in the digestive tract.

___ 12. In most respects, the actions of neurotransmitters and hormones on their respective target cells are distinctly different.

___ 13. After stimulation of their target receptors, hormones do not generally remain in the area and accumulate in the blood.
___ 14. To help excrete "old" steroid hormones in urine and in bile, the liver must first convert them into more polar, water-soluble metabolites.
___ 15. A "pharmacological" dose is one that results in an abnormally high concentration of a substance; more than would normally be present in the bloodstream.
___ 16. The priming effect of hormones may actually decrease the number of receptor proteins in their target cells, thereby causing a phenomenon called downregulation.

II. MECHANISMS OF HORMONE ACTION

Each hormone exerts its characteristic effects on target organs through the actions it has on the cells of these organs. The mechanisms of action are similar for hormones that have similar chemical natures. Lipid-soluble hormones pass through the target cell membrane, bind to intracellular receptor proteins, and act directly within the target cell. Polar hormones do not enter the target cells, but instead bind to receptors on the cell membrane. This results in the activation of intracellular second-messengers that mediate the actions of the hormone.

A. Multiple Choice

For questions 17-19, select the correct *location* (a, b, or c) for **hormone receptor proteins**.
　　a. within the nucleus of the target cell
　　b. within the cytoplasm of the target cell
　　c. on the outer surface of the target cell membrane
___ 17. The receptors for steroid hormones are found here.
___ 18. The receptors for thyroid hormones are found here.
___ 19. The receptors for catecholamine and polypeptide hormones are found here.
___ 20. Which statement about thyroxine is *false*?
　　a. It is the major hormone secreted by the thyroid gland; and also known as triiodothyronine, or T_3.
　　b. About 99.96% of thyroxine is attached to carrier proteins in the plasma and the rest is free or unbound.
　　c. Its carrier protein in the blood is named thyroxine-binding globulin (TBG) with a high affinity for thyroxine.
　　d. It is *not* the active thyroid hormone within the target cells.

For questions 21-23, match the *intracellular enzyme* involved with second messengers, to its best description.
　　a. protein kinase
　　b. phosphodiesterase
　　c. adenylate cyclase
___ 21. The membrane enzyme that is activated by G-protein subunits to catalyze the synthesis of cAMP as the second messenger of target cells.
___ 22. The normally inactive enzyme that is activated by newly formed cAMP - acting to stimulate the phosphorylation of proteins.
___ 23. The enzyme that inactivates the second messenger cAMP by hydrolyzing it into useless fragments.
___ 24. Which of the following does *not* describe *calmodulin*?
　　a. It is a protein found in the cytoplasm of specific target cells.
　　b. It activates transcription and directs the formation of new proteins in the target cells.
　　c. It is activated by Ca^{2+} entering the cytoplasm from the endoplasmic reticulum or from outside the cell.
　　d. It activates specific protein kinase enzymes that phosphorylate other proteins to affect target cell activity.
　　e. It is activated by the hormone insulin in adipose cells to direct the synthesis of fat.

B. True or False/Edit

___ 25. Hormones are delivered by the blood to every cell in the body, but only the target cells with specific receptor proteins for that hormone are able to respond.

___ 26. Hormones bind to receptor proteins with high capacity (receptors per target cell) and low affinity (bond strength).

___ 27. Because they are polar and thus water-soluble, steroid and thyroid hormones are transported bound to plasma carrier proteins.

___ 28. Steroid hormones attach to cytoplasmic receptor proteins of target cells that translocate to the nucleus to direct the production of specific new proteins through genetic transcription and translation.

___ 29. Cyclic AMP activates previously inactive protein kinase enzymes to modulate the activity of other enzymes already present in the target cell.

___ 30. Caffeine (in coffee) and theophylline (in tea) act as phosphodiesterase inhibitors that produce their effects by raising the cAMP concentrations within target tissue cells.

___ 31. The regulatory molecule nitric oxide (NO) can relax the smooth muscle of blood vessels by activating the second messenger, cyclic guanosine monophosphate (cGMP).

___ 32. Calcium ions (Ca^{2+}) may act as second messengers inside the cell, where very high intracellular concentrations are maintained by active transport membrane pumps.

___ 33. Two different hormones can act on the same target cell and produce different results; one activates cAMP production while the other activates the phospholipase C-IP_3-Ca^{2+}-calmodulin system.

III. PITUITARY GLAND

The pituitary gland includes the anterior pituitary and the posterior pituitary. The posterior pituitary secretes hormones that are actually produced by the hypothalamus, whereas the anterior pituitary produces and secretes its own hormones. The anterior pituitary, however, is regulated by hormones secreted by the hypothalamus, as well as by feedback influences exerted by hormones from other endocrine glands.

A. Multiple Choice

___ 34. Which of the following is *not* considered part of the adenohypophysis, or anterior pituitary gland?
   a. pars distalis
   b. pars nervosa
   c. pars tuberalis
   d. pars intermedia
   e. All of these are parts of the anterior pituitary.

___ 35. The pituitary hormone associated with dwarfism, gigantism, pituitary cachexia, and acromegaly is
   a. FSH
   b. GH
   c. ACTH
   d. TSH
   e. LH

___ 36. The supraoptic nuclei and paraventricular nuclei are clusters of neuron cell bodies located in the hypothalamus, responsible for secreting the hormones
   a. LH and FSH
   b. GH and ACTH
   c. TSH and prolactin
   d. oxytocin and ADH

___ 37. Which of the following is *not* a feature characteristic of the anterior pituitary?
   a. It synthesizes and releases tropic hormones that can regulate other endocrine glands.
   b. It is controlled by releasing and inhibiting hormones from the hypothalamus.

c. It serves as part of the hypothalamo-hypophyseal tract.
d. Its hormones may influence other endocrine glands.

___ 38. The two inhibiting hormones from the hypothalamus are
a. GnRH and PIH
b. TRH and CRH
c. GnRH and GRH
d. PIH and somatostatin
e. None of these are hypothalamic inhibiting hormones.

___ 39. A rare classic *positive* feedback effect is demonstrated by
a. increased TSH production during goiter
b. increased estradiol, causing the LH "surge" in females
c. increased GnRH and FSH following castration in males
d. increased ACTH, causing increased cortisol secretion

B. True or False/Edit

___ 40. The anterior pituitary develops as a downgrowth of the brain, while the posterior pituitary is derived from embryonic epithelium from Rathke's pouch.
___ 41. The anterior lobe of the pituitary is more a storage organ than a true gland.
___ 42. The hypothalamus rather than the anterior pituitary may be considered the true "master gland" in the body.
___ 43. Anterior pituitary secretion of ACTH, TSH, and the gonadotropins (FSH and LH) is controlled by negative feedback loops from hormones produced by target cells.
___ 44. During the menstrual cycle, rising levels of estradiol cause a temporary "surge" in the blood levels of LH that results in ovulation - an example of positive feedback control of target gland secretion.
___ 45. The synchronization of female menstrual cycles (the "dormitory effect") and circadian rhythms are good examples of the influence of higher brain centers on the anterior pituitary-adrenal axis.

C. Match 'n' Spell — Hormones

Match the letter of the following hormones listed on the right with the best description on the left. Write the selected letter in the numbered space and attempt to write out the *full name* of the hormone in the center space provided.

(*Note*: most hormones are identified by their acronyms, for example growth hormone is often written as GH)

___ 46. gonadotropic hormone — stimulates ovulation _____ a. GH
___ 47. active during labor and lactation in females _____ b. TSH
___ 48. stimulates glucocorticoid secretion (for example, cortisol) c. ACTH
     _____ d. FSH
___ 49. promotes amino acid uptake and protein synthesis_____ e. LH or ICSH
___ 50. stimulates sperm production in males _____ f. prolactin
___ 51. human function unknown, but causes darkening of the skin g. MSH
     of lower vertebrates _____ h. ADH
___ 52. stimulates the production and secretion of T_4 _____ i. oxytocin
___ 53. secreted by the pars intermedia and elsewhere _____ j. ß-endorphin
___ 54. acts on kidneys to retain water, concentrate urine _____ k. PIH
___ 55. stimulates milk production in females; has a supportive role l. CRH
     in male gonad and kidney function _____
___ 56. hypothalamic hormone - stimulates ACTH release _____
___ 57. inhibitory hormone from the hypothalamus _____

D. Label the Figure — Anterior Pituitary Hormones

Study the figure below and label the structures and the hormones indicated by the blank lines. Check your work *after* you finish by comparing your answers to those in figure 11.14 in your text.

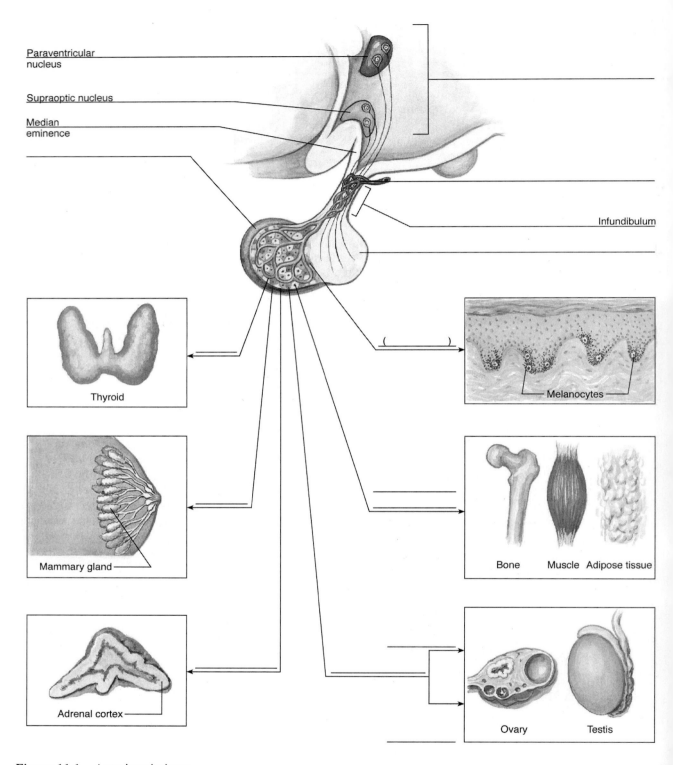

Figure 11.1 Anterior pituitary

IV. ADRENAL GLANDS

The adrenal cortex and adrenal medulla are structurally and functionally different. The adrenal medulla secretes catecholamine hormones, which complement the sympathetic nervous system in the "fight-or-flight" reaction. The adrenal cortex secretes steroid hormones, that participate in the regulation of mineral and energy balance.

A. Multiple Choice

____ 58. Which of the statements about the adrenal *cortex* is *false*?
   a. It is derived from mesoderm tissue in the embryo.
   b. It is stimulated by the hormone ACTH secreted by the anterior pituitary gland.
   c. It secretes the catecholamine hormones — mostly epinephrine.
   d. It is divided into three zones — an outer, middle, and inner zone, that appear to have different functions.
   e. All of these statements about the adrenal cortex are true.

____ 59. Which hormones are *not* secreted by the adrenal *cortex*?
   a. aldosterone and other mineralocorticoids
   b. sex steroids: weak androgens and some estrogens
   c. hydrocortisone and other glucocorticoids
   d. epinephrine and some norepinephrine catecholamines
   e. All of these are secreted by the adrenal cortex.

____ 60. Which statement about the hormone aldosterone is *false*?
   a. It is the most potent adrenal glucocorticoid hormone.
   b. It is secreted by the zona glomerulosa region of the adrenal cortex.
   c. Its secretion is controlled by alterations in blood volume and electrolyte balance.
   d. Its lack in Addison's disease may lead to electrolyte imbalance, dehydration, and death, if not treated.
   e. All of these statements about aldosterone are true.

____ 61. Hans Selye's general adaptation syndrome (GAS) does *not* include
   a. exhaustion, sickness, or death if adaptations or corrective changes aren't made
   b. activation of the pituitary-adrenal axis causing an initial alarm reaction
   c. the formation of a tumor of the adrenal medulla (pheochromocytoma) that secretes large amounts of epinephrine and norepinephrine
   d. a stage of resistance or readjustment to the demands of the stressors

____ 62. Which function of glucocorticoids (such as hydrocortisone), is best related to the suggestion that prolonged stress results in an increased incidence of cancer and other diseases?
   a. They stimulate an increase in heart rate and in cardiac output.
   b. They cause generalized vasoconstriction that elevates blood pressure.
   c. They stimulate the secretion of aldosterone hormones that regulates blood volume and electrolyte balance
   d. They can inhibit the ability of the immune system to protect against disease
   e. All of these statements regarding glucocorticoid function are true.

B. True or False/Edit

____ 63. The adrenal medulla is derived from embryonic mesoderm, whereas the adrenal cortex is derived from embryonic ectoderm (neural) tissue.

____ 64. *Adrenogenital syndrome* is caused by hypersecretion (or oversecretion) of the adrenal sex steroid hormones, such as androgens that can cause premature puberty and enlarged genitals.

____ 65. Under stressful conditions, there is increased secretion of ACTH and, thus, increased secretion of adrenal corticosteroids.

____ 66. Many pleasant life changes such as marriage, graduation, or job promotion can be forms of "stress" — activating the pituitary-adrenal axis and causing an increase in the secretions of ACTH and corticosteroids.

____ 67. Hormones secreted from the adrenal medulla are expected to increase cardiac rate and cardiac output, respiratory rate, and other major functions.

____ 68. Pheochromocytoma is a tumor of the adrenal cortex, releasing large quantities of epinephrine and norepinephrine.

V. THYROID AND PARATHYROID GLANDS

The thyroid secretes thyroxine (T_4) and triiodothyronine (T_3), which are needed for proper growth and development and which are primarily responsible for determining the basal metabolic rate (BMR). The parathyroid glands secrete parathyroid hormone, which helps to raise the blood Ca^{2+} concentration.

A. Multiple Choice

____ 69. Which statement about thyroid hormones is *false*?
  a. Thyroxine is synthesized by simple cuboidal epithelial cells called principal cells.
  b. The name, thyroxine, includes both the hormones T_4 and T_3.
  c. Calcitonin is a hormone produced by parafollicular cells located outside and between follicles.
  d. Thyroxine is formed from the amino acid tyrosine.
  e. Thyroxine is vital for normal central nervous system development and regulation of energy utilization by the body.

____ 70. The abnormal growth of the thyroid gland, called goiter, is
  a. caused by the oversecretion of thyroxine
  b. caused by abnormally high levels of TSH secretion
  c. successfully treated with radioactively labeled iodine
  d. caused by abnormally low levels of TRH secretion

____ 71. Which statement about the parathyroid glands is *false*?
  a. They usually include four small paired glands.
  b. They are embedded in the posterior surfaces of the lateral lobes of the thyroid gland.
  c. They secrete only one hormone called parathyroid hormone (PTH).
  d. PTH acts on tissues such as bone, kidney, and intestines to raise the levels of calcium in the blood.
  e. All of these statements regarding parathyroid glands are true.

B. True or False/Edit

____ 72. The thyroid is the largest of the endocrine glands, weighing between 20 and 25 grams.
____ 73. Basal metabolic rate (BMR) can be defined as the minimum number of calories burned or expended by the body each hour just to stay alive.
____ 74. Undersecretion of thyroxine (hypothyroidism) in infants results in myxedema, whereas hypothyroidism in adults causes cretinism.
____ 75. Graves' disease, or toxic goiter, is an autoimmune disease in which antibodies are made that function like TSH, resulting in overstimulation of the thyroid gland.
____ 76. The parafollicular cells of the thyroid gland secrete the hormone calcitonin.

VI. PANCREAS AND OTHER ENDOCRINE GLANDS

The islets of Langerhans in the pancreas secrete two hormones, insulin and glucagon. Insulin promotes the lowering of blood glucose and the storage of energy in the form of glycogen and fat. Glucagon has antagonistic effects that act to raise the blood glucose concentration. Additionally, many other organs secrete hormones that help regulate digestion, metabolism, growth, immune function, and reproduction.

A. Multiple Choice

____ 77. Which statement about *glucagon* is *false*?
  a. It is a hormone secreted by the alpha cells within the islets of Langerhans of the pancreas.
  b. It is a hormone that is secreted when blood glucose levels are low.
  c. As a hormone it stimulates both glycogen breakdown (glycogenolysis) and fat breakdown (lipolysis.)
  d. It is a hormone that is secreted during times of fasting (not eating.)
  e. All of these statements regarding glucagon are true.

____ 78. Which statement about *diabetes mellitus* is *false*?
  a. It is characterized by fasting hyperglycemia and the presence of glucose in the urine.
  b. Type I, or insulin-dependent diabetes is the more common form.

c. Type II, or non-insulin-dependent diabetes is caused by decreased tissue sensitivity to insulin so that more is required for normal effect.
  d. Type I diabetes is caused by the destruction of beta cells that produce insulin.
  e. Both types of diabetes mellitus are associated with abnormally high levels of glucagon secretion from the alpha cells of the islets of Langerhans.
___ 79. The hormone, insulin
  a. is secreted by the alpha cells of the pancreas
  b. promotes the entry of glucose and amino acids into tissue cells
  c. promotes the breakdown of glycogen (glycogenolysis) and fat (lipolysis)
  d. levels fall immediately after a meal is eaten
___ 80. Which statement about *melatonin* is *false*?
  a. It is secreted by the pineal gland, a small, cone-shaped gland located in the roof of the third ventricle.
  b. Its secretion is highest in children aged one to five and decreases thereafter.
  c. It may have an important role in the onset of puberty.
  d. More melatonin is secreted in the daytime than at night.
___ 81. Which statement about the *testes* is *false*?
  a. The seminiferous tubules produce sperm, the male gamete.
  b. The interstitial tissue (Leydig) cells secrete the primary androgen, testosterone.
  c. Testosterone is needed for the development of the male sex accessory organs, that include the prostate, seminal vesicles, epididymis, and ductus deferens.
  d. Testosterone is required for the development of male secondary sexual characteristics.
  e. All of these statements regarding the testes are true.
___ 82. During the menstrual cycle in females
  a. the hormone, progesterone is secreted by ovarian follicles
  b. many follicles within the ovary will undergo ovulation each month
  c. luteinizing hormone converts the empty follicle into a corpus luteum, which secretes progesterone and estradiol
  d. that critical event, ovulation, occurs near the end of the cycle
___ 83. Which hormone is *not* secreted by the endocrine tissues of the human placenta?
  a. prolactin
  b. estrogens
  c. progesterone
  d. human chorionic gonadotropin (hCG)
  e. somatomammotropin

B. True or False/Edit
___ 84. After a meal, glucagon secretion is increased and insulin secretion is decreased - an example of antagonistic action between these two hormones.
___ 85. The pineal gland is both an endocrine and an exocrine gland.
___ 86. After the age of seven, the pineal gland begins to shrink and in an adult appears as a thickened strand of fibrous tissue.
___ 87. The hormone melatonin may inhibit the pituitary-gonad axis in some species, and perhaps, be associated with a delay in the onset of reproductive maturity.
___ 88. After puberty, the thymus gland continues to shrink in size and reduce its secretions.
___ 89. The thymus gland serves as the site for production of B-type lymphocytes (B cells) that are involved in cell-mediated immunity.
___ 90. Both the stomach and small intestine secrete a number of hormones that act both locally on the gastrointestinal tract itself and remotely on tissues of the pancreas and gallbladder.
___ 91. *Somatomammotropin* is a hormone secreted by the placenta that is similar in its action to both growth hormone and prolactin.

VII. AUTOCRINE AND PARACRINE REGULATION

Many regulatory molecules produced throughout the body act within the organs that produce them. These molecules may regulate different cells within one tissue, or they may be produced within one tissue and regulate a different tissue within the same organ.

A. Multiple Choice

___ 92. Which of the following autocrine and paracrine regulators are produced by lymphocytes (WBC) and are involved in *specific immunity*?
   a. nitric oxide
   b. endothelins
   c. neurotrophins
   d. bradykinins
   e. interleukins

___ 93. Which statement about *prostaglandins* is *false*?
   a. They are twenty-carbon fatty acids with a five-membered carbon ring.
   b. They are derived from arachidonic acid molecules that are released from phospholipids located in the cell membrane.
   c. They are later converted into leukotrienes.
   d. They are made by the enzyme, cyclo-oxygenase, and others.

___ 94. Prostaglandins
   a. are produced by very specific tissues in the body
   b. are involved in only a few, very specific, regulatory functions
   c. may function specifically as vasoconstrictors while others may function specifically as vasodilators.
   d. always produce the same effects, even when acting on different tissues of the body

___ 95. Which of the following regulatory function does *not* involve prostaglandins?
   a. pain and fever control during the inflammatory response
   b. growth and development of skeletal muscles and long bones
   c. regulation of stomach secretions, intestinal motility, and fluid absorption in the gastrointestinal tract
   d. regulation of blood flow in the kidney and thus, some control of urine volume and content
   e. bronchiole dilation and constriction

B. True or False/Edit

___ 96. The major regulatory molecules in the body include hormones, neurotransmitters, and autocrine regulators such as prostaglandins and growth factors.

___ 97. All autocrine regulators in some ways control gene expression in their target cells that can, for example, result in the stimulation of cell division and proliferation of their target cells.

___ 98. Prostaglandins are the most diverse group of autocrine regulators.

___ 99. In the control of blood clotting, different prostaglandins can initiate antagonistic effects on the aggregation of platelets and the diameter of blood vessels.

___ 100. Aspirin is a nonsteroidal anti-inflammatory drug that works by stimulating the synthesis of prostaglandins such as those that cause pain.

CHAPTER REVIEW

A. Completion

101. Many hormones become active only after conversion from less active precursors called _____ — (pre/pro) hormones; whereas _____ — (pre/pro) hormones are inactive until activated by the target cells. The overall effects of hormones depend on their _____, where pharmacological doses are abnormally _____ (high/low). 102. Interaction between different hormones are described as _____, _____, or _____. 103. Steroid and thyroid hormones _____ (do/don't) enter their target cells, whereas amine, polypeptide, and _____ hormones _____ (do/don't) enter the target cells. Receptors for thyroid hormones are located in the _____, steroid hormone

receptors are located in the -_____, and protein-derived hormone receptors are located in the _____. 104. Many protein-derived hormones activate second messengers such as _____ _____, _____, or _____ to carry out the action of the hormone. 105. List the eight pituitary hormones (use their abbreviated spellings where applicable): _____, _____, _____, _____, _____, _____, _____ and _____. (On your own, can you spell out these abbreviations? Try it!) 106. Six of these are from the _____ pituitary and are controlled by releasing hormones from the _____, which flow along the hypothalamo-hypophyseal _____ system. 107. The adrenal _____ secretes mineralocorticoids such as _____; _____ such as cortisol; and _____ steroids (weak androgens). 108. The adrenal medulla secretes mainly _____ and lesser amounts of _____ hormones, which complement the action of _____ nervous system stimulation. 109. The major hormone of the thyroid is thyroxine or T_____ (3/4), which is synthesized within the _____ of the thyroid follicles. The parafollicular cells of the thyroid secrete the hormone _____, which may act to _____ (raise/lower) blood levels of _____. 110. Insulin is secreted by the _____ cells of the _____ of Langerhans, whereas the hormone _____ is secreted by the _____ cells. 111. Eating a meal _____ blood levels of glucose and stimulates the release of _____, which lowers blood glucose; whereas fasting stimulates _____ secretion, stimulating lipolysis and _____. 112. The pineal gland secretes _____, which may play a role in regulating _____ function. The thymus secretes hormones important in regulating the _____ system. 113. Testosterone is secreted by the _____ cells of the testes, whereas the _____ cells of the ovarian follicles secrete the hormone _____. Both progesterone and estrogen are secreted by the _____ and (if pregnant) the _____. 114. Prostaglandins are unique, twenty-carbon-long _____ acids produced by _____ (few/many) different tissues and appear to act within the organ in which they are produced.

B. Label the Figure — Negative Feedback Control of Gonadotropin Secretion

The endocrine system and the negative feedback control of hormone secretion is an excellent example of homeostasis. In figure 11.2 above, study the negative feedback control of gonadotropin secretion. Notice the hormonal connections between the hypothalamus, the anterior pituitary gland, and the gonads. Then on the blank lines provided label the proper hormones, their target organs, and the negative feedback pathways. After you have finished, check your work with figure 11.17 in your text and save this worksheet for review before the next examination.

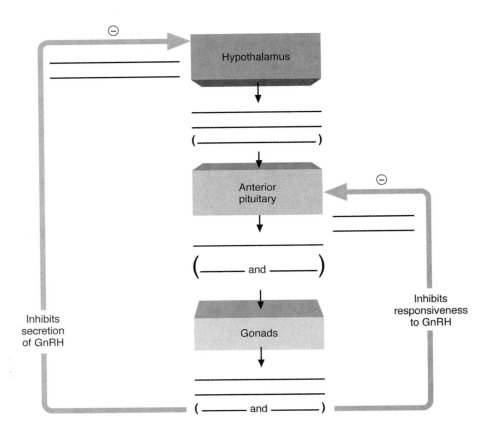

Figure 11.2 Negative feedback control of gonadotropin secretion.

C. Sequencer

115. In proper sequence, number the following seven events that occur when a hormone first arrives at the target cell membrane and begins the activation of cAMP as a second messenger molecule in the cytoplasm. *Note:* The first event has been done for you. When you have finished, check your work with table 11.4 in your text.

    ____ Cyclic AMP activates protein kinase enzymes that were already present in the cytoplasm in an inactive state.

    ____ The hormone binds to its receptor on the outer surface of the target cell membrane.

    _1_ The activity of specific enzymes is either increased or inhibited by phosphorylation.

    ____ Activated adenylate cyclase (enzyme) catalyzes the conversion of ATP to cyclic AMP (cAMP) within the cytoplasm.

    ____ Activated cAMP-dependent protein kinase transfers phosphate groups (phosphorylates) to other enzymes in the cytoplasm.

    ____ Altered enzyme activity mediates the target cell's response to the hormone.

    ____ Hormone-receptor interaction stimulates activation of adenylate cyclase on the cytoplasmic side of the membranes.

C. Essay

Essay Tutorial

This essay tutorial will answer the first essay question found in the "**Review Activities**" section of your *Human Physiology* textbook. Please look for *Essay Question* 1. at the end of chapter 11, read it carefully, and let me guide you through one possible answer. Watch for key terms in bold-face type, helpful tips and general suggestions on writing the essay or short-answer questions. Enjoy!

116. Explain how the **regulation** of the **neuro**hypophysis and adrenal **medulla** are related to their **embryonic origins**.

Note: One way to format an answer to this question is to first state the embryonic origins for each of the two tissues, then describe the regulation of these tissues based on what information you have provided related to embryonic origins.

Answer. The neurohypophysis, or pars nervosa, originates as neural tissue that grows down from the hypothalamic region of the brain. The hypothalamus has two important clusters of neurons, one called the supraoptic nuclei and the other, the paraventricular nuclei. The axons from these cell bodies project down the infundibulum stalk and terminate in the posterior pituitary where there respective hormones are stored in vesicles, awaiting release. The embryonic origin of the adrenal medulla is also from neural tissue, arising much like an enlarged ganglion at the end of preganglionic sympathetic neurons that emerge from the spinal cord.

Autonomic nerve activity regulates both of these glands. Sensory information sent to the hypothalamus (for example, from infant suckling) or the activation of receptors within the hypothalamus (for example, osmoreceptors by osmolality changes) stimulate reflex secretion of oxytocin and ADH hormones, respectively, which are released from vesicles into the posterior pituitary blood supply. Activation of the adrenal medulla (such as during stress) also starts from the hypothalamus as sympathetic nerve impulses which stimulate the release of epinephrine and norepinephrine catecholamine hormones into the bloodstream. This is part of the "fight-or-flight" response.

Alright! How did you do with this one? Do you see how this question could also be answered using a two-column table format using neurohypophysis and adrenal medulla as column headings?

Keep up the good work! If time permits, try a few more of mine, OK?

117. Compare the steroid hormones to the thyroid hormones with regard to entry, binding sites, and activation of the target cells.

118. Distinguish between the two major types of diabetes mellitus — and include the causes of each and the effects on both insulin and glucagon concentrations in the blood.

119. Suppose a person's immune system makes antibodies that mimic thyroid-stimulating hormone (TSH). What effects would you expect to see on the thyroid, its release of hormones, and target cell response? Can you name this autoimmune disease?

120. Construct a diagram to distinguish between the activation of protein kinase by cAMP in liver cells and activation of calmodulin in contracting skeletal muscle. (You can check your diagram against figure 11.10 in the text.)

Answers — Chapter 11

I. Endocrine Glands and Hormones
   A. 1. c, 2. e, 3. a, 4. b, 5. e, 6. c, 7. a, 8. b, 9. d
   B. 10. T, 11. T, 12. F—Neurotransmitter and hormone actions are very similar, 13. T, 14. T, 15. T, 16. F—Replace "decrease" with "increase," and "downregulation" with "upregulation"

II. Mechanisms of Hormone Action
   A. 17. b, 18. a, 19. c, 20. a, 21. c, 22. a, 23. b, 24. b
   B. 25. T, 26. F—Switch "high" and "low," 27. F—Replace "polar" with "nonpolar;" they are "not" water-soluble, 28. T, 29. T, 30. T, 31. T, 32. F—Replace "high" with "low", 33. T

III. Pituitary Gland
   A. 34. b, 35. b, 36. d, 37. c, 38. d, 39. b
   B. 40. F—Switch "anterior" and "posterior," 41. F—Replace "anterior" with "posterior," 42. T, 43. T, 44. T, 45. F—The "dormitory effect" is part of the pituitary-gonad axis (not adrenal)
   C. 46. e, 47. i, 48. c, 49. a, 50. d, 51. g, 52. b, 53. j, 54. h, 55. f, 56. l, 57. k
   D. Label the Figure—Anterior Pituitary See figure 11.14 in the text.

IV. Adrenal Glands
   A. 58. c, 59. d, 60. a, 61. c, 62. d
   B. 63. F—Switch "medulla" and "cortex," 64. T, 65. T, 66. T, 67. T, 68. F—Replace "cortex" with "medulla"

V. Thyroid and Parathyroids
   A. 69. b, 70. b, 71. e
   B. 72. T, 73. T, 74. F—Switch "infants" and "adults," 75. T, 76. T

VI. Pancreas and Other Endocrine Glands
   A. 77. e, 78. b, 79. b, 80. d, 81. e, 82. c, 83. a
   B. 84. F—Switch "glucagon" and "insulin," 85. F—Replace "pineal" with "pancreas," 86. T, 87. T, 88. T, 89. F—Replace "B" with "T," 90. T, 91. T

VII. Autocrine and Paracrine Regulation
   A. 92. e, 93. c, 94. c, 95. b
   B. 96. T, 97. 98. T, 99. T, 100. F—Replace "stimulating" with "inhibiting"

Chapter Review
   A. 101. pro, pre; concentration, high, 102. permissive, synergistic, antagonistic, 103. do, glycoprotein, don't; nucleus, cytoplasm, membrane, 104. cyclic AMP, cyclic GMP, Ca^{2+}, 105. GH, TSH, ACTH, FSH, LH, prolactin, ADH, oxytocin, 106. anterior, hypothalamus, portal, 107. cortex, aldosterone, glucocorticoids, sex, 108. epinephrine, norepinephrine, sympathetic, 109. 4, colloid; calcitonin, raise, calcium, 110. beta, islets, glucagon, alpha, 111. raises, insulin, glucagon, glycogenolysis, 112. melatonin, reproductive; immune, 113. Leydig, granulosa, estrogen; corpus luteum, placenta, 114. fatty, many
   B. Label the Figure—Negative Feedback Control of Gonadotropin Secretion See figure 11.17 in the text.
   C. Sequencer 115. 4,1,6,3,5,7,2

CHAPTER 12
MUSCLE: MECHANISMS OF CONTRACTION AND NEURAL CONTROL

CHAPTER SCOPE

Perhaps the most obvious body process is the voluntary movement of bones as skeletal muscles contract. Here is a chapter devoted to the complete description and analysis of this process. **Skeletal muscle** is uniquely composed of individual muscle cells, called *fibers*. Each individual fiber twitches or contracts following a precise sequence of events. In the sliding filament theory, muscle contraction occurs as *actin* and *myosin* protein filaments slide over one another, pulling the two ends of fiber toward the center. Skeletal muscle is controlled by voluntary nerve impulses that originate in the brain, travel along **somatic motor neurons**, and terminate on each fiber membrane. Skeletal muscle normally will not contract unless stimulated by action potentials from these efferent nerves. Keep in mind, however, that sensory input from **muscle spindles, Golgi tendon organs,** and **joint receptors** (collectively known as proprioceptors) flows continuously into the brain for assessment and modulation of motor output. Some of this sensory information need only travel to the spinal cord and back along a **spinal reflex** pathway. Other reflexes are more complex.

Recent research interest in exercise and muscular fitness has prompted an update on the structural and functional descriptions of slow-twitch, intermediate, and fast-twitch fibers, the muscle fatigue phenomenon, and the physiology of physical training. The last section summarizes the important differences in the structure and function of **cardiac muscle** with that of **smooth muscle**. The fundamental distinctions from each other and from skeletal muscle are highlighted. Cleverly, this final discussion serves as a nice introduction to the two chapters on the cardiovascular system that follow (chapters 13 and 14).

I. STRUCTURE AND ACTIONS OF SKELETAL MUSCLES

Skeletal muscles are composed of individual muscle fibers that contract when they are stimulated by a motor neuron. Each motor neuron branches to innervate a number of muscle fibers, and all of these fibers contract when their motor neuron is activated. Activation of varying numbers of motor neurons, and thus varying numbers of muscle fibers, results in gradations in the strength of contraction of the whole muscle.

A. Multiple Choice

____ 1. In a skeletal muscle contraction
   a. the origin is pulled toward the insertion
   b. flexor muscles increase the angle of a joint
   c. extensors and flexors may be found at the same joint
   d. abductor muscles move limbs inward toward the midline
   e. None of these statements regarding skeletal muscle contractions is correct.

____ 2. The "string" in cooked, stringy stew meat best describes this part of the muscle anatomy.
   a. epimysium
   b. fascicle
   c. perimysium
   d. myofiber
   e. endomysium

____ 3. The actual muscle cell, complete with such components as a nucleus, mitochondria, glycogen, and sarcoplasm is also known as a
   a. fascicle
   b. tendon
   c. myofiber

123

d. myofibril
e. None of these terms describe the actual muscle cell.

____ 4. When an isolated muscle is electrically stimulated outside of the body (*in vitro*), which of the following events does *not* occur?
a. Increasing the stimulus voltage increases the strength of the twitch.
b. Increasing the stimulus frequency may lead to consecutive twitches that "ride piggyback" and summate.
c. Increasing the stimulus frequency may lead to tetanus.
d. All of these events occur during electrical stimulation of an isolated muscle.

____ 5. Which of the following best demonstrates an *isometric* contraction?
a. lifting a chair up and over your head
b. sliding the chair horizontally across the room
c. sitting in the chair reading (and enjoying!) this text
d. gluing together the chair that just broke
e. None of these statements demonstrates an isometric contraction.

____ 6. Which statement about skeletal muscle fibers in the body (*in vivo*) is *false*?
a. The membranes of skeletal muscle fibers conducts action potentials just like those of neurons.
b. When activated, each individual muscle fiber contraction is an all-or-none twitch.
c. Activation of a single somatic motor neuron will activate every single muscle fiber in that motor unit only.
d. Contractions of whole muscles are produced with varying strength (graded) by increasing or decreasing the number of motor units that are activated.
e. All of these statements about skeletal muscle fibers are true.

____ 7. In the body (*in vivo*), each muscle fiber receives _____ axon(s) from a (an) _____ motor neuron, which always liberates the specific neurotransmitter _____.
a. one; somatic; ACh
b. many; autonomic; norepinephrine (NE)
c. many; somatic; norepinephrine (NE)
d. one; autonomic; ACh

____ 8. Which of the following muscles is controlled by the *greatest* number of small motor units, resulting in fine neural control over the strength of muscle contraction?
a. gastrocnemius
b. biceps brachii
c. deltoid
d. extraocular
e. gluteus

B. True or False/Edit

____ 9. Antagonistic muscle action occurs when flexors and extensors act on the same joint.
____ 10. A muscle that is contracting is called the *agonist* muscle.
____ 11. The connective tissue tendons, epimysium, perimysium, and endomysium are one continuous noncontractile unit within muscle.
____ 12. Like most other cells in the body, skeletal muscles have a single, centrally located nucleus as a control center.
____ 13. Complete muscle tetanus is the same as muscle tetany.
____ 14. The process of lifting a barbell up and over one's head is an example of an *isometric* muscle contraction.
____ 15. *Series elastic component* refers to noncontractile connective tissues of the muscle that are pulled tight first before muscles can shorten.
____ 16. An example of the series elastic component of muscle contraction is demonstrated by the elastic recoil of the thoracic structures during expiration.
____ 17. A single *motor unit* is composed of one somatic motor neuron and all of the muscle fibers innervated (excited) by the axon branches.

___ 18. All motor units to a given muscle (for example, gastrocnemius) innervate the same number of muscle fibers.

___ 19. Recruitment of larger motor units (with more fibers per unit) occurs when greater strength is needed.

II. MECHANISMS OF CONTRACTION

The A bands within each muscle fiber are composed of thick filaments and the I bands contain thin filaments. Movement of cross bridges that extend from the thick to the thin filaments causes sliding of the filaments, and thus muscle tension and shortening. The activity of the cross bridges is regulated by the availability of Ca^{2+}, which is increased by electrical stimulation of the muscle fiber. Electrical stimulation produces contraction of the muscle through the binding of Ca^{2+} to regulatory proteins within the thin filaments.

A. Multiple Choice

___ 20. The cytoplasm (sarcoplasm) of each muscle fiber (or cell) contains small, densely-packed parallel arrangements of subunits known as
   a. myofibrils
   b. fibers
   c. filaments
   d. fascicles
   e. None of these terms is correct.

___ 21. The I bands within a longitudinal section of a myofibril are seen as the _____ bands, composed primarily of the protein _____.
   a. dark; actin
   b. dark; myosin
   c. light; actin
   d. light; myosin

___ 22. That part of the myofibril striation pattern where actin and myosin filaments overlap is known as the
   a. A band.
   b. I band.
   c. H band.
   d. Z line (disc).
   e. sarcomere.

___ 23. During an isotonic muscle contraction, which statement about the shortening of adjoining sarcomeres is *false*?
   a. The distance between the two Z lines of each sarcomere appears to shorten.
   b. The A bands of adjoining sarcomeres appear to shorten in length.
   c. The I bands of adjoining sarcomeres appear to shorten in length.
   d. The H bands of adjoining sarcomeres appear to shorten.

___ 24. Which statement about the thin actin filaments is *false*?
   a. They are polymers of hundreds of globular G-actin subunits.
   b. They are also known as filament-actin or F-actin.
   c. They are arranged in a double row of subunits and twisted to form a helix.
   d. The grooves within the actin filaments contain the regulatory protein called troponin.
   e. All of these statements about actin filaments are true.

___ 25. Normal relaxation of skeletal muscle is most *directly* the result of
   a. a decrease in ATP concentrations within the sarcomere
   b. fewer action potentials on the muscle fiber membrane
   c. more acetylcholine (ACh) neurotransmitter molecules broken down in the synapse
   d. active transport of calcium ion (Ca^{2+}) out of the sarcoplasm and into the sarcoplasmic reticulum

___ 26. The *strength* of a muscle's contraction is affected by the
   a. number of muscle fibers within the muscle that are stimulated to contract

    b. thickness of each muscle fiber within the muscle
    c. initial length of the muscle fibers when they are at rest
    d. Only a and b are correct.
    e. All of these factors affect the strength of contraction.

B. True or False/Edit
___ 27. In the center of each A band is a thin, dark Z line (disc).
___ 28. The basic or smallest subunit of striated muscle contraction is the sarcomere.
___ 29. Shortening of the sarcomere is produced by shortening of the protein filaments called actin and myosin.
___ 30. Cross bridges are actually the globular "heads" of the myosin protein molecules that extend out toward the actin molecules.
___ 31. Splitting of ATP is required before myosin cross bridges attach to actin; and at the end of the power stroke, a new ATP must be attached to release the cross bridge.
___ 32. Each tropomyosin molecule covers a distance of approximately seven G-actin subunits within the groove of the longer F-actin molecule.
___ 33. When a muscle fiber is stimulated to contract, calcium ions (Ca^{2+}) are released that will bind directly to tropomyosin molecules located in the sacrcoplasm.
___ 34. Transverse tubules (or T tubules) are formed from, and continuous with, the muscle cell membrane and, therefore are capable of conducting action potentials.
___ 35. Perhaps with the help of the second messenger called *inositol triphosphate* (IP_3), action potentials along the transverse tubules cause the release of Ca^{2+} from the sarcoplasmic reticulum.
___ 36. Release of Ca^{2+} from the terminal cisternae of the sarcoplasmic reticulum is an active process, requiring the hydrolysis of ATP.
___ 37. Maximum muscle tension is produced at 100% of its normal (or "ideal") resting length, such that at 60% or less of this resting length, further contraction cannot occur.

C. Sequencer — Muscle Excitation-Contraction Coupling
38. Arrange the numbers the following events involved in stimulation of muscle contraction and relaxation (excitation-contraction coupling) in proper order from 1 to 10. *Note*: The first event has been done for you. If
    ___ you get stuck, sneak a peek at table 12.3 in the text.
    ___ action potentials are conducted along transverse tubules
    ___ cross-bridges are exposed as troponin moves tropomyosin
    ___ action potentials in the T tubules promote Ca^{2+} release
    _1_ somatic neuron action potentials release ACh molecules
    ___ with ATP, cross-bridges pull the thin over the thick filaments
    ___ without action potentials, Ca^{2+} is pumped away from troponin and into the sarcoplasmic reticulum
    ___ released Ca^{2+} binds to troponin, changing its structure
    ___ ACh binds to its sarcolemma receptors and produces new action potentials
    ___ contraction cycles continue as long as Ca^{2+} and fresh ATP are present in the sarcomere
    ___ ATP-activated myosin cross-bridges attach to actin

III. NEURAL CONTROL OF SKELETAL MUSCLES

Skeletal muscles contain stretch receptors called muscle spindles that stimulate the production of impulses in sensory neurons when the muscle is stretched. These sensory neurons can synapse with alpha motoneurons, which stimulate the muscle to contract in response to the stretch. Other motor neurons, called gamma motoneurons, stimulate the tightening of the spindles and thus increase their sensitivity.

A. Multiple Choice
___ 39. Lower motor neurons (motoneurons) that exit the spinal cord to stimulate skeletal muscle contraction are activated by all of the following influences *except*
    a. sensory feedback from the muscles and tendons

b. firing of autonomic motor neurons to skeletal muscles
c. excitatory effects from higher motor neurons
d. inhibitory effects from higher motor neurons

____ 40. The *Golgi tendon organs* are sensitive to muscle _____, while the *muscles spindle apparatus* is sensitive to muscle _____.
a. diameter; tension
b. length; diameter
c. tension; length (stretch)

____ 41. Which statement about the muscle spindle apparatus is *false*?
a. Nuclear bag fibers and nuclear chain fibers are intrafusal muscle fibers.
b. Sudden, rapid stretch of a muscle activates the secondary endings only.
c. Sudden, rapid stretch of a muscle results in a more powerful reflex contraction.
d. The frequency of action potentials produced in primary and secondary endings is proportional to the length of the muscle.

____ 42. Which statement about *gamma motoneurons* is *false*?
a. They innervate (stimulate) the intrafusal muscle fibers to contract.
b. They are thinner, more slowly conducting motoneurons than the alpha motoneurons.
c. Stimulation leads to tightening of the spindles and firing of action potentials along sensory neurons.
d. Stimulation directly causes visible muscle contraction and skeletal movements.
e. Stimulation results in only isometric contraction of the intrafusal fibers in the muscle spindles.

____ 43. Muscle stretch (monosynaptic) reflexes
a. are dependent on descending activation from higher motor neurons
b. involve sensory neurons, spinal cord interneurons and motor neurons only
c. are not present in all skeletal muscles
d. include the knee jerk reflex response to striking the patellar tendon
e. None of these statements regarding muscle stretch reflexes is correct.

____ 44. Which statement about Golgi tendon organs is *false*?
a. They continuously monitor tensions in the tendons during active contraction of, or passive stretching of, a muscle.
b. Their sensory neurons synapse with interneurons of the spinal cord.
c. They inhibit alpha motoneurons to the muscle involved via inhibitory postsynaptic potentials (IPSPs).
d. They are part of a disynaptic pathway of impulses from the receptor to the effector.
e. All of these statements about Golgi tendon organs are true.

____ 45. The major *extrapyramidal* tract(s) descending from higher brain centers is(are) the
a. reticulospinal tract
b. ventral corticospinal tract
c. lateral corticospinal tract
d. alpha and gamma motoneuron tracts

____ 46. Which higher center of the brain does *not* participate in the control of lower motor neurons?
a. basal ganglia (cerebral nuclei)
b. cerebellum
c. reticular formation (medulla oblongata and pons)
d. cerebral cortex (precentral gyrus)
e. All of these higher centers influence motor neuron control over lower motor neurons.

B. True or False/Edit

____ 47. Dorsal roots of spinal nerves contain sensory or efferent nerves, while ventral roots contain motor or afferent nerves.

____ 48. Most of the neurons in the spinal cord are sensory neurons.

____ 49. Those interneuron fibers that conduct impulses across the midline of the spinal cord to synapse on the opposite side are part of commissural tracts.

___ 50. Muscles that require the finest degree of control, such as the muscles of the hand, have the highest density of muscle spindles.

___ 51. Intrafusal fibers are located inside spindles, whereas extrafusal fibers are the stronger, more "ordinary" muscle fibers located outside the spindle.

___ 52. Primary (annulospiral) endings and secondary (flower-spray) endings are two types of motor (afferent) neuron endings found in muscle spindles.

___ 53. The effect of gamma motoneurons functions to tighten intrafusal fibers in the spindles, and thereby increase their sensitivity when the larger external muscle is passively stretched.

___ 54. About 90% of descending motor tracts synapse with interneurons in the spinal cord, with the remaining 10% forming synapses with alpha and gamma lower motoneurons.

___ 55. Upper motor neurons usually stimulate both alpha and gamma motoneurons to the agonist muscle simultaneously while inhibiting, via interneurons, both alpha and gamma motoneurons to the antagonistic muscle.

___ 56. Before exercise, slowly stretching your muscles can help avoid painful spasms by firing mostly the secondary endings in the muscle spindles and by activating the Golgi tendon organ reflex that promotes muscle relaxation.

___ 57. When the agonist muscles are stimulated to contract, simultaneously IPSPs are also formed by spinal cord interneurons that inhibit the antagonistic muscles involved in the action.

___ 58. All cerebellum control over the activity of lower motoneurons is indirect through other brain areas and is always inhibitory.

IV. ENERGY REQUIREMENTS OF SKELETAL MUSCLES

Skeletal muscles generate ATP through aerobic and anaerobic respiration and through the use of phosphate groups donated by creatine phosphate. The aerobic and anaerobic abilities of skeletal muscle fibers differ according to muscle fiber type. Slow-twitch (type I) fibers are adapted for aerobic respiration; fast-twitch (type II) fibers are adapted for anaerobic respiration.

A. Multiple Choice

___ 59. Skeletal muscle **at rest** obtains most of its energy from the breakdown, or catabolism of
  a. stored glycogen molecules within the muscle fiber
  b. imported glucose molecules extracted from the blood
  c. aerobic respiration of fatty acid molecules within the muscle fiber
  d. All of these sources of energy are used by resting muscle.

___ 60. During sustained muscle activity, the rapid regeneration of ATP molecules is accomplished mainly by the
  a. transfer of phosphate from high-energy phosphocreatine molecules in the muscle fiber
  b. hydrolysis of stored glycogen in the muscle fiber
  c. uptake and aerobic combustion of glucose molecules from the blood
  d. uptake and oxidation of free fatty acid molecules from the blood

___ 61. Slow-twitch skeletal muscle fibers
  a. are also known as type IIB fibers
  b. are found predominantly in the intraocular muscles of the eye
  c. are able to sustain contractions for long periods of time
  d. have fewer capillaries, mitochondria, and less total myoglobin
  e. All of these statements regarding slow-twitch muscle fibers are correct.

___ 62. Fast-twitch skeletal muscle fibers
  a. contain large amounts of the red pigment myoglobin
  b. respire anaerobically, primarily using glycogen for fuel
  c. can maintain contractions for long periods of time
  d. have lower than normal amounts of the enzyme myosin ATPase
  e. All of these statements regarding fast-twitch skeletal fibers are correct.

___ 63. Fatigue during moderate rhythmic exercise
  a. occurs as fast-twitch fibers deplete their reserve glycogen
  b. is the result of anaerobic respiration of glycogen in slow-twitch fibers

        c. occurs when lactic acid is produced, which lowers the pH of the muscle fibers
        d. results in an increase in ATP synthesis

___ 64. Which statement about the effects of endurance training on skeletal muscles is *false*? Endurance training results in
        a. an increase in the size and number of mitochondria
        b. less lactic acid is formed at a given level of exercise
        c. an increase in myoglobin content in the muscle
        d. an increase in the number of muscle fibers within the muscle
        e. an increase in the intramuscular triglyceride content and fat utilization

B. True or False/Edit

___ 65. After exercise has stopped, continued heavy breathing is necessary to repay the oxygen debt incurred primarily from losses to hemoglobin and myoglobin, and for metabolism of lactic acid.

___ 66. The enzyme creatine phosphokinase is also an isoenzyme since it is found in both heart and skeletal muscle, a fact that is used for clinical diagnoses.

___ 67. Myoglobin is a red pigment that is similar to hemoglobin in that both are vital for the delivery of oxygen mainly to the fast-twitch (type II) muscle fibers.

___ 68. The soleus muscle of the leg is a postural muscle composed predominantly of slow-twitch (type I) fibers.

___ 69. The conduction velocity of action potentials in motor neurons destined to slow-twitch muscle fibers is faster than those traveling to fast-twitch fibers.

___ 70. Since motor units are recruited from smaller numbers to larger numbers when increasing muscular effort is required, the smaller motor units with slow-twitch endurance fibers are used most often.

___ 71. Fatigue during maximal sustained contraction may be due to accumulation of extracellular K^+ - reducing the membrane potential of muscle fibers and interfering with their production of action potentials.

___ 72. True muscle fatigue usually starts with the accumulation of lactic acid and lowering of the pH, which reduces ATP synthesis—causing Ca^{2+} loss from the sarcoplasmic reticulum and fatigue.

V. CARDIAC AND SMOOTH MUSCLE

Cardiac muscle, like skeletal muscle, is striated and contains sarcomeres that shorten by sliding of thin and thick filaments. But while skeletal muscle requires nervous stimulation to contract, cardiac muscle can produce impulses and contract spontaneously. Smooth muscles lack sarcomeres, but they do contain actin and myosin that produce contractions in response to a unique regulatory mechanism.

A. Multiple Choice

___ 73. Which statement about cardiac and smooth muscle is *false*?
        a. Both are involuntary effectors.
        b. Both are regulated by autonomic motor neurons.
        c. Cardiac muscle, but not smooth muscle, contain sarcomeres.
        d. Ca^{2+} is involved in cardiac muscle but not smooth muscle excitation-contraction coupling.
        e. All of these statements regarding cardiac and smooth muscle are true.

___ 74. Smooth muscle
        a. contains actin and myosin filaments arranged in striations
        b. like skeletal muscle has a well-developed sarcoplasmic reticulum and sarcomeres
        c. when stretched eight times its resting length, may still contract
        d. contains 16:1 more thick myosin than thin actin filaments
        e. All of these statements regarding smooth muscle are correct.

___ 75. Which statement about smooth muscle *activation* is *false*?
        a. Ca^{2+} enters through voltage-sensitive calcium gates in the membrane.
        b. More membrane depolarization allows more Ca^{2+} entry, producing stronger smooth muscle contraction.

c. Ca²⁺ binds to *calmodulin* molecules inside the fibers to initiate the formation of cross-bridges.
   d. Smooth muscle cell activation leads to all-or-none muscle contractions.
   e. Smooth muscle cell contractions are slow due to slower ATPase and sustained because cross-bridges can enter a latch state.

___ 76. Which statement about *single-unit* or *multiunit* smooth muscles is *false*?
   a. Single-unit smooth muscles are intrinsically myogenic in that they contract in response to stretch.
   b. Single-unit smooth muscles display pacemaker activity in which certain cells stimulate others in the muscle.
   c. Multiunit smooth muscles have numerous gap junctions or electrical synapses.
   d. Multiunit muscle contractions require stimulation by separate nerve fibers.

B. True or False/Edit

___ 77. Cardiac muscle intercalated discs are actually electrical synapses, or gap junctions.
___ 78. Unlike the contraction of skeletal muscle that is all-or-none, cardiac muscle contraction strength is graded based on the number of muscle cells stimulated.
___ 79. Smooth muscle is commonly found arranged in a circular or longitudinal pattern around tubes, vessels, and hollow organs.
___ 80. *Myosin light chain kinase* is an enzyme in smooth muscle that helps catalyze the formation of myosin cross bridges between actin and myosin molecules during contraction.

CHAPTER REVIEW

A. Crossword Puzzle — Muscle: Mechanisms of Contraction and Neural Control

Across
1. type II skeletal muscle fiber twitch speed
4. higher brain center for muscle action, the basa_____
5. series_____ component
9. muscle filament composition of the I band
12. simple knee jerk reflex neuron pathway
14. all-or-_____
17. motor neurons traveling to skeletal muscles
18. neurotransmitter released from all motor axons
20. "piggyback" of a twitch on top of another, stronger twitch
22. contraction during which the muscle does shorten
23. one single muscle cell
24. nuclear_____ fibers are loose in the muscle spindle apparatus
25. color of slow-twitch fibers due to myoglobin pigmentation
27. another name for a reflex pathway
30. innervation to the antagonist muscles while agonists contract
33. descending tracts controlling fine voluntary movements
34. name for the muscle being moved
35. the smallest unit of muscle contraction
36. actin or myosin, for example

Down
2. sustained muscle contraction
3. high-energy phosphate molecule required for contraction and relaxation of muscles
4. tendon organs inhibiting the agonist muscle contractions
6. the ion required for muscle excitation-contraction coupling
7. includes the brain and spinal cord
8. name of motoneurons to muscle spindles
10. the appearance of actin molecules
11. contractions during which the muscle does not shorten
13. excitation of both alpha and gamma motoneurons simultaneously
15. muscle whose contractions open the angle of joints
16. one complete contraction-relaxation cycle of a muscle
19. collective name for descending higher motor neurons involving many brain nuclei is _____ pyramidal
20. the sensory apparatus within the muscle responding to the stretch of a muscle
21. efferent
26. motoneurons innervating the extrafusal muscle fibers
28. actin and myosin form cross-_____

29. inability to maintain muscle tension any longer — perhaps due to a lack of ATP
31. thick sarcomere filament
32. Ca^{2+} is stored in the terminal cisternae of the _____ plasmic reticulum

B. Essay

Essay Tutorial

This essay tutorial will answer the first essay question found in the "**Review Activities**" section of your *Human Physiology* textbook. Please look for *Essay Question* 1. at the end of chapter 12, read it carefully, and let me guide you through one possible answer. Watch for key terms in bold-face type, helpful tips and general suggestions on writing the essay or short-answer questions. Enjoy!

81. Using the concept of **motor units,** explain how skeletal muscles *in vivo* produce **graded** and **sustained** contractions.

Note: First define motor units, since our question is centered around them, and then define graded and sustained while we progress through the answer.

Answer. A motor unit is one somatic motor neuron together with all of its axon collaterals and muscle fibers innervated (stimulated) by these collaterals. Motor units may be small with only a few fibers per motor neuron, or large with one neuron innervating thousands of muscle fibers to contract. Larger motor units produce more powerful contractions, so that to some degree muscle contractions are graded based on the size of the motor unit fired. Usually smaller units are fired first, with larger units activated when greater strength is required. *In vivo* (in the body), graded contractions of whole muscle are produced by variations in the **number** of motor units that are activated, and the smooth, sustained contractions (called tetanus) are produced by rapid, asynchronous stimulation of **different** motor units, both large and small.

This wasn't so bad was it? Here are a few of mine.

82. Explain the statement, "one muscle fiber is one muscle cell." As best you can, draw and completely label one muscle fiber. (When you have done your best, refer to figure 12.8 in the text to complete your drawing.)

83. Go into the muscle sarcomere and describe a cross bridge between actin and myosin, revealing as much as possible about their chemical structures and interactions with ATP.

84. Describe the various components of the muscle spindle apparatus. Distinguish among the parts that are contractile and noncontractile; and those that are sensory and motor. (*Hint*: Could we use a table format here?)

85. Draw the pathway that action potentials take from Golgi tendon organs to the spinal cord and back to the muscle undergoing rapid contraction. (*Hint*: This is a disynaptic reflex.)

86. Explain why slow-twitch fibers are red, adapted for aerobic respiration, and resistant to fatigue; whereas fast-twitch fibers are white, adapted for anaerobic respiration, and susceptible to fatigue.

87. On a piece of paper make three columns with headings **skeletal muscle**, **smooth muscle**, and **cardiac muscle**. List the structural and functional characteristics of smooth muscle and note which are in common with characteristics of the other muscle types.

Answers — Chapter 12

I. Structure and Actions of Skeletal Muscles
   A. 1. c, 2. b, 3. c, 4. d, 5. c, 6. e, 7. a, 8. d
   B. 9. T, 10. T, 11. T, 12. F—Skeletal fibers are multinucleate, 13. F—Tetany is a painful state of muscle contracture, 14. F—Replace "isometric" with "isotonic," 15. T, 16. T, 17. T, 18. F—Motor units vary in size, even within the same muscle, 19. T

II. Mechanisms of Contraction
   A. 20. a, 21. c, 22. a, 23. b, 24. d, 25. d, 26. e
   B. 27. F—Replace "A" with "I," 28. T, 29. F—Shortening occurs as actin and myosin filaments slide over one another, 30. T, 31. T, 32. T, 33. F—Replace "tropomyosin" with "troponin," 34. T, 35. T, 36. F—The uptake of Ca^{2+} is active; its release is passive as action potentials pass by, 37. T

   C. 38. 3, 6, 4, 1, 8, 10, 5, 2, 9, 7

III. Neural Control of Skeletal Muscles
   A. A. 39. b, 40. c, 41. b, 42. d, 43. d, 44. e, 45. a, 46. e
   B. 47. F—Switch "efferent "and "afferent," 48. F—Replace "sensory" with "interneurons," 49. T, 50. T, 51. T, 52. F—Replace "motor" with "sensory," 53. T, 54. T, 55. T, 56. T, 57. T, 58. T

IV. Energy Requirements of Skeletal Muscle
   A. 59. c, 60. a, 61. c, 62. b, 63. c, 64. d
   B. 65. T, 66. T, 67. F—Replace "fast-twitch (type II)" with "slow-twitch (type I) ," 68. T, 69. F—Switch "slow-" and "fast-," 70. T, 71. T, 72. T

V. Cardiac and Smooth Muscle
   A. 73. d, 74. c, 75. d, 76. c
   B. 77. T, 78. F—Switch "skeletal" and "cardiac," 79. T, 80. T

Chapter Review
   A. Crossword Puzzle

	1F	A	2S	T			3A			4G	A	N	G	L	I	A		
			5E	L	A	S	T	I	6C	O							7C	
		8G		T			P		A		L		9A	C	10T	I	N	
		A		A	11I						G				H		S	
		12M	O	N	O	S	Y	N	A	P	T	I	13C			I		
		M		U			O						O		14N	O	N	15E	16T
		A		17S	O	M	A	T	I	C			A					X	W
							E					18A	C	H		19E		T	I
20S	U	21M	M	A	T	I	O	N				T				X		E	T
P		O			R						22I	S	O	T	O	N	I	C
I		T		23F	I	B	E	R			V			R		S		H
N		O			C					24B	A	G		A		O	
D		25R	E	D				26A		T			27A	R	C		
L						28B		L		I		29F					
E					30R	E	C	I	P	R	O	C	A	L		31M	
			32S		I			H		N		T				Y	
33P	Y	R	A	M	I	D	A	L		A		I				O	
			R		G							34A	G	O	N	I	S	T
35S	A	R	C	O	M	E	R	E				U				I	
			O		S			36F	I	L	A	M	E	N	T	

134

CHAPTER 13
HEART AND CIRCULATION

CHAPTER SCOPE

Lub-dub, lub-dub, lub-dub! Seventy beats each minute, 4,200 beats each hour, 100,800 beats each day your heart contracts, ejecting blood into elastic blood vessels for distribution around the body. **Blood** is mostly water and proteins, with millions of red blood cells (*erythrocytes*) carrying oxygen, white blood cells (*leukocytes*) defending against infections, and platelets (*thrombocytes*) plugging vascular leaks. Platelets are intimately involved in blood clotting, or **coagulation** — a rapid series of complex *positive feedback* events that serve to stop bleeding. With the bleeding stopped, the disturbance has been corrected (*negative feedback*) and homeostasis has been restored.

The **heart** has blood receiving chambers (*atria*) and blood pumping chambers (*ventricles*) with valves at each exit to ensure the continuous flow of blood. Each complete cardiac cycle starts with a spontaneous electrical excitation followed shortly by a mechanical contraction of the myocardium. The *electrical* cycle originates from the pacemaker region and spreads throughout the heart, as recorded on the **electrocardiogram** (**ECG**). The *mechanical* cycle is characterized by pressure and volume changes within the heart that result in the ejection of blood and the formation of two valve sounds (lub-dub) that can be heard with a *stethoscope*.

Blood is forced out of the heart and into large **arteries**, which branch into smaller and smaller **arterioles**. Beyond arterioles, the exchange of gases and nutrients for wastes is accomplished by miles of **capillaries** running near all cells. After this exchange, blood is drained away from tissue capillaries through **venules** and then larger **veins**, returning to the heart for another boost around the vascular network.

Since some fluid and other materials are forced out of capillaries, and others are released from neighboring cells, the lymph system vessels (**lymphatics**) provide a beautifully designed drainage system for the filtering and recycling of extracellular fluid that eventually returns to the blood. In the next chapter, the focus is on the arterioles, where blood pressure and the distribution of blood flow to various parts of the body such as the kidney, skin, and brain is regulated. These two chapters combine to provide a circulatory theme that helps us to better understand the following chapters that discuss the respiratory (chapter 15), urinary (chapter 16), digestive (chapters 17 and 18), and endocrine (chapters 11 and 20) systems.

I. FUNCTIONS AND COMPONENTS OF THE CIRCULATORY SYSTEM

Blood serves numerous functions, including the transport of respiratory gases, nutritive molecules, metabolic wastes, and hormones. Blood is transported through the body in a system of vessels leading from and returning to the heart.

A. Multiple Choice

____ 1. Which of the following is *not* a function of the circulatory system?
   a. respiration
   b. transportation
   c. regulation
   d. protection
   e. All of these are functions of the circulatory system.

____ 2. Which substances involved in cellular metabolism are not normally transported by the circulatory system?
   a. respiratory gas molecules, such as oxygen and carbon dioxide
   b. absorbed products of digestion
   c. Krebs cycle enzymes

       d. metabolic wastes
       e. water and ions
  3. How many liters of blood does the adult heart pump each minute?
       a. three
       b. five
       c. seven
       d. nine
       e. twelve
  4. The thinnest and most numerous of all blood vessels are the
       a. arteries
       b. arterioles
       c. capillaries
       d. venules
       e. veins

B. True or False/Edit

  5. As blood flows through capillaries, the *hydrostatic* pressure of the blood forces some fluid out of the capillary walls and into the tissue spaces.
  6. Tissue fluid is the same as interstitial fluid; and may form lymph, returning to the venous blood through lymphatic vessels.
  7. The lymph nodes within the lymphatic system are considered part of the excretory system.

II. COMPOSITION OF BLOOD

Blood consists of formed elements that are suspended and carried in the plasma. These formed elements and their major functions include erythrocytes (oxygen transport), leukocytes (immune defense), and platelets (blood clotting). Plasma contains different types of proteins and many water-soluble molecules.

A. Multiple Choice

  8. A normal hematocrit of 45 means that
       a. 45% of the formed elements are erythrocytes.
       b. there are 45 million formed elements per milliliter of blood.
       c. 45% of the total blood volume is formed elements.
       d. 45 milliliters of plasma is the standard volume measured.
  9. Much like extracellular fluid (ECF), the major solute dissolved in the plasma portion of the blood is
       a. glucose
       b. Na^+
       c. K^+
       d. albumin
       e. Ca^{2+}
  10. Which of the following proteins is *not* considered a plasma protein?
       a. globulin
       b. insulin
       c. albumin
       d. fibrinogen
  11. Which statement about erythrocytes is *false*?
       a. They lack both a nucleus and mitochondria.
       b. They outnumber leukocytes by a large margin.
       c. They require dietary iron and vitamin B_{12}.
       d. Their circulating life span is about twelve months.
       e. All of these statements regarding erythrocytes are true.
  12. Which of the following is *not* a granular leukocyte?
       a. neutrophil
       b. basophil

c. lymphocyte
d. eosinophil
e. All of these are granular leukocytes.

___ 13. Which statement about platelets is *false*?
a. They have a life span of about 120 days.
b. They are the smallest of the formed elements, derived originally from megakaryocytes.
c. During blood clotting, they release a chemical called serotonin that constricts blood vessels in the injured area.
d. Phospholipids in their membranes activate clotting factors in the plasma.
e. They lack nuclei but are capable of ameboid movement.

___ 14. Which of the following cells has the *shortest* life span? (*Hint*: see table 13.2 in your text.)
a. erythrocytes
b. platelets
c. agranular leukocytes
d. granular leukocytes

___ 15. In the **ABO system** of red blood cell typing, which of the following genotypes is *not* possible?
a. ii
b. I^AI
c. I^Bi
d. I^AI^B
e. All of these genotypes are possible.

___ 16. A person whose blood type is BO has red blood cells with membrane-bound ____ antigens and anti-____ antibodies in the plasma.
a. B; B
b. B; A
c. A; A
d. A; B

___ 17. In *erythroblastosis fetalis* (hemolytic disease of the newborn), the
a. baby is Rh positive and the mother is Rh negative.
b. mother has made antibodies against th Rh factor present on the baby's red blood cells.
c. baby has abnormally low numbers of red blood cells (anemia).
d. mother should have been given RhoGAM (antibodies) by injection.
e. All of these statements regarding erythroblastosis fetalis are correct.

___ 18. Which of the following events does *not* occur during *hemostasis* within an injured vessel?
a. The endothelial lining is damaged, exposing collagen proteins to the blood.
b. The injured blood vessel is constricted by newly released chemicals.
c. Platelets become "sticky" and a platelet plug is formed near the injury.
d. A web of fibrin protein strands interweave the platelet plug.
e. All of these events occur during hemostasis.

___ 19. The endothelial cells of the damaged blood vessel secrete two important chemicals involved in hemostasis - *prostacyclin* and _____.
a. serotonin
b. von Willebrand factor
c. ADP
d. thromboxane A_2
e. None of these chemicals is secreted by damaged endothelial cells.

___ 20. The ion most involved in blood clotting sequences, is
a. Na^+.
b. Ca^{2+}.
c. K^+.
d. H^+.
e. Fe^{+++}.

___ 21. The final step in blood clot formation is the conversion of
   a. factor XII to factor XI.
   b. factor VII to factor X.
   c. fibrinogen to fibrin.
   d. prothrombin to thrombin.

___ 22. The vitamin that converts glutamate ammino acids in clotting factor proteins into gamma-carboxyglutamate, that effectively binds to Ca^{2+} during blood clotting is vitamin _____.
   a. K
   b. C
   c. B_{12}
   d. D
   e. A

___ 23. Which of the following chemicals is *not* an anticoagulant?
   a. citrate
   b. EDTA (chelator)
   c. heparin
   d. bradykinin
   e. coumarin

B. True or False/Edit

___ 24. Oxyhemoglobin is the combination of oxygen with hemoglobin inside the erythrocytes, giving venous blood its blue color.

___ 25. Normal blood pH ranges from 7.35 to 7.45.

___ 26. The most common plasma protein is albumin, whose primary function is to draw water from the extracellular fluid (ECF) into the capillary plasma.

___ 27. Alpha, beta, and gamma globulins are all plasma proteins produced by the liver that all function as antibodies in immunity.

___ 28. Diapedesis is the amoeba-like movement of leukocytes (white blood cells) through pores in capillary walls to reach sites of infection.

___ 29. The most abundant type of leukocyte, comprising 50% to 70% of all white blood cells is the lymphocyte.

___ 30. Plasma cells are actually enlarged monocytes that produce and secrete large amounts of antibodies into the blood.

___ 31. Polycythemia is to anemia what leukocytosis is to leukemia.

___ 32. Red bone marrow (myeloid tissue) produces all of the different types of blood cells, while lymphoid tissue makes lymphocytes.

___ 33. Erythropoietin is a hormone secreted by the kidneys in response to lowered blood oxygen concentrations, thus stimulating erythrocyte stem cells in bone marrow to divide.

___ 34. People who are blood type O (or ii), have both anti-A and anti-B antibodies in their plasma.

___ 35. A and B antigens on red blood cells are sometimes called agglutinogens, and the plasma antibodies made against them are called agglutinins.

___ 36. A prostaglandin derivative that normally prevents platelets from sticking to each other and to the lining of healthy blood vessels is thromboxane A_2.

___ 37. Aspirin is an inhibitor of prostaglandin synthesis and therefore would be expected to slow the clotting sequence.

___ 38. Plasma is actually serum without the clotting factor called fibrinogen.

___ 39. When repairs have been made to the vessel, the activated plasma enzyme that digests fibrin and dissolves the clot is called plasmin.

III. ACID-BASE BALANCE OF THE BLOOD

The pH of blood plasma is maintained very constant through the functions of the lungs and kidneys. The lungs regulate the carbon dioxide concentration of the blood, and the kidneys regulate the bicarbonate concentration.

___ 40. Which statement regarding acid-base balance in the body is *false*?
   a. Bicarbonate ion (HCO_3^-) is the major buffer in the blood plasma.
   b. The lungs and kidneys are the two organs most responsible for maintaining a constant body pH.
   c. Normal blood plasma pH is maintained near 7.4 within the range of 7.35 to 7.45.
   d. All acids in the body are considered nonvolatile acids.

___ 41. In metabolic acidosis,
   a. the production of nonvolatile acids is abnormally increased.
   b. CO_2 production exceeds CO_2 loss through ventilation at the lungs.
   c. the cause can be attributed to a decrease in respirations (hypoventilation).
   d. the cause can be attributed to an increase in bicarbonate ion concentration in the blood.
   e. severe vomiting is usually evident.

___ 42. In *respiratory alkalosis*,
   a. the blood pH usually falls below 7.35.
   b. the rate of respirations are abnormally increased (hyperventilation).
   c. both the blood levels of P_{CO_2} and HCO_3^- levels are unusually high.
   d. the cause can be attributed to prolonged breathholding maneuvers.
   e. severe vomiting is usually evident.

B. True or False/Edit

___ 43. The kidneys regulate the carbon dioxide concentration of the blood and the lungs regulate the bicarbonate concentration of the blood.

___ 44. Carbonic acid is referred to as a volatile acid because it can be converted into a gas; and, thus, its blood concentration can be altered by changes in ventilation.

___ 45. Uncontrolled diabetes mellitus is a clinical condition that can result in a metabolic alkalosis.

___ 46. The Henderson-Hasselbalch equation can be used to demonstrate the relationship between abnormal levels of bicarbonate and respiratory acidosis or alkalosis.

IV. STRUCTURE OF THE HEART

The heart contains four chambers: two upper atria, which receive venous blood, and two lower ventricles, which eject blood into arteries. The right ventricle pumps blood to the lungs, where the blood becomes oxygenated; the left ventricle pumps oxygenated blood to the entire body. The proper flow of blood within the heart is aided by two pairs of one-way valves.

A. Multiple Choice

___ 47. In the pulmonary circulation, the
   a. pulmonary artery carries oxygen-poor blood.
   b. pulmonary vein carries blood toward the lung capillaries.
   c. blood returning to the left atrium of the heart is oxygen-poor.
   d. oxygen from the blood diffuses into the air sacs (alveoli) of the lungs.
   e. blood leaves the left ventricle and returns to the right atrium.

___ 48. The atrioventricular *(AV) valve*
   a. between the right atrium and ventricle is the bicuspid.
   b. between the left atrium and ventricel is the tricuspid.
   c. called the mitral valve, is also known as the bicuspid valve.
   d. normally prevents blood flow from the atria to the ventricles.

___ 49. The semilunar valves
   a. prevent the backward flow of blood into the atria of the heart.
   b. are open during relaxation of the ventricles.
   c. are held tightly by papillary muscles and chordae tendinae.
   d. direct blood ejected from the ventricles into the pulmonary artery and the aorta.

B. True or False/Edit

___ 50. A muscular wall called a septum prevents the mixture of blood between the left and right sides of the heart.

___ 51. The myocardial cells of the atria and ventricles are structurally and functionally separated from each other.

___ 52. The work performed by the right ventricle is five to seven times greater than that performed by the left ventricle.

___ 53. The cardiac valves open and close due to changes in pressure on either side of the valves.

C. Sequencer - Pathway of Circulating Blood

54. You are a red blood cell entering the heart from the superior vena cava! Test your understanding of cardiac structures by tracing your route through the entire heart, past the valves, and into the aorta. Starting with number 1, write the numerical sequence of the following structures on the left in the spaces provided. On the right side of the page, write out the name of the structure that corresponds to the numerical sequence from 1 to 12 that you have chosen. The last one, number 12 (aorta), has been done for you. Notice that the pulmonary circulation is included. Completion of the next figure should be of further help in learning these structures.

Notice that the pulmonary circulation is included. Now label the figure in the next section.

___ pulmonary capillary
___ mitral valve
___ aortic semilunar valve
___ tricuspid valve
___ pulmonary vein
_12_ aorta
___ left ventricle
___ right ventricle
___ right atrium
___ pulmonary semilunar valve
___ left atrium
___ pulmonary artery

1. _____
2. _____
3. _____
4. _____
5. _____
6. _____
7. _____
8. _____
9. _____
10. _____
11. _____
12. _____aorta_____

D. Label the Figure — The Heart

Study figure 13.1 below and label all structures of the heart, including the four valves. When finished, check your work with figure 13.8 in your text.

V. CARDIAC CYCLE AND HEART SOUNDS

The two atria fill with blood and then contract simultaneously. This is followed by simultaneous contraction of both ventricles, which sends blood through the pulmonary and systemic circulations. Contraction of the ventricles closes the AV valves and opens the semilunar valves; relaxation of the ventricles allows the semilunar valves to close. The closing of first the AV valves and then the semilunar valves produces the "lub-dub" sounds heard with a stethoscope.

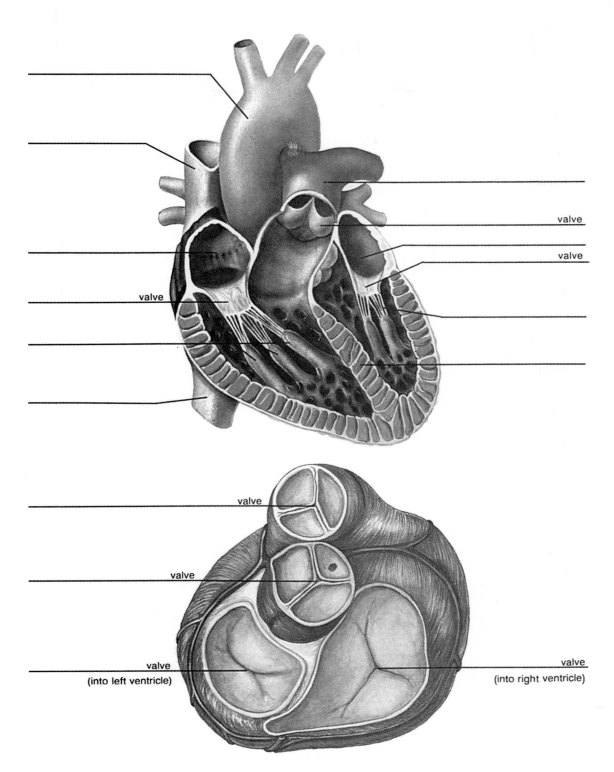

Figure 13.1 The structure of the heart and valves.

A. Multiple Choice

_____ 55. The terms *systole* and *diastole* refer, respectively, to the
   a. contraction phase and relaxation phase of the atria.
   b. relaxation phase and contraction phase of the atria.

141

c. contraction phase and relaxation phase of the ventricles.
d. relaxation phase and contraction phase of the ventricles.
e. the simultaneous contraction and relaxation phases of both the atria and the ventricles.

___ 56. During normal ventricular contraction, what *fraction* of the end-diastolic volume is ejected as the stroke volume?
a. one-fourth
b. one-third
c. one-half
d. two-thirds
e. three-fourths

___ 57. At rest, each cardiac cycle lasts about 0.8 seconds; of which systole lasts ___ seconds, and diastole lasts ____ seconds.
a. 0.3; 0.5
b. 0.4; 0.4
c. 0.1; 0.7
d. 0.6; 0.2
e. 0.2; 0.6

___ 58. During one cardiac cycle, the major difference between the left and the right halves of the heart is that the
a. left heart pumps a greater volume of blood than the right heart.
b. right heart contracts shortly before the left heart.
c. right heart pumps blood with less force (at lower pressure) than the left heart.
d. left heart has a shorter cardiac cycle duration than the right heart.

___ 59. The *first* heart sound results from vibrations generated by the
a. opening of the AV valves.
b. closing of the AV valves.
c. opening of the semilunar valves.
d. closing of the semilunar valves.
e. Both b and d are correct.

B. True or False/Edit

___ 60. Normally, both atria contract at the same time, followed shortly by both ventricles contracting at the same time.

___ 61. Venous blood returning to fill the heart (venous return) is greatest during systole.

___ 62. The contraction of both atria is essential for life because it delivers about 80% of the total volume of blood to the ventricles for subsequent ejection.

___ 63. During both isovolumetric contraction and isovolumetric relaxation phases, all four valves in the heart (2 AV and 2 semilunar) are closed.

___ 64. During inhalation particularly, the first heart sound may be "split" into two separate sounds as the tricuspid and mitral heart valves close individually.

___ 65. A streptococcus bacterial throat infection in susceptible persons may lead to rheumatic fever and rheumatic endocarditis, resulting in damage to the heart valves and detectable murmurs.

___ 66. Simple septal defects are usually congenital (from birth), resulting in the flow of blood from the right side of the heart to the left side of the heart since the pressure is higher on the right side.

VI. ELECTRICAL ACTIVITY OF THE HEART AND ELECTROCARDIOGRAM

The pacemaker region of the heart (SA node) exhibits a spontaneous depolarization that causes action potentials and results in the automatic beating of the heart. Electrical impulses are conducted by myocardial cells in the atria and are transmitted to the ventricles by specialized conducting tissue. Electrocardiogram waves correspond to the electrical events in the heart as follows: P wave (depolarization of the atria); QRS wave (depolarization of the ventricles); and T wave (repolarization of the ventricles).

A. Multiple Choice

___ 67. The sinoatrial (SA) node region of the right atrium is the normal pacemaker of the heart because this region
   a. demonstrates spontaneous electrical activity.
   b. depolarizes to threshold before other cardiac regions.
   c. has Ca^{2+} diffusing first through slow and then fast Ca^{2+} channels.
   d. develops pacemaker potentials during diastole.
   e. All of these statements are correct.

___ 68. Action potentials in myocardial cells have a characteristic *plateau phase*, which is caused primarily by the
   a. slow outward diffusion of Na^+.
   b. fast inward diffusion of Na^+.
   c. fast outward diffusion of Ca^{2+}.
   d. slow inward diffusion of Ca^{2+}.

___ 69. Which statement about the normal *electrocardiogram* (ECG) tracing is *false*?
   a. Lead I is a recording from the right arm to the left arm.
   b. The unipolar leads are found only on the chest.
   c. There are a total of twelve standard ECG leads that "view" the changing pattern of the heart's electrical activity.
   d. There are six unipolar chest leads.
   e. Lead III is a recording from the left arm to the left leg.

___ 70. Which statement about the normal *electrocardiogram* (ECG) tracing is *false*?
   a. The T wave represents depolarization of the atria.
   b. The QRS wave represents depolarization of the ventricles.
   c. The repolarization of the atria is hidden by the QRS wave.
   d. The P wave occurs shortly before the QRS wave.
   e. All of these statements about the ECG are true.

___ 71. The *second* heart sound (S_2) is heard while the corresponding ECG is recording the
   a. P wave.
   b. P-R interval.
   c. QRS wave.
   d. T wave.
   e. S-T segment.

B. True or False/Edit

___ 72. An ectopic pacemaker (or ectopic focus) is a cluster of myocardial cells located away from the SA node that take over and regulate the cardiac pace.

___ 73. The rate of impulse conduction from the SA node is slowed through the AV node, causing a time delay before the ventricles are excited.

___ 74. Unlike skeletal muscles, heart muscle cannot maintain a sustained maximal contraction (tetany).

___ 75. The summation of myocardial cell contractions is prevented by their relatively short refractory period.

___ 76. The body is a good conductor of electricity because tissue fluids contain a high concentration of ions that move in response to changes in the membrane potentials.

___ 77. The electrocardiogram (ECG) wave patterns designated P, QRS, and T are recordings of action potentials from specific regions in the heart.

C. Label the Figure — The Conduction System of the Heart

Study the drawing of the electrical conduction pathway of the heart in figure 13.2 below. Then write the words that best describe the conduction pathway structures indicated by the blank lines on the figure. Remember this is the pathway for *electrical* excitation — the *mechanical* contraction of cardiac muscle fibers will follow shortly. See figure 13.17 in the text to check your work.

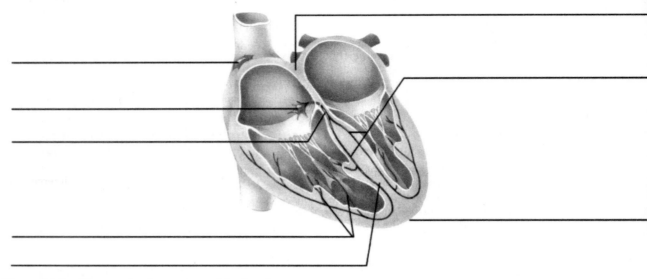

Figure 13.2 The conduction system of the heart.

VII. BLOOD VESSELS

The thick muscle layer of arteries allows them to transmit blood ejected from the heart under high pressure, and the elastic recoil of the large arteries further contributes to blood flow. The thinner muscle layer of veins allows them to distend when an increased amount of blood enters them, and their one-way valves ensure that blood flows back to the heart. Capillaries are composed of only a single layer of endothelium, which allows water and other molecules to move across the capillary walls and thus permits exchanges between the blood and tissue fluid.

A. Multiple Choice

___ 78. The blood vessel layer composed primarily of smooth muscle is called the tunica
   a. externa
   b. media
   c. interna
   d. endothelium

___ 79. Which of the following statements about arteries and veins is *false*?
   a. Arteries have more smooth muscle than comparable veins.
   b. Arteries carry blood under higher pressure.
   c. Veins have one-way valves, promoting flow in only one direction.
   d. Veins collapse providing the greatest resistance to blood flow in the circulatory system.
   e. All of these statements regarding arteries and veins are true.

___ 80. The "business ends" of the circulatory system in which the exchanges of gases and nutrients occur, are blood vessels known as
   a. arteries
   b. arterioles
   c. capillaries
   d. venules
   e. veins

___ 81. In the central nervous system (CNS), the type of capillary that lacks intercellular channels and helps form the blood-brain barrier, is called a
   a. continuous capillary.
   b. discontinuous capillary.
   c. fenestrated capillary.

___ 82. Which of the following mechanisms is *not* an important part of the normal return of venous blood to the heart?
   a. the inhalation phase of normal breathing
   b. skeletal muscle contractions (pump)
   c. the higher average hydrostatic pressure in the veins than that found in the heart
   d. standing upright, perfectly still

B. True or False/Edit

___ 83. Compared to larger arteries, smaller arteries and arterioles are less elastic and have a thicker layer of smooth muscle.
___ 84. In skeletal muscle at rest, precapillary sphincter muscles are open and permit blood flow in only 5%-10% of the capillary beds; with the remaining 90%-95% of the capillary beds closed.
___ 85. *Fenestrated capillaries* of the kidneys, endocrine glands, and intestines have wide intercellular pores, or "windows," that are covered by a layer of mucoprotein, serving as a diaphragm.
___ 86. Varicose veins result from extra blood accumulating in large veins over a long period of time, thereby stretching these vessels and making the valves incompetent — no longer able to prevent blood from flowing backwards.

VIII. ATHEROSCLEROSIS AND CARDIAC ARRHYTHMIAS

Atherosclerosis is a disease process that can lead to obstruction of coronary blood flow. As a result, the electrical properties of the heart and its ability to function as a pump may be seriously compromised. Abnormal cardiac rhythms, or arrhythmias, can be detected by the abnormal electrocardiogram patterns they produce.

A. Multiple Choice

___ 87. Which of the following events is *not* considered part of the progression that occurs during the development of long-term atherosclerosis?
   a. Monocytes, attracted to the tunica intima region of the damaged endothelium, engulf lipids and take on a "foamy cells" appearance.
   b. Gray-white "fatty streaks" formed by lipid-filled macrophages, protrude into the lumen of arteries and thus reduce blood flow.
   c. White blood cells (phagocytes) attempt to attack and reject the developing atheroma as a foreign substance.
   d. Fibrous plaques may form, composed of accumulated lipids, white blood cells, and debris, covered by a cap of connective tissue and smooth muscle cells.
   e. All of these events are part of the long-term progression in atherosclerosis.
___ 88. Which of the following is *not* considered a risk factor in the development of atherosclerosis?
   a. advanced age
   b. smoking
   c. high blood HDL — cholesterol
   d. hypertension
   e. high blood LDL — cholesterol
___ 89. Which of the following statements about low-density lipoproteins (LDL) is *false*?
   a. In the liver, LDL consists of a core of cholesterol surrounded by an outer layer of phospholipid and protein molecules.
   b. LDL levels are higher in females and in exercising males than in those who are inactive.
   c. Floating past certain organ cells, LDL is recognized by specific receptors and engulfed by the process known as receptor-mediated endocytosis.
   d. Persons with high blood LDL levels usually have a low number of LDL receptors in their livers.
   e. LDL blood levels rise in persons with high cholesterol, in those eating high-fat diets, and in people with familial hypercholesteremia.

___ 90. Which of the following statements about *myocardial infarction* (MI) is *false*?
   a. An MI is commonly referred to by the general public as a "heart attack."
   b. An MI may be detected by changes in the S-T segment of the ECG.
   c. Since myocardial cells are adapted to respire anaerobically for several hours, an MI takes time to develop.
   d. An MI can be diagnosed by the abnormal release of creatine phosphokinase (CPK) and lactate dehydrogenase enzymes released from the infarcted cells.
   e. All of these statements regarding an MI are true.

B. True or False/Edit

___ 91. Atherosclerosis, accompanied by heart disease and stroke, is responsible for about 50% of the deaths in the United States, Europe, and Japan.
___ 92. "Fatty streaks" are gray-white areas that protrude from the tunica intima into the lumen of arteries; and are even present in children to a small degree in the aorta and coronary arteries of children aged 10 to 14.
___ 93. In the progression of atherosclerosis, lymphocytes may engulf lipids while passing through the endothelium of arteries, developing into "foamy cells."
___ 94. Platelets contribute to atherosclerosis and the occlusion of blood flow as they adhere to damaged subendothelial tissue.
___ 95. Persons having higher plasma LDL-cholesterol concentrations and lower plasma HDL-cholesterol concentrations appear to have a lower risk of developing atherosclerosis.
___ 96. About 40%-58% of the calories eaten in a typical fast-food meal are derived from the ingestion of fat.
___ 97. *Ischemia* is an inadequate flow of blood (and an inadequate supply of oxygen) to any tissue.

C. Matching — Arrhythmias of the Heart

Match the letter of the cardiac arrhythmia on the right with the best description on the left.

___ 98. life-threatening ventricular condition
___ 99. cardiac rates over 100 bpm
___ 100. atria and ventricles beat separately; may require an artificial pacemaker
___ 101. parasympathetic SA node slowing (under 60 bpm)
___ 102. P-R interval exceeding 0.2 seconds
___ 103. myocardial excitation without refractory periods
___ 104. rapid, yet coordinated atrial or ventricular contractions
___ 105. not every P wave is followed by a QRS wave (one normal QRS every two or three beats)

a. bradycardia
b. tachycardia
c. flutter
d. fibrillation
e. circus rhythms
f. first degree AV node block
g. second degree AV node block
h. third degree AV node block

IX. LYMPHATIC SYSTEM

Lymphatic vessels absorb excess tissue fluid and transport this fluid — now called lymph — to ducts that drain into veins. Lymph nodes, and lymphoid tissue in the thymus, spleen, and tonsils produce lymphocytes, which are white blood cells involved in immunity.

A. Multiple Choice

___ 106. Which of the following is *not* a basic function of the lymphatic system?
   a. transport interstitial (tissue) fluid back to the blood
   b. transport lymph to the right and left subclavian veins
   c. transport fat absorbed from the gut to the blood
   d. help in the immune defense against disease-causing agents
   e. All of these are lymphatic system functions.
___ 107. Due to the unique structure of lymph capillaries, lymph contains all of the following substances, *except*
   a. interstitial proteins

        b. interstitial microorganisms
        c. interstitial RBCs and WBCs
        d. interstitial fluid
        e. absorbed fat
___ 108. Lymph fluid from around the body eventually flows into lymphatics that merge and drain directly into the
        a. right and left subclavian veins
        b. superior and inferior vena cavae
        c. aorta
        d. right atrium
        e. right and left pulmonary veins
___ 109. Which of the following is *not* considered a lymphoid organ since it does *not* contain phagocytic cells and germinal centers for the production of lymphocytes?
        a. the thymus gland
        b. the thyroid gland
        c. the tonsils
        d. the spleen
        e. All of these are considered lymphoid organs.

B. True or False/Edit

___ 110. Like veins, lymphatic vessels have the same three vessel layers and one-way valves to prevent the backward flow of lymph.
___ 111. Lymph is formed by the filtration of plasma from blood capillaries; returning later to the blood to complete the cycle.
___ 112. Lymph node germinal centers are sites of pathogen removal by resident phagocytes in the lymphatic system.

CHAPTER REVIEW

B. Essay

Essay Tutorial

This essay tutorial will answer the first essay question found in the "**Review Activities**" section of your *Human Physiology* textbook. Please look for *Essay Question* 1. at the end of chapter 13, read it carefully, and let me guide you through one possible answer. Watch for key terms in bold-face type, helpful tips and general suggestions on writing the essay or short-answer questions. Enjoy!

113. Explain why the beat of the heart is **automatic** and why the SA node functions as the normal **pacemaker**.

Answer. The term "automatic" refers to the inherent property of myocardial cells to continue beating as long as they are alive; and can beat without the assistance of nerves or hormones. This property is known as *automaticity*. The sinoatrial (SA) node region is the pacemaker responsible for initiating each heart beat because the myocardial cells in this region depolarize spontaneously, reaching threshold and firing the action potentials characteristic of the most excitable myocardium cells. Since all myocardial cells are connected by gap junctions, SA node depolarization waves spread rapidly along conduction pathways to the other regions of the heart. These other areas of the heart are capable of producing pacemaker potentials, but normally do not because their rate of spontaneous depolarization is slower than that of the

SA node. Consequently, the pace of the heart is established by the fastest depolarizing cells in the heart (the SA node region) while the others fire when stimulated by the arrival of depolarization wave.

OK, now that wasn't so hard was it? Here are some more.

114. Draw and label two consecutive heart beats as recorded on the electrocardiogram (ECG). Describe each electrical event in sequence. (*Hint*: this is a favorite test question!)

115. In three columns, compare and contrast the structure and related functions of (a) arteries, (b) veins, and (c) lymph vessels. (*Hint*: Use a table format here, OK?)

116. Describe the first two events that occur when blood begins to clot along the *intrinsic* pathway and the *extrinsic* pathway. State the differences in these two pathways. Write the final two enzymatic steps in the formation of a fibrin clot (notice that these last steps are the same for both pathways).

117. Trace the recycling pathway of plasma fluid from capillary blood, through the extracellular (interstitial) spaces, its conversion to lymph fluid, and transport through lymph vessels to become part of blood once again. Name all structures involved and the forces (or pressures) that keep the fluids moving continuously. (Hint: Work slowly, this is difficult, but the result will give you an excellent overview of the lymphatic system.)

118. Describe the *ABO blood typing system* — including the genotypes responsible, the synthesis of A and B antigens from the DNA code, and the differences between the antibodies which are found in the plasma and the A and B antigens which are found on the red blood cell membrane.

Answers — Chapter 13

I. Functions and Components of the Circulatory System
   A. 1.a 2.c 3.b 4.c
   B. 5.T 6.T 7.F—Replace "excretory" with "circulatory"

II. Composition of the Blood
   A. 8.c 9.b 10.b 11.d 12.c 13.a 14.d 15.e 16.b 17.e 18.e 19.b 20.b 21.c 22.a 23.d
   B. 24.F—Replace "venous" with "arterial" and "blue" with "red" 25.T 26.T 27.F—Only gamma globulins are antibodies; alphas and betas transport lipids 28.T 29.F—Replace "lymphocyte" with "neutrophil" 30.F—Replace "monocytes" with "lymphocytes," 31.F—Leukemia represents abnormal WBCs 32.T 33.T 34.T 35.T 36.F—Replace "thromboxane A_s" with "prostacyclin" 37.T 38.F—Switch "plasma" and "serum" 39.T

III. Acid-Base Balance of the Blood
   A. 40.d 41.a 42.b
   B. 43.F—Switch "kidneys" and "lungs" 44.T 45.F—Replace "alkalosis" with "acidosis" 46.F—Replace "bicarbonate" with "carbon dioxide"

IV. Structure of the Heart
   A. 47.a 48.c 49.d
   B. 50.T 51.T 52.F—Switch "right" and "left," 53.T
   C. 54.- 6, 9, 11, 2, 7, 12, 10, 3, 1, 4, 8, 5
   D. Label the Figure — The Heart; See figure 13.8 in the text.

V. The Cardiac Cycle and the Heart Sounds
   A. 55.c 56.d 57.a 58.c 59.b
   B. 60.T 61.F—Replace "systole" with "diastole" 62.F—Atrial contraction is *not* essential for life 63.T 64.T 65.T 66.F—Switch "right" and "left;" replace "higher" with "lower"

VI. Electrical Activity of the Heart and the Electrocardiogram
   A. 67.e 68.d 69.b 70.a 71.d
   B. 72.T 73.T 74.T 75.F—Replace "short" with "long" 76.T 77.F—The ECG represents total potential changes of *all* myocardial cells in the heart
   C. Label the Figure—The Conduction System of the Heart; See figure 13.17 in the text.

VII. Blood Vessels
   A. 78.b 79.d 80.c 81.a 82.d
   B. 83.T 84.T 85.T 86.T

VIII. Atherosclerosis and Cardiac Arrhythmias
   A. 87.c 88.c 89.b 90.e
   B. 91.T 92.T 93.F—Replace "lymphocytes" with "monocytes" 94.T 95.F—Switch "LDL" and "HDL" 96.T 97.T
   C. 98.d 99.b 100.h 101.a 102.f 103.e 104.c 105.g

IX. Lymphatic System
   A. 106.b 107.c 108.a 109.b
   B. 110.T 111.T 112.F—Germinal centers produce lymphocytes

CHAPTER 14
CARDIAC OUTPUT, BLOOD FLOW, AND BLOOD PRESSURE

CHAPTER SCOPE

The last chapter introduced blood, the structure and function of the heart and the blood vessels. This chapter follows with descriptions of the many complex factors that specifically control **cardiac output**; and the normal regulation of **blood flow** and **blood pressure** throughout the body. As we shall see, blood will always flow from blood vessels in areas of higher *pressure* toward those in areas of lower pressure. Blood flow is also related to the *volume* of blood pumped from the heart each minute (cardiac output) and the degree of vascular constriction, or **peripheral resistance,** that circulating blood encounters as it spurts away from the heart. A thorough knowledge of these cardiovascular dynamics can help form the basis for proper diagnosis and treatment of conditions when blood flow and blood pressures are not normal. Such abnormal conditions occur in *hypertension, circulatory shock*, and *congestive heart failure*.

I. CARDIAC OUTPUT

The pumping ability of the heart is a function of the beats per minute (cardiac rate) and the volume of blood ejected per beat (stroke volume). The cardiac rate and stroke volume are regulated by autonomic nerves and by mechanisms that are intrinsic to the cardiovascular system.

A. Multiple Choice

____ 1. With a cardiac rate of 70 bpm and a stroke volume of 70 ml, the *cardiac output* is equal to
   a. 70 ml per minute
   b. 140 ml per minute
   c. 1400 ml per minute
   d. 4900 ml per minute

____ 2. The total blood volume (in liters) of an adult is approximately
   a. 3 L
   b. 6 L
   c. 9 L
   d. 12 L
   e. 15 L

____ 3. Which chemical has a *negative* chronotropic effect on the cardiac rate by hyperpolarizing the sinoatrial (SA) node and thus decreasing the rate of its spontaneous firing?
   a. acetylcholine (ACh)
   b. norepinephrine (NE)
   c. epinephrine
   d. None of these chemicals slows the heart in this manner.

____ 4. The cardiac control centers are located in the
   a. hypothalamus region of the brain
   b. medulla oblongata of the brainstem
   c. cerebral cortex
   d. pituitary gland
   e. cerebellum region of the brain

____ 5. Which of the following variables does *not* contribute directly to the stroke volume ejected from the ventricle?
   a. the end-diastolic volume (EDV) of blood in the ventricle before systole
   b. the total peripheral resistance or impedance to the flow of blood through the arteries
   c. the increase in parasympathetic (vagus) nerve stimulation of the SA node and myocardium
   d. the contractility or strength of ventricular contraction

___ 6. The *Frank-Starling law* of the heart states that the
   a. cardiac rate times stroke volume equals cardiac output
   b. afterload is proportional to the total peripheral resistance
   c. stroke volume is proportional to the end-diastolic volume (EDV)
   d. cardiac output varies directly with the blood pressure
___ 7. The volume of blood pumped from the left ventricle through the systemic circulation is _____ that pumped from the right ventricle through the pulmonary circulation.
   a. greater than
   b. equal to
   c. less than
___ 8. A *positive* inotropic effect would cause a(n)
   a. increase in the contractility of the heart
   b. decrease in the cardiac rate
   c. increase in the end-diastolic volume (EDV)
   d. increase in the flow of K^+ into the myocardium
___ 9. Which statement about veins is *false*?
   a. Veins contain about 66% (two-thirds) of the total circulating blood volume.
   b. Venous pressure averages about 100 mm Hg.
   c. Sympathetic stimulation can contract the smooth muscles located in the walls of veins.
   d. Due to the structure of the walls, veins have a higher compliance than the walls of arteries.
   e. Veins are called capacitance vessels due to their capacity to expand and hold more blood.

B. True or False/Edit

___ 10. A *positive* chronotropic effect is one caused by excitatory chemicals, which depolarize the SA node membranes and thus result in an increase in the cardiac rate.
___ 11. In exercise, the initial cardiac rate increase occurs because the vagus nerve inhibition of the SA node is decreased.
___ 12. Sensory feedback information from pressure receptors located in the carotid sinus and the aortic arch is interpreted by the cardiac control centers.
___ 13. *Preload* refers to the total peripheral resistance opposing the ejection of blood out of the ventricle.
___ 14. The lower the peripheral resistance, the lower the stroke volume (that is, they are directly proportional).
___ 15. The *Frank-Starling law of the heart* describes the built-in, or intrinsic property of heart muscle in which changes in the end-diastolic volume produce changes in the strength of ventricular contraction.
___ 16. Parasympathetic (vagal) stimulation of the heart has a *negative* chronotropic effect, but it has no direct inotropic effect.
___ 17. Contraction of the diaphragm during inhalation lowers the pressure in the chest and in the heart; thereby increasing the return of venous blood to the heart.

II. BLOOD VOLUME

Fluid in the extracellular environment of the body is distributed between the blood and the tissue fluid compartments by filtration and osmotic forces acting across the walls of capillaries. The function of the kidneys influences blood volume because urine is derived from blood plasma. The hormones ADH and aldosterone act on the kidneys to help regulate the blood volume.

A. Multiple Choice

___ 18. Most of the water in the body (two-thirds) is found in the
   a. intracellular compartment
   b. blood plasma
   c. extracellular environment
   d. interstitial fluid

___ 19. Which statement about *colloid osmotic pressure* of the plasma is *false*?
   a. It is the osmotic pressure exerted by the presence of plasma proteins.
   b. It is normally a very high pressure if measured in the tissue fluid.
   c. It is essentially equal to the oncotic pressure of the plasma.
   d. It has been estimated to be 25 mm Hg.
   e. It usually favors the movement of water by osmosis into capillaries.

___ 20. *Starling forces* refer to the
   a. ejection pressures exerted by the heart during contraction
   b. pressures exerted by the peripheral resistance blood vessels that dilate and constrict, affecting the cardiac output
   c. opposing hydrostatic and colloid osmotic pressures that determine the distribution of fluid across the capillary wall
   d. pressures that influence the return of venous blood to the heart

___ 21. Which of the following is *not* a cause of *edema*?
   a. high blood pressure in the arteries
   b. blood congestion or obstruction in the veins
   c. an increase in capillary permeability causing plasma proteins to leak into tissue fluid
   d. liver disease or kidney disease which results in a drop in the levels of plasma proteins
   e. All of these are causes of edema.

___ 22. Both the blood volume and the urine volume are regulated ultimately by the amount of glomerular filtrate reabsorbed in the kidney, which, in turn, is normally adjusted by the
   a. amount of fluid consumed during the day
   b. action of specific hormones on the kidneys
   c. neuron control of bladder function
   d. frequency of micturition (urination)

___ 23. Which statement about *antidiuretic hormone* (ADH) is *false*?
   a. ADH is a hormone also known as vasopressin.
   b. ADH is synthesized by neurons located in the hypothalamus.
   c. Receptors (osmoreceptors) release ADH when the plasma osmolality rises.
   d. ADH decreases water reabsorption from the glomerular filtrate and increases water loss in the form of urine.
   e. All of these statements regarding ADH are true.

___ 24. Which of the following statements about *aldosterone* is *false*?
   a. It is a steroid hormone.
   b. It is secreted by the cortex region of the adrenal gland.
   c. It promotes the excretion of both salt and water in proportionate amounts from the kidneys.
   d. Its secretion is stimulated during salt deprivation, when the blood volume and pressure are reduced.
   e. Unlike ADH, aldosterone does not act to dilute the blood.

___ 25. The *juxtaglomerular apparatus* (JGA) of the kidney
   a. is stimulated by increased blood flow and blood pressure in the renal arterioles
   b. secretes the enzyme called renin into the blood
   c. secretes the angiotensin converting enzyme (ACE)
   d. filters blood and reabsorbs water

___ 26. Which of the following actions is *not* used by angiotensin II to produce a rise in blood pressure?
   a. vasoconstriction of smooth muscle in the walls of small arteries
   b. stimulation of thirst centers located in the hypothalamus to drink more water
   c. stimulation of the heart, causing an increase in myocardial contractility
   d. stimulation of the adrenal cortex to secrete aldosterone, which then acts to reabsorb salt from the kidney

___ 27. *Atrial natriuretic factor* (ANF) is a hormone that
   a. is secreted from the atria of the heart when blood volume is high
   b. works to oppose the action of aldosterone on the kidneys

c. promotes the excretion of salt (and water follows) from the kidneys
d. antagonizes the various actions of angiotensin II, resulting in both a decrease in the secretion of aldosterone and vasodilation.
e. All of these statements describe the ANF.

B. True or False/Edit

___ 28. The blood pressure that is exerted against the inner wall of the capillary, causing the filtration of plasma and the formation of tissue fluid is called hydrostatic pressure.
___ 29. Hydrostatic pressure can also be the pressure measured in the tissues outside the capillary which opposes the filtration pressure of the blood.
___ 30. The protein concentration of tissue fluid (ECF) is greater than the protein concentration of blood plasma.
___ 31. A positive value for the net Starling forces at the venule end of a capillary favors the return of fluid into that portion of the capillary.
___ 32. About 15% of fluid filtered from the arteriolar end of the capillary (amounting to at least 2 L per day) is returned to the blood as lymph rather than being absorbed into the venular end of the capillary.
___ 33. Capillaries of the kidney that filter plasma and begin the formation of urine, are called glomeruli.
___ 34. After drinking several large glasses of water, your plasma osmolality would decrease, stimulating osmoreceptors, that, in turn, stimulate the release of ADH from the posterior pituitary.
___ 35. Water is a diuretic substance because water intake inhibits the secretion of antidiuretic hormone (ADH) and causes a larger volume of urine to be excreted.
___ 36. Very high blood volume stimulates specialized stretch receptors located in the left atrium of the heart, that, in turn, send signals to inhibit ADH secretion, ultimately reducing the blood volume.
___ 37. A drug inhibiting *angiotensin-converting enzyme* (ACE) would be expected to cause an increase in both the total peripheral resistance and blood pressure.

C. Label the Figure — The Renin-Angiotensin-Aldosterone System

Figure 14.11 in the text is a very important flow diagram. It summarizes the renin-angiotensin-aldosterone system and its negative feedback control over blood flow and blood pressure. **Before** looking up the figure in the text, give yourself a pretest by attempting to complete the empty flow diagram shown below in figure 14.1. Later, correct or complete your work using the text. If you erase your answers, this diagram can also help prepare for the next exam! Don't worry if you have difficulty following the flow of this outline because this important concept will also be discussed again later in the kidney chapter (chapter 17).

III. VASCULAR RESISTANCE TO BLOOD FLOW

The rate of blood flow to an organ is related to the resistance to flow in the small arteries and arterioles that serve the organ. Vasodilation decreases resistance and increases flow, whereas vasoconstriction increases resistance and decreases flow. Vasodilation and vasoconstriction occur in response to intrinsic and extrinsic regulatory mechanisms.

A. Multiple Choice

___ 38. From the following list, which of these tissues receives the *least* amount of blood under resting conditions?
a. coronary arteries of the heart
b. liver
c. kidneys
d. skeletal muscles
e. brain

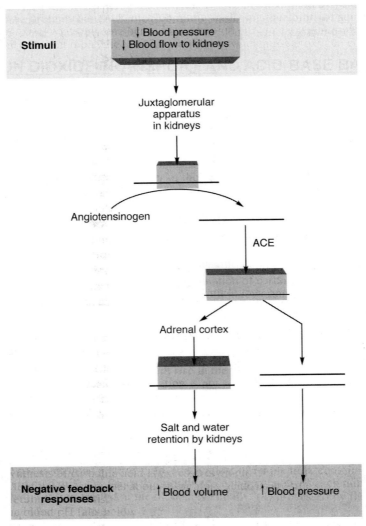

Figure 14.1 The negative feedback control of blood volume and pressure by the renin-angiotensin-aldosterone system. ACE = angiotensin converting enzyme.

___ 39. Which factor does *not* result in an increase in the resistance to blood flow through a vessel?
   a. a vessel with longer length
   b. "thicker" blood with higher viscosity
   c. blood flowing at a higher velocity
   d. decrease in the radius of the blood vessel
   e. All of these factors increase the resistance to blood flow.

___ 40. The blood vessel that can become narrower through vasoconstriction and thereby provide the greatest resistance to the flow of blood, is the
   a. artery
   b. arteriole
   c. capillary
   d. venule
   e. vein

___ 41. Vasodilation of skeletal muscles that occurs during "fight-or-flight" reactions is caused mainly by the
   a. alpha-adrenergic stimulation of vascular smooth muscle, primarily with norepinephrine (NE) as the neurotransmitter.
   b. cholinergic sympathetic stimulation of vascular smooth muscle with acetylcholine (ACh) as the neurotransmitter
   c. beta-adrenergic stimulation of vascular smooth muscle with epinephrine from the adrenal medulla as the hormone
   d. adrenergic parasympathetic stimulation of vascular smooth muscle with norepinephrine as the neurotransmitter
   e. Both b and c result in vasodilation of skeletal muscles.

___ 42. Two organs that use both *myogenic* and *metabolic* **intrinsic** mechanisms to help maintain relatively constant flow rates despite wide fluctuations in blood pressures are the
   a. heart and brain
   b. liver and kidneys
   c. genitals and skin
   d. brain and kidneys

___ 43. Which metabolic or chemical condition produced by local cell activity does *not* promote vasodilation within that organ?
   a. a decrease in oxygen concentrations
   b. an increase in carbon dioxide concentrations
   c. an increase in the tissue pH
   d. an increase in the release of adenosine or K^+
   e. All of these chemical conditions promote vasodilation.

B. True or False/Edit

___ 44. The rate of blood flow through a blood vessel is proportional to the pressure difference between the upstream and downstream regions of the blood vessel.

___ 45. As the frictional resistance to blood flow through blood vessels increases, the blood flow itself will decrease.

___ 46. The flow of blood to tissues can be decreased by dilation of its arterioles and increased by constriction of its arterioles.

___ 47. The endothelium of the tunica intima produces nitric oxide, bradykinin, and prostacyclin — all chemicals that promote vascular smooth muscle contraction (*vasoconstriction*).

___ 48. *Autoregulation* is the ability of organs to use both myogenic and metabolic intrinsic mechanisms to maintain the blood flow rates relatively constant through these organs.

___ 49. The myogenic response of cerebral vessels to excessively high blood pressure results in vasoconstriction that may prevent a cerebrovascular accident (stroke) in the brain.

___ 50. The increase in blood flow to skeletal muscles and other organs (vasodilation) that occurs during physical exercise; and that is due to the increase in metabolism and the accumulation of metabolic products, is called *reactive hyperemia*.

IV. BLOOD FLOW TO THE HEART AND SKELETAL MUSCLES

Blood flow to the heart and skeletal muscles is regulated by both extrinsic and intrinsic mechanisms. These mechanisms provide increased rates of blood flow when the metabolic requirements of these tissues are raised during exercise.

A. Multiple Choice

___ 51. Which of the following is *not* an adaptation of the heart to stress?
   a. Heart muscle contains large amounts of the oxygen-binding pigment, myoglobin.
   b. Heart muscle has large amounts of stored enzymes for metabolism when anaerobic.
   c. Heart muscle has large numbers of mitochondria.
   d. Heart muscle capillaries run very close to each myocardial fiber for rapid gas exchange.
   e. All of these are adaptations of the heart to stress.

___ 52. Which of the following local products of metabolism would *not* dilate the smooth muscle of coronary blood vessels during exercise?
   a. increased carbon dioxide levels
   b. decreased pH levels
   c. decreased oxygen levels
   d. increased extracellular K⁺ and the secretion of adenosine
   e. All of these metabolic products would cause dilation of coronary blood vessels during exercise.

___ 53. Which of the following changes is *not* responsible for the increase in blood flow to skeletal muscle during progressively intense exercise?
   a. increase in total blood flow (cardiac output)
   b. metabolic (intrinsic) vasodilation in the exercising muscles
   c. diversion of blood away from the viscera and skin
   d. diversion of blood away from the heart and brain
   e. All of these increase blood flow in exercising muscle.

___ 54. During *heavy* exercise, the
   a. stroke volume usually decreases
   b. end-diastolic ventricular volume usually decreases
   c. afterload (peripheral resistance) usually increases, especially in the skeletal muscles
   d. proportion of blood volume ejected per stroke (ejection fraction) is increased
   e. cardiac output stays relatively constant

B. True or False/Edit

___ 55. The enormous density of coronary capillaries within the heart myocardium brings blood flow within 10 Tm of each myocardial fiber, promoting the rapid diffusion of gases between the capillary blood and each heart cell.

___ 56. Unlike blood flow in most other organs, the flow of blood in the coronary vessels decreases during systole and increases during diastole.

___ 57. During exercise, *most* dilation of the coronary vessels is produced by the sympathoadrenal activation of beta-adrenergic receptors.

___ 58. Pain and fatigue occur much more quickly during rhythmic isotonic skeletal muscle contractions than would occur during sustained isometric contractions.

___ 59. During the "fight-or-flight" response to stress, the combined stimulation of cholinergic receptors by ACh and beta-adrenergic receptors by epinephrine in skeletal muscle results in profound vasodilation and an increase in blood flow.

___ 60. As the vascular resistance in blood vessels is decreased, the rate of blood flow is increased.

___ 61. During exercise, the five-fold increase in cardiac output (from 5 L per minute to about 25 L per minute) is primarily due to an increase in cardiac stroke volume, not cardiac rate.

___ 62. Only 8 days of endurance training is needed to increase the blood volume by as much as 0.5 L; thus raising the cardiac output and delivery of oxygen to skeletal muscles.

V. BLOOD FLOW TO THE BRAIN AND SKIN

Intrinsic control mechanisms help to maintain a relatively constant blood flow to the brain. Blood flow to the skin, in contrast, can vary tremendously in response to regulation by sympathetic nerves.

A. Multiple Choice

___ 63. Which statement about blood flow to the brain (cerebral flow) and skin (cutaneous flow) is *false?*
   a. Cerebral blood flow normally remains remarkably constant at about 750 ml per minute.
   b. The brain can not tolerate low rates of blood flow.
   c. Blood flow through the skin can fluctuate dramatically.
   d. The skin can tolerate low rates of blood flow.

___ 64. During inadequate ventilation, such as *hypoventilation,* the
   a. blood carbon dioxide concentration rises

      b. cerebral arterioles constrict
      c. pH of the cerebrospinal fluid (CSF) goes up, and becomes a larger number
      d. blood flow to the brain decreases

___ 65. Which event in the skin does *not* occur when the ambient (outside) temperature is cold?
      a. Sympathetic nerve activity will stimulate vasoconstriction in cutaneous blood vessels, reducing blood flow to the skin.
      b. Arteriovenous anastomoses constrict, bypassing the skin surface; yet diverting small amounts of blood to superficial capillary loops and causing "rosy cheeks."
      c. Total cutaneous blood flow rises, causing generalized redness throughout the skin surfaces.
      d. Inner body temperatures are maintained relatively constant as less heat is lost.

___ 66. Sweat glands secrete the polypeptide *bradykinin*, that
      a. stimulates vasodilation and increased blood flow in the skin
      b. reduces sweat production and heat loss through evaporation
      c. lubricates the skin and hair follicles
      d. causes the "blanching" of skin during extreme cold
      e. gives concentrated sweat its normal salty taste

B. True or False/Edit

___ 67. Blood flow through the brain is regulated primarily by intrinsic (local, autoregulation) mechanisms; whereas blood flow through the skin is regulated mainly by extrinsic (from outside) mechanisms.

___ 68. Those brain regions that are most active and have the highest metabolic activity accumulate chemicals locally, resulting in the delivery of more blood to that area.

___ 69. The great tolerance of the skin to very low ambient temperatures is partly due to the fact that such temperatures reduce the metabolic rate in the tissues of cold skin.

___ 70. Control centers in the medulla oblongata mediate changes in sympathetic nerve activity; and are responsible for both the blushing (vasoconstriction) and "cold sweat" (vasodilation) responses of cutaneous blood vessels.

VI. BLOOD PRESSURE

The pressure of the arterial blood is regulated by the blood volume, total peripheral resistance, and the cardiac rate. Regulatory mechanisms adjust these factors in a negative feedback manner to compensate for deviations. Arterial pressure rises and falls as the heart goes through systole and diastole.

A. Multiple Choice

___ 71. The blood vessel with the greatest total cross-sectional area is the
      a. artery
      b. arteriole
      c. capillary
      d. venule
      e. vein

___ 72. Which of the following is *not* one of the three most important variables affecting blood pressure?
      a. cardiac rate
      b. stroke volume (blood volume)
      c. total peripheral resistance
      d. coronary artery vasodilation

___ 73. Increased activity of the *sympathoadrenal* system
      a. causes vasodilation in the arterioles
      b. causes cardiac output to fall
      c. raises total peripheral resistance
      d. ultimately increases renal blood flow and urine output

___ 74. *Baroreceptors* increase the *frequency* of action potentials to the medulla oblongata control centers, when the
   a. blood pressure falls in the aorta and carotid arteries
   b. aortic arch and carotid sinus walls are stretched
   c. cardiac rate and the cardiac output decreases
   d. arterial blood gas concentrations are too high

___ 75. Which statement about the **medulla oblongata** region of the brainstem, is *false?*
   a. It receives sensory nerve action potentials from the baroreceptors located in the carotid sinus and aortic arch.
   b. It uses autonomic nerves to direct various target tissues.
   c. It helps regulate vasoconstriction and vasodilation of blood vessels, and thus total peripheral resistance.
   d. It houses cardiac control centers for the regulation of heart rate.
   e. All of these statements regarding the medulla oblongata region of the brainstem are true.

___ 76. Which statement about the *left atrial stretch receptors* is *false*?
   a. They respond to an increase in venous return to the heart.
   b. They stimulate sympathetic nerve activity, causing a reflex tachycardia.
   c. They inhibit ADH secretion from the hypothalamus, resulting in a decrease in blood volume.
   d. They cause vasoconstriction in peripheral arterioles.
   e. They stimulate the increased secretion of atrial natriuretic factor (ANF), resulting in an increase in urinary salt and water excretion.

___ 77. Which statement about the **sounds of Korotkoff** is *false?*
   a. They are heard when vibrations occur in the arterial walls as blood flows noisily through a pinched artery.
   b. They are used to detect defects in the cardiac valves that produce the "lub-dub" sounds.
   c. They are only present when blood pressures are between the high systolic and the low diastolic pressure extremes.
   d. The quality of these sounds is different in persons with high blood pressure than in those with low blood pressure.
   e. The last sound occurs when the cuff pressure is equal to the diastolic pressure.

___ 78. A person whose blood pressure is 135/85 mmHg has a *pulse pressure* of _____ mmHg.
   a. 35
   b. 50
   c. 60
   d. 85
   e. 135

___ 79. The mean arterial pressure (MAP) in a person whose blood pressure reads 135/85 mmHg is approximately _____ mmHg?
   a. 98
   b. 100
   c. 102
   d. 110
   e. 120

B. True or False/Edit

___ 80. The *greatest* resistance to blood flow in the arterial system is found in the capillaries.

___ 81. Vasodilation of arterioles downstream (away from the heart) decreases the peripheral resistance and results in a lower arterial blood pressure upstream (closer to the heart).

___ 82. Baroreceptors are stretch receptors located in the aortic arch and carotid sinuses regions, monitoring the degree of stretch in the walls of these arteries as pressure changes.

___ 83. The vagus and glossopharyngeal nerves carry sensory action potentials from baroreceptors to the vasomotor control center in the pons region of the brainstem.

____ 84. Manual massage of the carotid sinus regions can mimic high blood pressure and thereby, through the baroreceptor reflex, can slow any existing tachycardia and lower blood pressure.

____ 85. Antidiuretic hormone (ADH) and aldosterone increase blood pressure by increasing blood volume, while angiotensin II increases blood pressure by stimulating vasoconstriction.

____ 86. Nothing is heard through a stethoscope when listening to normal blood flow through an artery because normal flow is smooth or laminar (in layers).

____ 87. The *first* sound of Korotkoff is heard when pressure in the cuff equals the pressure in the artery during the diastole phase of the heart.

____ 88. The *mean arterial pressure* is simply the average pressure, calculated as halfway between the systolic and diastolic pressures.

VII. HYPERTENSION, SHOCK, AND CONGESTIVE HEART FAILURE

An understanding of the normal physiology of the cardiovascular system is prerequisite to the study of its pathophysiology, or mechanisms of abnormal function. Since the mechanisms that regulate cardiac output, blood flow, and blood pressure are highlighted in particular disease states, a study of pathophysiology at this time can strengthen your understanding of the mechanisms involved in normal function.

A. Multiple Choice

____ 89. Which of the following is *not* a cause of **hypertension**?
   a. sustained high stress, activating the sympathetic nervous system
   b. myocardial infarction (MI)
   c. kidney disease or renal artery disease
   d. high-salt diet

____ 90. Which mode of treatment would *not* be used to treat hypertension?
   a. angiotensin II to help constrict peripheral arterioles
   b. various diuretics to decrease blood volume and increase urine volume
   c. beta-adrenergic blocking drugs to decrease cardiac rate
   d. ACE inhibitors, calcium antagonists, and various vasodilators to decrease peripheral resistance
   e. lifestyle changes: stop smoking, limit alcohol intake, weight reduction, reduce salt ingestion, and regular physical exercise

____ 91. Dangerously low blood volume can lead to *hypovolemic shock*, a condition that
   a. activates the sympathoadrenal system and the baroreceptor reflex, resulting in peripheral vasoconstriction and tachycardia
   b. activates the renin-angiotensin-aldosterone system, resulting in salt and water retention
   c. results in decreased cardiac output and lowered blood pressure
   d. results in a person with low blood pressure, rapid pulse, cold and clammy skin, and little urine excretion
   e. All of these statements describe hypovolemic shock.

____ 92. The vasodilator substance released during anaphylactic shock that may follow a severe allergic reaction, for example to penicillin or bee stings, is
   a. aldosterone
   b. angiotensin II
   c. histamine
   d. antidiuretic hormone (ADH)
   e. nitric oxide

B. True or False/Edit

____ 93. About 90% of the hypertensive population in the United States have *secondary* hypertension that is the result of complex and poorly understood processes.

____ 94. The majority of people with hypertension have what is also, somewhat illogically, known as essential hypertension.

___ 95. Circulatory shock occurs when there is inadequate blood flow and/or oxygen utilization by the tissues.

___ 96. Congestive heart failure (CHF) is heart failure that occurs when the cardiac output is insufficient leading to the accumulation of fluid within the myocardial fibers of the heart.

CHAPTER REVIEW

A. Completion

97. Cardiac rate is _____ (increased/decreased) by sympathoadrenal stimulation and _____ (increased/decreased) by parasympathetic stimulation of the SA node (pacemaker) region of the heart. The end-diastolic volume is also known as the _____ load (pre/after), while the _____ load (pre/after) refers to the total peripheral resistance to blood flow in the arterioles. An increased venous return _____ (increases/decreases) preload, and will ultimately _____ (increase/decrease) the contractility of the ventricles that will eject more blood from the heart. 98. The organ most responsible for regulating the total blood volume is the _____. Tissue fluid (ECF) is formed from _____ and roughly 85% will return to the _____. The pressure that forces fluid out of the arteriolar end of capillaries is called _____ pressure, while the _____ _____ pressure of the plasma encourages the return of fluid to the venular end of capillaries. 99. Any extra tissue fluid (the remaining 15%) becomes _____ fluid and is returned to the blood via _____ vessels or remains in the tissues, causing swelling or _____. 100. Reabsorption of water from the kidney filtrate is regulated by _____ hormone made by the hypothalamus, while the hormone _____ is secreted by the adrenal _____ (cortex/medulla) to promote the _____ (loss/retention) of salt (and water). 101. The law relating the vascular and the resistance to the flow of blood in blood vessels is _____ law. Vasoconstriction of arterioles usually occurs due to stimulation by the _____ branch of the autonomic nervous system, whereas the local myogenic response to _____ (high/low) blood pressure would also cause vasoconstriction. 102. The heart normally respires _____ because its capillary supply, myoglobin, and enzyme content are all _____ (high/low); consequently, during exercise the coronary arteries dilate due to _____ (intrinsic/extrinsic) or accumulated metabolic factors. 103. The heart rate increases due to the _____ (increased/decreased) activity of the vagus nerve and the _____ (increased/decreased) activity of the sympathetic nerves to the SA node. Cardiac rate multiplied by _____ volume equals cardiac _____. 104. High blood pressure to the brain causes cerebral vessels to _____ (constrict/dilate), while accumulation of metabolites causes local _____ (constriction/dilation). As body temperature falls, _____ nerve fibers cause cutaneous arterioles and shunts called arteriovenous _____ to _____ (constrict/dilate). 105. Baroreceptors located in the _____ _____ and _____ _____ send sensory action potentials to the cardiac control centers in the _____ _____, which regulates both cardiac _____ and peripheral _____ through efferent nerves of the _____ nervous system. 106. Normal blood flow is smooth or _____, yet compression by a sphygmomanometer cuff causes _____ flow, which is heard as the sounds of _____. 107. If systolic pressure is 122 and diastolic pressure is 74 mmHg, then pulse pressure = _____ mmHg and mean arterial pressure = _____ mmHg. Essential hypertension or _____ hypertension may be the result of many factors, whereas _____ hypertension is the direct result of known, specific, diseases. 108. Circulatory shock occurs when there is inadequate delivery of _____ to the organs of the body. This is also seen in congestive heart failure where "congestion" refers to the accumulation of _____ (arterial/venous) blood surrounding the heart that has failed.

B. Crossword Puzzle — Cardiac Output, Blood Flow, and Blood Pressure

Across
1. another common term for a heart attack
4. the vagus nerve, for example
6. *first* heart sound (AV valves close)
9. one activity that can increase the return of venous blood to the heart

11. very important oxygen-carrying molecules found in cardiac fibers
13. measure of the total number of particles in plasma — exerting pressure for water to move
14. trace element in the body — also used to make kettles
17. the kind of resistance most responsible for regulating blood pressure
18. organs most responsible for the regulation of fluid and electrolytes in the blood
20. pressure of the blood forcing fluid from the arteriolar ends of capillaries to tissues
22. another student in your class, for example
23. vibrational sounds heard with a stethoscope over partially constricted blood vessels
25. maximum pressure generated by the contraction of the ventricles
26. dietary ingredient that, when restricted, can lower blood pressure
28. type of breathing common in dogs to assist in temperature regulation
29. a courtroom experience; or a bout of exercise
30. property of "self" control some organs have over blood flow
32. accumulation of extracellular fluid (ECF) in the tissue spaces
33. vasodilation control due to the accumulation of local chemicals around blood vessels
36. hormone causing vasoconstriction and the release of aldosterone from the adrenal cortex
37. your mental condition required to conquer this puzzle
39. that part of the adrenal gland that secretes aldosterone
40. also known as *primary* hypertension; it is the most common type
42. description of a person at risk for heart disease
43. abbreviation for the average driving force required for blood flow through the arterial system
45. the Frank-_____ law of the heart
46. osmotic pressure due to the presence of proteins in the blood or tissue spaces
49. pressure equal to the difference between systolic and diastolic pressures
51. heart rate **X** stroke volume = _____ output
52. blood vessel action that can raise blood pressure
53. if successful in an athletic contest, you have _____
54. end-diastolic volume (EDV) present in the ventricles prior to systole

Down
2. enzyme from the juxtaglomerular apparatus of the kidneys [it reduces urinary salt and water excretion]
3. body tissue where arteriovenous anastomoses operate to shunt blood away from capillary beds
5. hormone synthesized by the hypothalamus but released from the posterior pituitary
7. stretch receptors located in the carotid sinus and aortic arch
8. the law describing the effects of pressure difference and vessel resistance on blood flow
10. a condition of high blood pressure
12. not tight
15. muscle used as "pumps" to assist the return of venous blood to the heart
16. abbreviation for the hormone also known as vasopressin
19. heart sound caused by closure of the semilunar valves
21. pressure in the aorta following a beat that acts to reduce the stroke volume
24. abbreviation for the pacemaker node of the heart
26. autonomic nerves that speed up the heart rate and increase the force of ventricular contractions
27. artery whose sinuses contain baroreceptors
30. the division of the nervous system that regulates the heart and blood vessel diameters
31. blood vessel action that reduces peripheral resistance
34. pressure recorded when Korotkoff sounds just disappear
35. one circulatory region of the body that can regulate its own blood flow both metabolically and myogenically
38. anaphylactic or neurogenic are examples
41. name for extracellular fluid that returns to the blood via the thoracic duct
44. major blood vessel, the arch of which contains baroreceptors
47. the capacitance blood vessels
48. following vasoconstriction, blood pressure usually will
50. Frank-Starling _____ of the heart

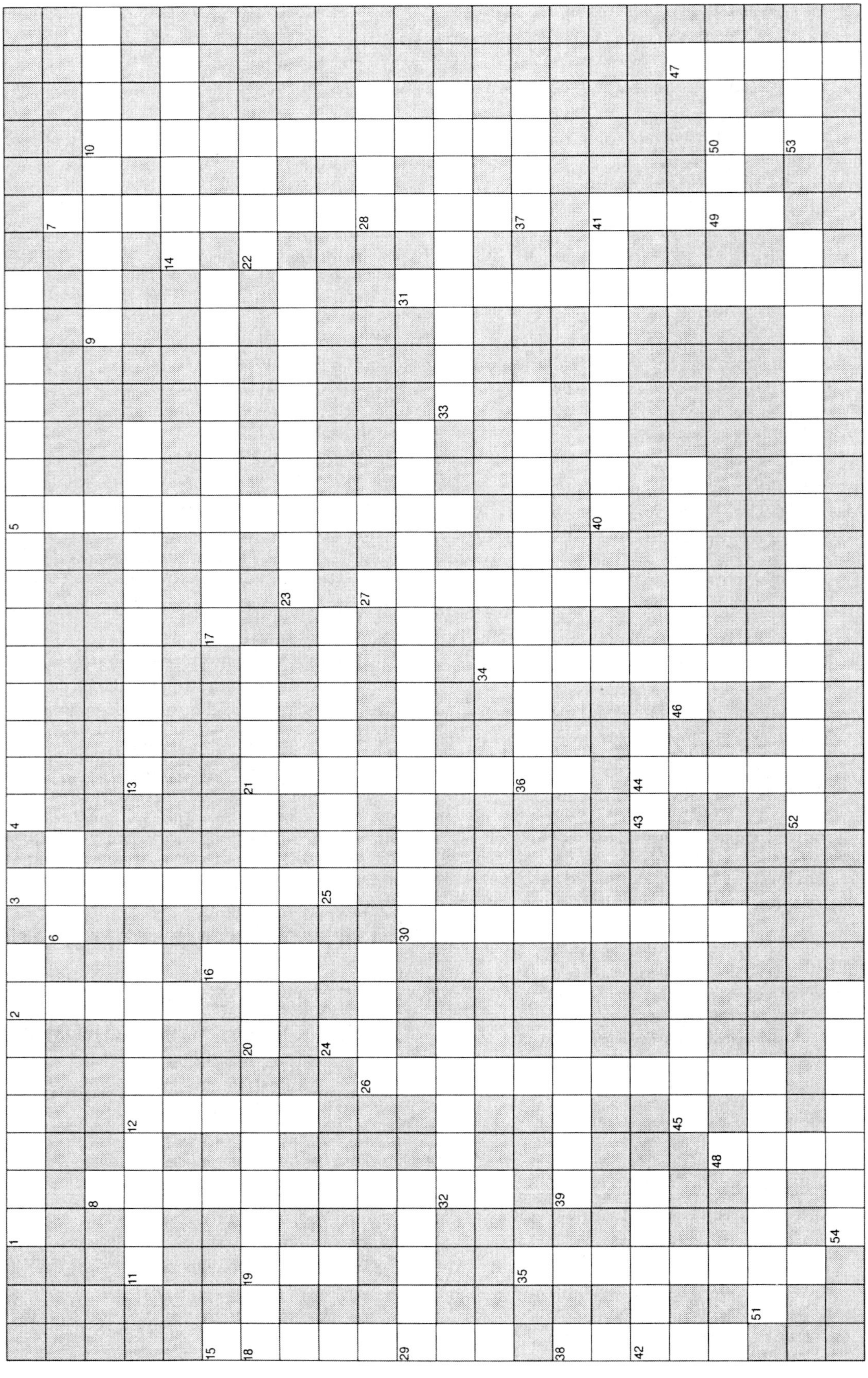

C. Essay

Essay Tutorial

This essay tutorial will answer the first essay question found in the "**Review Activities**" section of your *Human Physiology* textbook. Please look for *Essay Question* 1. at the end of chapter 14, read it carefully, and let me guide you through one possible answer. Watch for key terms in bold-face type, helpful tips and general suggestions on writing the essay or short-answer questions. Enjoy!

109. **Define** the terms *contractility, preload,* and *afterload,* and **explain** how these factors affect the cardiac output.

Answer. Contractility refers to the *strength* of a ventricular contraction. The greater the contractility, the more force is applied to the blood in the ventricles and the greater volume of blood is ejected from the heart. **Preload** refers to the *amount of work* the heart has to perform to eject the blood present in the ventricles immediately *prior* to contraction. Because ventricular contraction (systole) has not yet occurred, this volume of blood is called the end-diastolic volume. **Afterload** is the total resistance to the ejection of blood from the ventricle that the heart has to overcome to successfully deliver blood to the tissues. *Cardiac output* is stroke volume multiplied times cardiac rate. Therefore, as ventricular contractility increases, stroke volume increases and cardiac output will increase. As preload (end-diastolic volume) increases, the Frank-Starling law of the heart states that the stroke volume will increase, also increasing cardiac output. As the afterload increases, however, stroke volume decreases and cardiac output falls. A decrease in afterload or stroke volume will have the opposite effect, thus raising the cardiac output.

How did you do on this one? Don't give up. Keep on trying!

110. Define *hydrostatic* and *osmotic* pressures, explain the role they play in the formation of tissue fluid from blood, and list the various factors that can cause the excess accumulation of tissue fluid (edema).

111. Describe the role each of the following substances has on the kidney regulation of *blood volume*: (1) antidiuretic hormone (ADH), (2) aldosterone, (3) angiotensin II, and (4) atrial natriuretic factor.

112. Explain how the *baroreceptor reflex* operates to compensate for cardiovascular changes that occur upon rising from bed in the morning to a standing position. Note that this represents another example of negative feedback regulation of homeostasis.

Answers — Chapter 14

I. Cardiac Output
   A. 1. d, 2. b, 3. a, 4. b, 5. c, 6. c, 7. b, 8. a, 9. b
   B. 10. T, 11. T, 12. T, 13. F—Replace "preload" with "afterload," 14. F—When one is "lower," the other is "higher" (they are inversely proportional), 15. T, 16. T, 17. T

II. Blood Volume
   A. 18. a, 19. b, 20. c, 21. e, 22. b, 23. d, 24. c, 25. b, 26. c, 27. e
   B. 28. T, 29. T, 30. F—Replace "greater" with "less," 31. F—Replace "positive" with "negative," 32. T, 33. T, 34. F—Osmoreceptors would stop firing and ADH levels would decrease, 35. T, 36. T, 37. F—Replace "increase" with "decrease"
   C. Label the Figure— The Renin-Angiotensin-Aldosterone System   See figure 14.11 in the text

III. Vascular Resistance and Blood Flow
   A. 38. a, 39. c, 40. b, 41. e, 42. d, 43. c
   B. 44. T, 45. T, 46. F—Switch "increased" and "decreased," 47. F—Replace "contraction (vasoconstriction)" with "relaxation (vasodilation)," 48. T, 49. T, 50. F—Replace "reactive" with "active"

IV. Blood Flow to the Heart and Skeletal Muscles
   A. 51. b, 52. e, 53. d, 54. d
   B. 55. T, 56. T, 57. F—Intrinsic (local) metabolites are primarily responsible for vasodilation, 58. F—Switch "rhythmic isotonic" and "sustained isometric," 59. T, 60. T, 61. F—Switch "stroke volume" and "cardiac rate," 62. T

V. Blood Flow to the Brain and Skin
   A. 63. e, 64. a, 65. c, 66. a
   B. 67. T, 68. T, 69. T, 70. F—Switch "vasoconstriction" and "vasodilation"

VI. Blood Pressure
   A. 71. c, 72. d, 73. c, 74. b, 75. e, 76. d, 77. b, 78. b, 79. c
   B. 80. F—Replace "capillaries" with "arterioles," 81. T, 82. T, 83. F—Replace "pons" with "medulla oblongata," 84. T, 85. T, 86. T, 87. F—Replace "diastole" with "systole," 88. F—Mean systemic arterial pressure = 1/3 pulse pressure + diastolic pressure

VII. Hypertension, Shock, and Congestive Heart Failure
   A. 89. b, 90. a, 91. e, 92. c
   B. 93. F—Replace "secondary" with "primary," 94. T, 95. T, 96. F—Congestive heart failure occurs when fluids accumulate just outside the entrance to the "failed" side of the heart

Chapter Review
   A. 97. increased, decreased, pre, after; increases, increases, 98. kidney, blood, blood; hydrostatic, colloid osmotic, 99. lymph, lymphatic, edema, 100. antidiuretic, aldosterone, cortex, retention, 101. Poiseuille's; sympathetic, high, 02. aerobically, high, intrinsic, 103. decreased, increased; stroke, output, 104. constrict, dilation; sympathetic, anastomoses, constrict, 105. carotid sinus, aortic arch, medulla oblongata, rate, resistance, autonomic, 106. laminar, turbulent, Korotkoff, 107. 48, 90; primary, secondary, 108. oxygen, venous

B. Crossword Puzzle

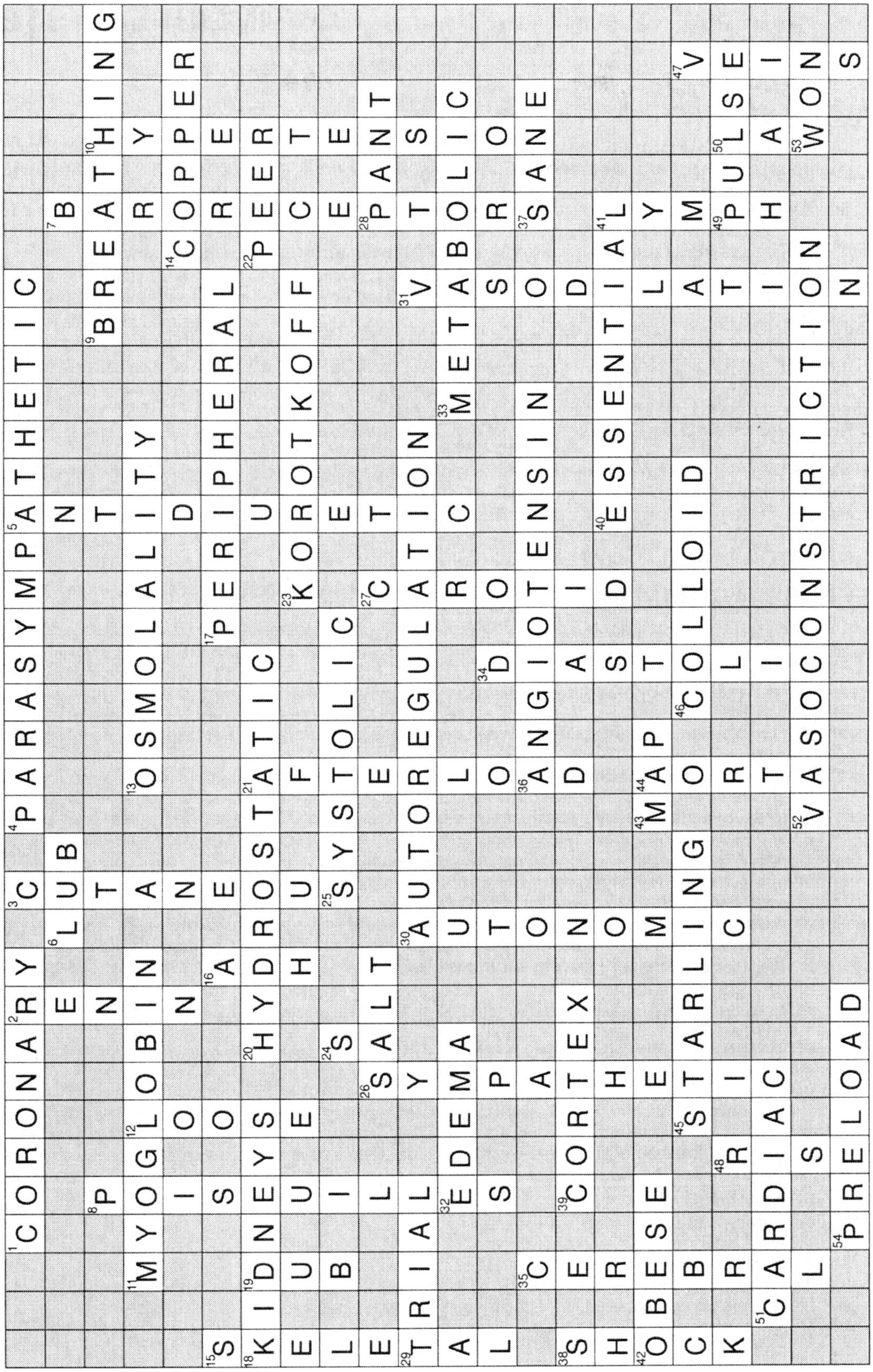

CHAPTER 15
THE IMMUNE SYSTEM

CHAPTER SCOPE

An efficient and effective **immune system** that can defend the body against invading pathogens, mediate local inflammatory responses, reject tissue transplants, and provide immunological surveillance against cancer, requires the cooperation and complex interaction of many tissues. In this chapter, many of the circulating *leukocytes* initially introduced with blood in chapter 13 will play *direct* defense roles calling for actual contact with and destruction of potentially disease causing foreign particles (phagocytosis). In addition, certain cell populations such as the **T** and **B lymphocytes**, and the **monocytes** (that, when activated become *macrophages*) participate in body defense. The defensive role of these cells is *indirect* since the activation of each cell type produces specific chemicals such as **antibodies** and **lymphokines** that operate to provide immune protection.

To help explain the complex communication network between the various cell types and the logistical details that must exist to carry out this immune defense, many new concepts are described. Some of the concepts presented here include *nonspecific* and *specific* forms of *immunity, antigen-antibody reactions, immunological tolerance, active and passive immunity, clonal selection theory, monoclonal antibody formation, tumor immunology, and autoimmunity*. The last section discusses specific diseases caused by immune system disorders. These clinical cases of breakdown in the immune system's formidable defensive methods will serve as a teaching tool to help clarify some of these complex interactions required to keep us healthy. Like many other examples of homeostasis in the body such as heart rate, blood pH, and breathing, these defensive actions of the immune system largely go unnoticed. Since most of us are exposed daily to many potentially pathogenic substances, it seems truly remarkable that our immune system seldom malfunctions, with illness as the result.

I. DEFENSE MECHANISMS

Nonspecific immune protection is provided by such mechanisms as phagocytosis, fever, and the release of interferons. Specific immunity involves the functions of lymphocytes and is directed at specific molecules, or parts of molecules, known as antigens.

A. Multiple Choice

____ 1. Which defense mechanism is *not* in either the external or the internal category of *nonspecific* immunity?
   a. epithelial membranes (skin) that cover the body surfaces
   b. strong acidity of gastric juice (pH of 1 to 2)
   c. phagocytosis of unwanted substances
   d. activation of lymphocyte cell populations
   e. All of these defense mechanisms are nonspecific.

____ 2. Which cell type does *not* participate in phagocytosis?
   a. neutrophils within the blood and tissues
   b. monocytes within the blood
   c. macrophages within the connective tissues
   d. Kupffer cells that are "fixed" within the liver
   e. lymphocytes within the blood

____ 3. The highly mobile cells that are the first to arrive at the site of an infection, are the
   a. neutrophils
   b. monocytes
   c. macrophages
   d. basophils
   e. lymphocytes

____ 4. Which organelle contains powerful digestive enzymes and participates directly in the process of phagocytosis?
   a. nucleus
   b. mitochondrion
   c. endoplasmic reticulum
   d. lysosome
   e. Golgi apparatus

____ 5. The thermoregulatory control center or "thermostat" that regulates the body's response to changes in temperature such as during a fever, is located in the
   a. hypothalamus
   b. pituitary

c. cerebral cortex
   d. adrenal gland
   e. thyroid gland
___ 6. Which statement about *haptens* is *false*?
   a. They are small organic molecules that are not antigenic by themselves.
   b. Bonded to protein, haptens can become antigenic.
   c. Bonded to protein, haptens are available for research or diagnostic purposes.
   d. They are able to attract phagocytes (chemotaxis).
   e. All of these statements about haptens are true.
___ 7. The clumping of antigen-to-antibody particles during an immunoassay such as the modern pregnancy test, is known as
   a. clustering
   b. agglutination
   c. chemotaxis
   d. diapedesis
   e. hapten formation
___ 8. Populations of lymphocytes known as **B lymphocytes**
   a. secrete antibodies into blood and lymph fluids
   b. are said to provide cell-mediated immunity
   c. attack host cells infected with viruses, fungi, or cancer cells
   d. are originally derived from the thymus gland
   e. must come into close contact with infected cells to destroy them

B. True or False/Edit
___ 9. The process of phagocytosis is an integral part of both specific and nonspecific immune defense activities.
___ 10. *Specific* immune response refers to the selective action of lymphocytes that is acquired after a prior exposure to a particular disease-causing agent (pathogen).
___ 11. Blood flowing through capillaries of the liver and spleen encounter "fixed" phagocytic cells that remove invading pathogens, rendering the blood sterile after a few passes through those organs.
___ 12. *Chemotaxis* refers to the movement of erythrocytes to the site of an infection, lured by chemical attractants.
___ 13. *Macrophages* are neutrophils that have transformed and become phagocytic after exposure to some foreign substance at the site of an infection.
___ 14. *Diapedesis* refers to the movement of large phagocytic cells from the capillary blood as they squeeze between adjacent endothelial cells and into the tissue spaces.
___ 15. Many fevers result from exposure to certain bacteria that release *endogenous pyrogens* that, in turn, stimulate leukocytes to release chemicals known as *endotoxins*.
___ 16. *Interferons* are polypeptides produced in small amounts by host cells infected with one virus, which can then interfere with the ability of a second, unrelated strain of virus to infect other cells in the same host.
___ 17. There are three major categories of short-acting, nonspecific *interferons*: alpha, beta, and gamma.
___ 18. Most antigens are polysaccharides because of their large size and their complex structure.
___ 19. Each antigen molecule triggers the formation of one and only one type of antibody molecule that is specific for that antigen.
___ 20. About 65% to 85% of circulating lymphocytes in the blood and most of the lymphocytes in the germinal centers of lymph nodes and spleen are **B lymphocytes**.

II. FUNCTIONS OF B LYMPHOCYTES

B lymphocytes secrete antibodies that can bond in a specific fashion with antigens. Binding of these secreted antibodies to antigens stimulates a cascade of reactions whereby a system of proteins in the plasma called complement is activated. Some of these activated complement proteins kill the cells containing the antigen; others promote phagocytosis and other activity, resulting in a more effective defense against pathogens.

A. Multiple Choice
___ 21. Which plasma protein does *not* form a distinct band in the *globulin* class during electrophoresis of blood?
   a. fibrinogen
   b. albumin
   c. alpha-1 globulin
   d. beta globulin
   e. gamma globulin

___ 22. Which is *not* a subclass of *immunoglobulins*?
   a. IgA
   b. IgB
   c. IgD
   d. IgE
   e. IgM
___ 23. Which subclass of immunoglobulin molecules mediates allergic reactions?
   a. IgA
   b. IgB
   c. IgD
   d. IgE
   e. IgM
___ 24. Which statement about *complement* proteins is *false*?
   a. Complements are normally present in an inactive state in body fluids.
   b. C1 complement proteins are involved in antibody recognition and activation of enzymes.
   c. C4, C2, and C3 are involved in the specific attack, creating large holes that actually kill the victim cell.
   d. Complement proteins C1 through C5 function primarily as enzymes operating at the victim cell membrane.
   e. Complement fragments that are not fixed but instead are released into the surrounding fluid have a number of important effects.
___ 25. Which substance is released from tissue mast cells and plasma basophils to dilate blood vessels and increase capillary permeability?
   a. complements C5 through C9
   b. histamine
   c. IgG
   d. complements C2 through C4
   e. gamma globulin
___ 26. Which event best represents the *nonspecific* mechanism of an inflammatory reaction following the entry of bacteria through a break in the skin?
   a. the activation of B lymphocytes to produce specific antibodies
   b. histamine vasodilation and increased capillary permeability
   c. hagocytosis by neutrophils and macrophages; and the activation of complement proteins
   d. chemotaxis and diapedesis of new phagocytes to the infected area
   e. opsonization or "buttering" of foreign cells such as bacteria with antibodies
___ 27. Which symptom is *not* characteristic of local inflammation?
   a. redness
   b. warmth
   c. swelling (edema)
   d. pus formation
   e. All of these are characteristic of local inflammation.

B. True or False/Edit

___ 28. *B lymphocytes* exposed to antigens can transform into *plasma cells* — cell factories that live for about a week, releasing about two thousand specific antibody proteins per second.
___ 29. Most of the immunoglobulins in serum are in the IgA subclass, whereas most of the antibodies in external secretions, such as saliva and milk, are in the IgG subclass.
___ 30. All antibodies have a "Y" shape composed of four interconnected protein chains, with the "fork" region serving as antigen-binding fragment and the "stalk" region the crystallizable fragment.
___ 31. That portion of the antibody that binds specifically to the antigen is the called the F_{ab} region or the constant stalk region of the antibody molecule.
___ 32. As part of the attack phase, complement proteins C5 through C9 open large pores in membranes of the victim cells allowing water to enter; and causing these cells to swell and burst.
___ 33. Histamine causes vasodilation and increased capillary permeability allowing plasma proteins to leak out and into the tissue fluid, causing localized swelling or edema.
___ 34. Untreated local infections may result in a fever when *endogenous* pyrogen molecules are released from leukocytes and macrophages.

C. Label the Figure — The Local Inflammatory Reaction

A wood sliver, a bug bite, a scratch, or scrape — all of us have experienced a local inflammatory reaction. Study the sequence of events that occur following the entry of bacteria through a cut in the skin, producing the local inflammatory reaction. Notice the reaction occurs in the dermis, outside the capillary yet many of the cells involved are recruited from the blood. Name the cells that produce antibodies and those that secrete histamine. Refer to figure 15.11 in your text for help, OK?

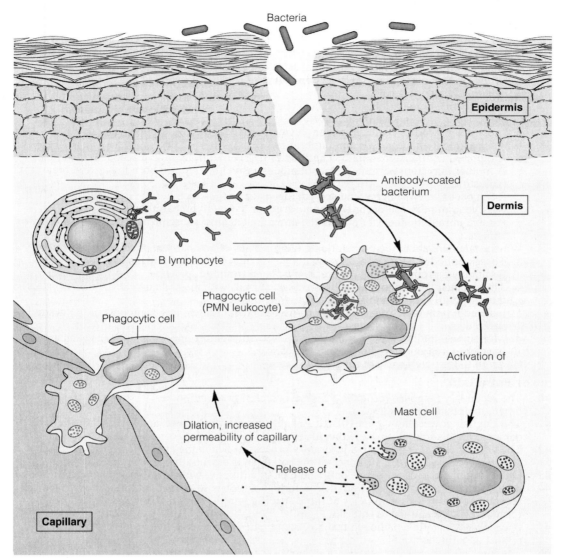

Figure 15.1 The entry of bacteria through a cut in the skin produces a local inflammatory reaction. In this reaction, antigens on the bacterial surface are coated with antibodies and ingested by phagocytic cells. Symptoms of inflammation are produced by the release of lysosomal enzymes and by the secretion of histamine and other chemicals from tissue mast cells.

III. ACTIVE AND PASSIVE IMMUNITY

When a person is first exposed to a pathogen, the immune response may be insufficient to combat the disease. In the process, however, the lymphocytes that have specificity for those antigens are stimulated to divide many times and produce a clone. This is active immunity, and it can protect the person from getting the disease upon subsequent exposures.

A. Multiple Choice

___ 35. Which of the following descriptions is a characteristic part of the *secondary* response?
    a. It represents the response to an initial exposure of that pathogen.
    b. The latent period between the secondary exposure and the appearance of antibodies is about 5-10 days.
    c. Antibody concentrations during this response reach a plateau in a few days and decline after a few weeks.
    d. The production of antibody can reach a maximum in less than two hours and is maintained for a long time.

___ 36. The *clonal selection theory* helps to explain
   a. the primary immune response
   b. the secondary immune response
   c. the secretion of monoclonal antibodies
   d. passive immunity
   e. None of these helps explain the clonal selection theory.

___ 37. A "**clone**" is best described as a large population of
   a. genetically identical cells
   b. antibody or immunoglobulin molecules belonging to the same subtype
   c. cancer cells growing within a tumor
   d. specific antigen molecules found on the membrane surface of lymphocytes

___ 38. Which statement about *passive* immunity is *false*?
   a. A mother may transfer some IgG antibodies passively through the placenta to the fetus.
   b. A mother may transfer some IgA antibodies passively to the newborn in her first breast milk (colostrum).
   c. It can occur when either attenuated pathogens or similar vaccines are injected.
   d. Passive immunity can occur when antiserum or antitoxin preparations are injected.
   e. Passive immunity does not protect the individual against subsequent exposure to the same antigen.

___ 39. Which statement about the preparation and properties of *monoclonal antibodies* is *false*?
   a. These antibodies are raised when an antigen is injected into animals to activate B lymphocyte production, which are then isolated from the spleen.
   b. The selected B lymphocytes are hybridized (fused) with multiple myeloma (cancer) cells so that they will survive and reproduce in large numbers.
   c. Isolated lymphocyte-myeloma fusions (hybridomas) secrete large amounts of the desired antibodies.
   d. Monoclonal antibodies are clinically very specific against important antigens such as interferon, reproductive hormones, and cancer.
   e. All of these statements are true.

B. True or False/Edit

___ 40. The secondary response results in the greater secretion of antibodies — sooner, faster, and with longer maintained protection.

___ 41. The English physician who inoculated a healthy boy with cowpox; and later, with smallpox to demonstrate his immunity was Edward Jenner.

___ 42. The term *attenuation* refers to a laboratory process in which the antigens present on a pathogen are greatly altered yet the virulence of the pathogen is essentially unchanged.

___ 43. One B lymphocyte can produce only one type of antibody, with specificity for one antigen.

___ 44. According to the clonal selection theory, foreign antigens select and interact with surface receptors only on the membranes of those specific lymphocytes that are genetically capable of responding with antibody synthesis.

___ 45. A vaccine is usually a pathogen that has been treated to reduce or destroy its antigenicity but retains its virulence.

___ 46. The injected Salk vaccine and the oral Sabin vaccine were both developed to sensitize individuals against the smallpox virus and its antigens.

___ 47. Identical monoclonal antibodies are produced by specific B lymphocyte-cancer cell hybridoma clones against one specific antigen.

IV. FUNCTIONS OF T LYMPHOCYTES

T cells assist all aspects of the immune system, including cell-mediated destruction by killer T cells and supporting roles by helper and suppressor T cells. T cells are activated only by antigens presented to them on the surface of particular antigen-presenting cells. Activated helper T cells produce lymphokines that stimulate other cells of the immune system.

A. Multiple Choice

___ 48. The gland most responsible for maturation, storage, and formation of T lymphocytes is the
   a. thymus
   b. thyroid
   c. spleen
   d. liver
   e. None of these choices is correct.

___ 49. Which of the following is *not* a thymus gland hormone?
   a. thymopoietin I
   b. thymopoietin II
   c. thyroxine

        d. thymosin
        e. All of these are thymus gland hormones.
___ 50. Which function is *not* characteristic of T lymphocytes?
        a. attacking virus and fungal infections
        b. stimulating the direct formation of antibodies
        c. carrying out rejection of transplants
        d. patrolling the body as defense against cancer
        e. All of these are T lymphocyte functions.
___ 51. The subpopulation of T lymphocytes that is attacked by the human immunodeficiency virus (HIV) in persons with AIDS is the
        a. helper T cells
        b. suppressor T cells
        c. cytotoxic T cells
        d. killer T cells
___ 52. The term used to describe autocrine proteins secreted by T lymphocytes that are often referred to as the cytokines of lymphocytes, is
        a. interleukins
        b. interferons
        c. lymphokines
        d. antibodies
___ 53. The two cell types that are most responsible for engulfing and presenting foreign antigens together with surface histocompatibility antigens on the membrane for the activation of helper T lymphocytes, are macrophages and
        a. B lymphocytes
        b. dendritic cells
        c. platelets
        d. neutrophils
        e. mast cells
___ 54. The membrane surface molecules that are carefully matched between a donor and the recipient to avoid organ transplantation rejection, are called
        a. histocompatibility antigens
        b. lymphokines
        c. interleukins
        d. interferons
        e. antibodies
___ 55. Genes labeled A, B, C, and D, located on chromosome number 6, are unique, in that they
        a. comprise the major histocompatibility complex (MHC)
        b. produce two classes of human leukocyte antigens (HLA), called class-1 and class-2 antigens
        c. genetically mark the membrane surface of all tissue cells in the body (except mature red blood cells) with characteristic antigens
        d. are involved in activating macrophages, B lymphocytes, T cells, and other cells of the immune system
        e. All of these statements are correct regarding the genes.
___ 56. Which specific type of molecule is *not* secreted by helper T cells following their activation by antigen-presenting macrophages?
        a. macrophage colony-stimulating factor
        b. gamma interferon
        c. tumor necrosis factor
        d. interleukin-2
        e. All of these molecules are secreted by activated helper T cells.
___ 57. Antibodies made against self-antigens are called
        a. immunoglobulins
        b. autoantibodies
        c. gamma globulins
        d. transplant antigens

B. True or False/Edit
___ 58. Unlike T cells, B lymphocytes provide specific immune protection without secreting antibodies.
___ 59. Unlike the short five-day to seven-day life span of the B lymphocyte, the small T lymphocyte, especially those that have not yet been stimulated by antigens, have a long life that spans months or perhaps years.
___ 60. Most bacterial infections are fought by antibodies from B cells (humoral) rather than direct cell-mediated contact by T lymphocytes (one exception: attack on the tubercle bacilli).
___ 61. The activity of B cells and cytotoxic T cells is decreased by helper T lymphocytes and increased by suppressor T lymphocytes.

___ 62. Acquired immune deficiency syndrome (AIDS) appears to caused by a virus that specifically attacks and destroys the killer T lymphocyte subpopulations.

___ 63. The T lymphocytes secrete lymphokines and other cells such as macrophages secrete other proteins called cytokines that help regulate many aspects of the immune system.

___ 64. There appears to be two subtypes of *helper* T lymphocytes — the T_H1 subtype that secretes lymphokines that activate killer T cells and promotes humoral immunity; and the T_H2 subtype that stimulates B lymphocyte to promote cell-mediated immunity.

___ 65. In order for a *helper* T lymphocyte to respond to a foreign antigen, that antigen must be attached to the membrane of another cell such as a macrophage or a dendritic cell, and thereby be "presented" to the *helper* T lymphocyte.

___ 66. Synthesis of the histocompatibility antigens is directed by a group of four genes labeled A, B, C, and D that are located on chromosome number 6; and are known as the *major histocompatibility complex* (MHC).

___ 67. *Class-2* MHC molecules are protein molecules coded for by histocompatibility genes A, B, C, and D that are ultimately placed on the plasma membrane of all cells in the body except those of mature red blood cells.

___ 68. The coreceptor protein known as **CD8** is associated with the killer T lymphocyte membrane receptor and the coreceptor protein known as **CD4** is associated with the helper T lymphocyte membrane receptor.

___ 69. *Helper* T lymphocytes are normally activated by contact with macrophages "presenting" both the foreign antigens and the local class-2 MHC antigens already present on their membrane surfaces.

___ 70. *Interleukin-2* secreted by activated helper T lymphocytes stimulates macrophages to secrete *tumor necrosis factor*, an agent which is particularly effective in killing cancer cells.

___ 71. The *glucocorticoids* such as *cortisone* inhibit the secretion of cytokines and thus are used clinically to treat inflammatory disorders and to inhibit the rejection of transplanted organs.

___ 72. *Immune tolerance* is more complete and longer lasting when antigens are exposed to the weak immune system of a fetus or newborn than when exposed to that of adults.

___ 73. Two general proposals to help explain the mechanisms of immune tolerance are the *clonal deletion theory* in which lymphocytes with self-antigens are destroyed and the *clonal anergy* ("without working") *theory* in which these lymphocytes are permanently inactivated.

V. TUMOR IMMUNOLOGY

Tumor cells can reveal antigens that activate an immune reaction that destroys the tumor. When cancers develop, this immunological surveillance system — primarily the function of T cells and natural killer cells--has failed to prevent the growth and metastasis of the tumor.

A. Multiple Choice

___ 74. *Dedifferentiation* is a term that refers to the process by which tumor cells become
  a. relatively unspecialized and similar to the less specialized cells of an embryo
  b. more specialized and thus similar to the more complex cells of the adult
  c. stimulated to divide erratically with less inhibitory control than that seen in normal cells
  d. altered by mutations that interfere with the normal expression of MHC antigens

___ 75. Which of the following cytokines has *not* recently proved useful in the treatment of cancer or is *not* currently undergoing experimental investigation?
  a. interleukin-2 (IL-2)
  b. alpha-fetoprotein
  c. gamma interferon
  d. interleukin-12 (IL-12)

___ 76. Which statement about *natural killer* (NK) cells is *false*?
  a. NK cells are not processed (matured) by the thymus gland.
  b. NK cells can attack and destroy tumor cells
  c. NK cells provide a first line of cell-mediated defense, destroying tumors in a nonspecific fashion.
  d. NK cells must first be activated by macrophages that present foreign tumor antigens.
  e. NK cells and killer T cells can interact as part of the immune response to the presence of tumors.

___ 77. Which statement about cancer is *false*?
  a. Cancer can be caused by a virus.
  b. The risk of cancer increases with age as lymphocytes age and thymus hormone production declines.
  c. Cancer grows faster when corticosteroid hormone levels in the bloodstream are lowered by stressful conditions.
  d. Cancer normally develops from tumor cells that escape the body's immunological surveillance system.
  e. Burkitt's lymphoma and Kaposi's sarcoma are examples of cancer.

B. True or False/Edit

___ 78. *Oncology* is the study of tumors or clones of single cells that have become transformed.
___ 79. Most tumors appear to be specific cell clones that escape the normal inhibitory controls and behave in a relatively more unspecialized way.
___ 80. Killer T cells are identical to natural killer (NK) cells.
___ 81. Tumors are usually described as either benign or metastatic.
___ 82. *Carcinoembryonic antigen* helps in the diagnosis of liver cancer and *alpha-fetoprotein* aids in the diagnosis of colon cancer.
___ 83. Although the production of human interferons has not proved to be the "magic bullet" against cancer, interferons have been used effectively in certain forms of lymphomas, renal carcinoma, melanoma, Kaposi's sarcoma, and breast cancer.
___ 84. The risk of developing cancer increases with age partly because aging lymphocytes appear to accumulate genetic errors over the years that decrease their effectiveness.

VI. DISEASES CAUSED BY THE IMMUNE SYSTEM

Immune mechanisms that normally protect the body are very complex and subject to errors that can result in diseases. Autoimmune diseases and allergies are two categories of disease that are not caused by an invading pathogen, but rather by a derangement in the normal functions of the immune system.

A. Multiple Choice

___ 85. The autoimmune disease characterized by the abnormal production of IgM antibodies that attack IgG type antibodies, is called
   a. Hashimoto's thyroiditis
   b. sympathetic ophthalmia
   c. thrombocytopenia
   d. rheumatoid arthritis
   e. rheumatic fever

___ 86. In Graves' autoimmune disease
   a. normally "hidden" antigens escape and stimulate the autoimmune response
   b. self-antigens combine with circulating drugs to produce new antigens that stimulate the autoimmune response
   c. class-2 MHC molecules unexpectedly appear in tissues that stimulate autoantibody production
   d. self-antigens cross-react with foreign antigens, causing inflammation and damage

___ 87. Which statement about *systemic lupus erythematosus* (SLE) is *false*?
   a. SLE results from the abnormal combination of self-antigens and autoantibodies.
   b. SLE victims produce antibodies against their own DNA and nuclear protein.
   c. SLE is an autoimmune disease that results in the formation of immune complexes throughout the body.
   d. SLE is characterized by unexpected immediate hypersensitivity reactions.
   e. All of these statements about SLE are true.

___ 88. Which of the following conditions belongs to that form of allergy known as *delayed* hypersensitivity?
   a. allergic rhinitis (runny or stuffy nose)
   b. conjunctivitis (red eyes)
   c. allergic asthma (difficulty breathing)
   d. contact dermatitis (poison ivy)
   e. atopic dermatitis (skin hives)

___ 89. Which immunoglobulin is most responsible for the symptoms of *immediate* hypersensitivity?
   a. IgG
   b. IgE
   c. IgM
   d. IgD
   e. IgA

___ 90. The chemical released during an *immediate* hypersensitivity response, such as hay fever, that is most responsible for the itching, sneezing, tearing, and runny nose, is
   a. histamine
   b. prostaglandins
   c. leukotrienes
   d. serotonin
   e. bradykinin

___ 91. Which statement about *delayed* hypersensitivity is *false*?
   a. It is a cell-mediated T cell response, rather than a B cell humoral response involving antibodies.
   b. Its symptoms are caused primarily by the action of various secreted lymphokines.
   c. Both the tuberculosis tine test and the Mantoux test are examples.

d. Antihistamines are clinically effective as treatment in sufferers of delayed hypersensitivity.
e. A relatively longer time is required for the development of symptoms (hours to days).

B. True or False/Edit

___ 92. Diseases that are *not* caused by foreign pathogens but by abnormal responses of the immune system, are the autoimmune diseases, the immune complex diseases, and the allergies or hypersensitivities.

___ 93. Autoimmune diseases result in the production of autoantibodies by B cells to self-antigens, which may result in inflammation and organ death.

___ 94. *Rheumatoid arthritis* and *rheumatic fever* are two autoimmune diseases that are caused by similar defects in the immune system.

___ 95. Type I diabetes mellitus is an autoimmune disease in which class-2 MHC molecules mistakenly appear on the beta cells of the pancreas, resulting in autoimmune destruction of these insulin-producing cells.

___ 96. The formation of immune complexes activates complement proteins in the bloodstream which promote inflammation and phagocytosis.

___ 97. *Immediate* hypersensitivity is caused by an abnormal T lymphocyte response to an allergen, whereas *delayed* hypersensitivity is due to an abnormal B lymphocyte response.

___ 98. Allergy and hypersensitivity refer to the same abnormal response by the immune system to the presence of antigens (or allergens).

___ 99. *Asthma*, caused by an allergic reaction, results in inflammation and smooth muscle constriction in the bronchioles of the lungs that is due to the release of leukotrienes and other molecules.

___ 100. In the typical flare-and-wheal reaction, the flare is due to local edema, and the wheal results from vasodilation of blood vessels.

CHAPTER REVIEW

A. Completion

101. Certain pathogens that enter the body are engulfed by _____ in a nonspecific way. Viral infections are often limited by polypeptides called _____, which help protect other cells from subsequent viral infection. _____ immune responses usually begin with large, complex, and foreign molecules called _____ that stimulate _____ lymphocytes to secrete _____ molecules.

102. Since these antibodies are released into the blood, they provide _____ immunity, whereas T lymphocytes require cell contact known as _____-_____ immunity.

103. There are _____ (number) subclasses of antibodies, or _____, which are identified by these capital letters that follow Ig: _____ _____ _____ _____ _____.

104. They differ in the polypeptides that make up the constant region of their _____ chains, whereas the two _____ regions of each antibody combine with specific _____.

105. Opsonization is the process of combining _____ with _____, resulting in phagocytosis. Destruction of foreign cells may also be accomplished by the _____ system of plasma proteins which are activated by _____-_____ complexes.

106. These free-floating proteins promote opsonization and _____, attracting other leukocytes to the area and promoting the release of _____ from mast cells.

107. During the primary immune response, Ig _____ antibodies are produced _____ (quickly/slowly) and the person may get sick. During the secondary response, Ig _____ antibodies are produced _____ (quickly/slowly) by large numbers of identical _____ (B/T) lymphocytes known as _____, which provides the person with resistance to the pathogen.

108. A person receiving antibody protection made by another organism, such as the antibodies a fetus receives from its mother or a victim receives from antiserum injections, is an example of _____ immunity. Monoclonal antibodies are made by artificially fusing _____ lymphocytes with _____ _____ cells, forming specific antibody "factories" known as _____.

109. T lymphocytes are processed by the _____ gland, which also secretes hormones. There are _____ (number) subtypes of T lymphocytes. The _____ subtype of T lymphocytes requires _____ with the fungus, virus, or certain bacteria to kill these invaders or to reject _____ tissues or organs.

110. Helper T lymphocytes _____ — and suppressor T lymphocytes _____ — the function of B lymphocytes and _____ T lymphocytes. Important chemicals secreted by T lymphocytes which participate in the immune response are known as _____, such as interleukin-2.

111. HLA or _____ antigens must combine with proteins on the _____ lymphocyte and the foreign antigen for activation. The immune cell most responsible for "presenting" these antigens is the _____, which partially digests the invader alerting the _____ T lymphocytes, which secrete interleukin-2.

112. Interleukin-2 also may stimulate _____ T lymphocytes, which proliferate slowly, providing a(an) _____ feedback control of the immune system and stimulate B lymphocytes to synthesize and to secrete _____ in response to the specific foreign _____.

113. Immunological surveillance against cancer is provided mainly by the _____ T lymphocytes that participate in specific immune attacks and the _____ _____ cells that are more involved in _____ immune defense. Psychological or physical stress seems to _____ (strengthen/weaken) the body's immunological surveillance mechanisms.
114. Autoimmune diseases are caused by the production of _____ antibodies against _____-antigens, resulting in inflammation and destruction of specific tissues. Immediate and delayed hypersensitivity are two types of _____.
115. Immediate hypersensitivity stimulates the synthesis of specific Ig _____ antibodies from _____ lymphocytes; these antibodies attach to _____ cells and basophils, which in turn secrete specialized chemicals such as _____, _____, and _____.
116. Delayed hypersensitivity is a _____ lymphocyte or _____-mediated immune response, resulting in the release of proteins known as _____ that produce the symptoms seen in the allergy sufferer.

B. Label the Figure — The Formation of B-lymphocyte and T-lymphocyte Clones

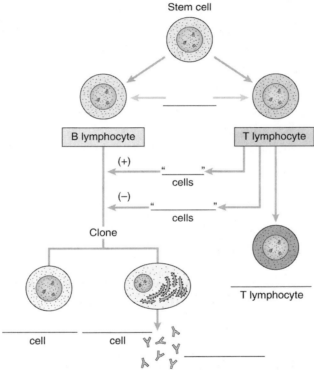

Study figure 15.2 carefully. Any one antigen can stimulate the formation of *both* B and T lymphocyte clones. Notice the influence of *helper* and *suppressor* T lymphocytes. **Label**: antigen, helper cells, suppressor cells, antibodies, cytotoxic "killer" T lymphocyte, memory cell, and plasma cell. As always, try to identify as many as possible before looking up figure 15.17 in your text.

C. Essay

Essay Tutorial

This essay tutorial will answer the first essay question found in the "**Review Activities**" section of your *Human Physiology* textbook. Please look for *Essay Question* 1. at the end of chapter 15, read it carefully, and let me guide you through one possible answer. Watch for key terms in bold-face type, helpful tips and general suggestions on writing the essay or short-answer questions. Enjoy!

117. Explain how *antibodies* help destroy invading bacterial cells.

Answer. Antibodies are specific polypeptides secreted in large numbers by transformed B lymphocytes known as *plasma* cells in response to the presence of antigens. These Y-shaped antibodies combine with the antigens and serve to identify the targets for immunological attack and to activate nonspecific immune processes that destroy the invader. For example, bacteria "buttered" with antibodies are better targets for phagocytosis by roving neutrophils and macrophages recruited from the blood. This process of promoting phagocytosis using antibodies is called *opsonization*.

In addition, antigen-antibody combinations trigger *complement fixation*, whereby normally inactive plasma proteins (complements) attach themselves to the bacterial cell membrane and can indirectly destroy the cell by puncturing large holes in the membrane. Other complement proteins that are not fixed (or are free-floating) lead to bacterial destruction by such mechanisms as chemotaxis, opsonization, and histamine release from mast cells.

Are you getting better at spotting key words in the question and directing your answer around these words? How about the organization of your answers? Remember, your essay skills will improve with practice, so how about practicing with a few of mine?

118. Distinguish between the sequence of *nonspecific* and *specific* immune events that follow local inflammation when bacteria enter through a break in the skin. (*Hint*: use a table format.)

119. Describe the source of *histocompatibility* (MHC) *antigens* and the roles the two classes of MHC antigens play in immune defense.

120. Distinguish between the *primary* and the *secondary* response of an individual's immune system following the entry of a pathogen into the body.

121. Define **autoimmune disease** and describe *three* mechanisms by which these diseases may disrupt the immune system by discussing examples of autoimmune diseases from your text.

122. Distinguish between *immediate* and *delayed hypersensitivity*. Include the cell types involved, the time involved, the chemicals that cause the symptoms, and suggestions for treatment.

Answers — Chapter 15

I. Defense Mechanisms
   A. 1. d, 2. e, 3. a, 4. d, 5. a, 6. d, 7. b, 8 a
   B. 9. T, 10. T, 11. T, 12. F—Replace "erythrocytes" with "leukocytes," 13. F—Replace "neutrophils" with "monocytes", 14. T, 15. F—Switch "endogenous pyrogens" with "endotoxins," 16. T, 17. T, 18. F—Replace "polysaccharides" with "proteins," 19. F—Antigens may have many antigenic determinant sites per molecule, with each site responsible for making specific antibodies, 20. F—Replace "B" with "T"

II. Functions of B Lymphocytes
   A. 21. a, 22. b, 23. d, 24. c, 25. b, 26. c, 27. e
   B. 28. T, 29. F—Switch "IgA" and "IgG", 30. T, 31. F—Replace "constant stalk" with "variable fork", 32. T, 33. T, 34. T
   C. Label the Figure — The Local Inflammatory Reaction; See figure 15.11 in the text.

III. Active and Passive Immunity
   A. 35. d, 36. b, 37. a, 38. c, 39. e
   B. 40. T, 41. T, 42. F—In attenuation, the virulence is reduced yet the antigens are unaffected, 43. T, 44. T, 45. F—Switch "antigenicity" and "virulence," 46. F—Replace "smallpox" with "polio," 47. T

IV. Functions of T Lymphocytes
   A. 48. a, 49. c, 50. b, 51. a, 52. c, 53. b, 54. a, 55. e, 56. c, 57. b
   B. 58. F—Switch "T" and "B", 59. T, 60. T, 61. F—Switch "decreased"and "increased," 62. F—Replace "killer" with "helper," 63. T, 64. F—Switch "humoral" and "cell-mediated," 65. T, 66. T, 67. F—Replace "2" with "1," 68. T, 69. T, 70. T, 71. T, 72. T, 73. T

V. Tumor Immunology
   A. 74. a, 75. b, 76. d, 77. c
   B. 78. T, 79. T, 80. F—Killer T cells are specific; NK cells are nonspecific, 81. F—Replace "metastatic" with "malignant," 82. F—Switch "liver" and "colon," 83. T, 84. T

VI. Diseases Caused by the Immune System
   A. 85. d, 86. c, 87. d, 88. d, 89. b, 90. a, 91. d
   B. 92. T, 93. T. 94. F—Replace "similar" with "different," 95. T, 96. T, 97. F—Switch "T" and "B," 98. T, 99. T, 100. F—Switch "flare" and with "wheal"

Chapter Review
   A. 101. phagocytes; interferons; Specific, antigens B, antibody, 102. humoral, cell-mediated, 103. five, immunoglobulins, G, A, M, D, E, 104. heavy, variable, antigens, 105. antigens, antibodies; complement, antigen-antibody, 106. chemotaxis, histamine, 107. M, slowly; G, quickly, B, clone, 108. passive; B, multiple myeloma, hybridomas, 109. thymus; three; killer, contact, transplanted, 110. stimulate, suppress, killer; lymphokines, 111. histocompatibility, T; macrophage, helper, 112. suppressor, negative, antibodies, antigen, 113. killer, natural killer, nonspecific; weaken, 114. auto, self; allergy, 115. E, B, mast, histamine, prostaglandins, leukotrienes, 116. T, cell, lymphokines
   B. Label the Figure — The Formation of B-lymphocyte and T-lymphocyte Clones; See figure 15.17 in the text.

CHAPTER 16
RESPIRATORY PHYSIOLOGY

CHAPTER SCOPE

The respiratory system regulates the process of breathing and monitors the behavior of **oxygen (O_2)** and **carbon dioxide (CO_2)** gases in the body. The thoracic cavity is the ideal sealed enclosure for the **lungs** (and the heart, in between), playing an important role in the mechanics of breathing. Of primary importance is the exchange of O_2 and CO_2 both in the **air sacs (alveoli)** of the lungs and around the body at the various tissue cells where metabolic reactions are consuming oxygen and producing carbon dioxide (can you describe these metabolic reactions? Perhaps, a review of metabolism in chapter 5 would help?).

Since breathing continues with or without our conscious thought there must nerve endings sensitive to the gases and other chemicals in the blood that signal the **respiratory centers** in the control of ventilation. These nerve sensors or chemoreceptors are located in the *carotid sinus* and *aortic arch* regions, sending nerve impulses to the brainstem region. In the medulla oblongata, the respiratory centers interpret this incoming sensory information and respond most vigorously to a *rise* in plasma carbon dioxide concentrations or a *fall* in acid-base or pH levels. Interestingly, your brain is more sensitive to rising CO_2 levels than it is to falling O_2 levels! Furthermore, since we can voluntarily alter our breathing, there must be some conscious control that descends from higher cortical regions of our brain to affect the rate and depth of our respirations.

Perhaps the most remarkable molecule in the body is **hemoglobin.** Featuring an *iron* atom core that attracts oxygen, thousands of hemoglobin-O_2 molecules are transported in the cytoplasm of each *erythrocyte* (red blood cell) past every cell in the body. As erythrocytes tumble single file through the tissue capillaries, the rate of oxygen release or *dissociation* from the flexible framework of hemoglobin is determined by the unique influence of pH, temperature, and concentration of 2,3-DPG.

Carbon dioxide is produced within the cytoplasm and mitochondria of cells during the catabolism (breakdown) of fuels such as glucose and triglyceride molecules. Considered a waste product of metabolism, CO_2 is delivered to the lungs for exhalation. (Do you remember glycolysis and the Krebs cycle — chapter 5?) Blood transports CO_2 in three different forms — let's see if you can find them. Since carbon dioxide concentration is directly related to H^+ formation, the CO_2 levels in blood play a major role in the overall acid-base balance of the body. Under conditions of exercise and acclimatization to high altitudes, the normal exchange of oxygen and carbon dioxide becomes altered in unusual, but predictable ways.

I. THE RESPIRATORY SYSTEM

The respiratory system is divided into a respiratory zone, which is the site of gas exchange between air and blood, and a conducting zone, which conducts the air to the respiratory zone. The exchange of gases between air and blood occurs across the walls of tiny air sacs called alveoli, which are only a single cell layer thick to permit very rapid rates of gas diffusion.

A. Multiple Choice

____ 1. Which function is *not* part of *respiration*?
    a. ventilation of air into and out of the lungs(breathing)
    b. gas exchange at the lungs and at the tissues
    c. oxygen utilization by the tissue mitochondria
    d. immune defense against the invasion of foreign pathogens

____ 2. Gas exchange between the air and blood occurs entirely by the process of
    a. simple diffusion
    b. facilitated diffusion
    c. active transport
    d. co-transport (secondary active transport)

____ 3. Which of the following locations is *not* part of the *conducting zone* of the respiratory system?
    a. pharynx
    b. larynx
    c. trachea
    d. terminal bronchiole
    e. alveolus

____ 4. Which of the following is *not* a function of the respiratory system?
    a. air conduction into the respiratory zone
    b. air warming
    c. air humidification (moistening the air)

        d. air filtration and cleaning
        e. All of these are functions of the respiratory system.
    ___ 5. Which structure is *not* located within the thoracic cavity?
        a. heart
        b. spleen
        c. esophagus
        d. thymus gland
        e. large blood vessels

B. True or False/Edit

___ 6. Respiration is the mechanical process that moves air into and out of the lungs.
___ 7. The diffusion rate of gases is very fast, partly because only two thin squamous cells separate the air swirling in the alveoli from that flowing with the blood of the capillary.
___ 8. Gas exchanges can occur anywhere along the conducting passageways of the respiratory system.
___ 9. Both the visceral and the parietal pleural membranes are wet epithelial membranes that come together in the central region of the thoracic cavity and surround the heart.
___ 10. Under normal conditions of ventilation, there exists only a "potential" space, known as the *intrapleural space*, that exists between the two wet pleural membranes.

C. Label the Figure —The Thoracic Cavity

Study the cross section of the thoracic cavity shown in figure 16.1 below. In the spaces provided, identify and label the following important thoracic cavity structures: parietal pericardium, visceral pericardium, lung, bronchus, anterior mediastinum, posterior mediastinum, parietal pleura, and visceral pleura. When finished, check your work with figure 16.8 in the text.

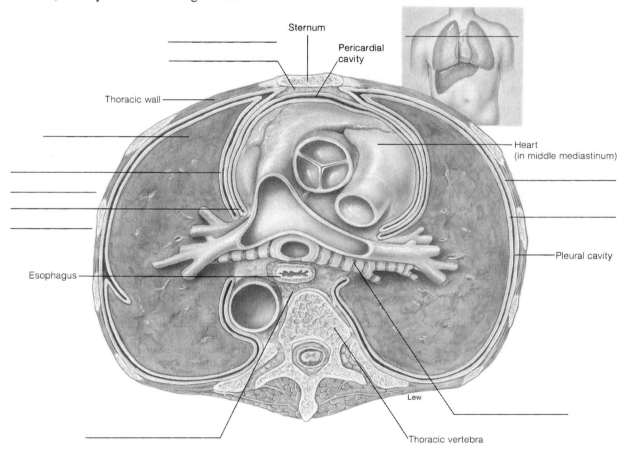

Figure 16.1 · A cross section of the thoracic cavity showing the mediastinum and pleural membranes.

179

II. PHYSICAL ASPECTS OF VENTILATION

The movement of air into and out of the lungs occurs as a result of pressure differences induced by changes in lung volumes. Ventilation is thus influenced by the physical properties of the lungs, including their compliance, elasticity, and surface tension.

A. Multiple Choice

___ 11. Air flow through the bronchioles, like blood flow through arterioles, is *inversely proportional* to the
   a. frictional resistance to air flow
   b. volume of air in the lungs
   c. pressure difference upstream versus downstream
   d. diameter of the airway

___ 12. The *transpulmonary* pressure can best be described as
   a. the pressure measured within the lungs during inhalation only
   b. the pressure in the intrapleural space that rises during expiration only
   c. the difference between the intrapulmonary pressure and the intrapleural pressures
   d. the difference between the intrapleural pressure and the atmospheric pressure

___ 13. **Boyle's law** states that for a given quantity of gas, the gas
   a. volume is directly proportional to gas temperature
   b. pressure is inversely proportional to gas volume
   c. solubility is directly proportional to gas pressure
   d. pressure is inversely proportional to gas temperature

___ 14. Which statement about lung *compliance* is *false*?
   a. Compliance can be measured as the change in lung volume per unit change in transpulmonary pressure.
   b. Compliance can also be described as lung distensibility (capable of being stretched).
   c. Compliance decreases in abnormal conditions such as pulmonary fibrosis.
   d. During ventilation, compliance is aided by the property of fluid in the alveoli, known as surface tension.
   e. All of these statements regarding compliance are true.

___ 15. Which statement about lung *elasticity* is *false*?
   a. Elasticity describes the physical recoil property of lung tissue.
   b. Since the lungs are normally stuck to the chest wall, they are always under a state of elastic tension.
   c. Elasticity aids in pushing the air out of the lung during expiration.
   d. Elasticity is abnormal due to a genetic defect in patients with cystic fibrosis.
   e. All of these statements regarding elasticity are true.

___ 16. The law demonstrating that the *pressure* in an alveolus is directly proportional to the *surface tension* of its fluid and inversely proportional to the size (*radius*) of that alveolus, is known as
   a. the Law of LaPlace
   b. Boyle's law
   c. Graham's law
   d. Dalton's law
   e. Henry's law

___ 17. Which statement about **respiratory distress syndrome (RDS)**, is *false*?
   a. It is normally seen in premature infants born before their eighth month.
   b. It is also known as hyaline membrane disease.
   c. In this condition the surface tension within the alveoli is abnormally low.
   d. In this condition the type II alveolar cells are not yet functioning properly.
   e. This condition appears to be related to certain hormone activity and to possible genetic factors.

B. True or False/Edit

___ 18. Air flow through lung bronchioles follows the same basic principles as blood flow through arteriole blood vessels.

___ 19. *Inspiration* occurs when the intrapulmonary (alveolar) pressure is greater than the intrapleural pressure or the atmospheric pressure outside the body.

___ 20. Compliance and elasticity refer to the same physical property of the lungs.

___ 21. Lung elasticity is the primary force that exists to return the lungs to their original shape during exhalation.

___ 22. Surface tension exerted by the thin film of water lining all alveoli opposes the expansion (or compliance) of alveoli during inspiration.

___ 23. Surfactant molecules are phospholipid molecules related to lecithin that serve to raise the surface tension of fluids in the alveoli.

III. MECHANICS OF BREATHING

Normal, quiet inspiration results from muscle contraction, and normal expiration from muscle relaxation and elastic recoil. These actions can be forced by contractions of the accessory respiratory muscles. The amount of air inspired and expired can be measured in a number of ways to test pulmonary function.

A. Multiple Choice

___ 24. Which of the following statements best describes the *vital capacity* of the lung?
   a. the volume of gas inspired or expired in an unforced respiratory cycle
   b. the volume of gas remaining in the lungs after a maximum expiration
   c. the total amount of gas in the lungs at the end of a maximum inspiration
   d. the maximum amount of gas that can be expired after a maximum inspiration
   e. the maximum amount of gas that can be inspired at the end of a tidal expiration

___ 25. Which of the following statements best describes the *tidal volume* of the lung?
   a. the volume of gas inspired or expired in an unforced respiratory cycle
   b. the volume of gas remaining in the lungs after a maximum expiration
   c. the total amount of gas in the lungs at the end of a maximum inspiration
   d. the maximum amount of gas that can be expired after a maximum inspiration
   e. the maximum amount of gas that can be inspired at the end of a tidal expiration

___ 26. Multiplying the tidal volume at rest by the number of breaths per minute, yields a number called the
   a. residual volume
   b. inspiratory reserve volume
   c. total lung capacity
   d. total minute volume
   e. vital capacity

___ 27. Which statement about *asthma* is *false*?
   a. It is an obstructive lung disease.
   b. Damage to the lung damage does not normally occur.
   c. Inspiration becomes relatively more difficult than expiration.
   d. The vital capacity is usually measured as normal.
   e. Bronchoconstriction increases the resistance to air flow.

___ 28. Which statement about *epinephrine* is *false*?
   a. Epinephrine acts on beta-adrenergic receptors in the bronchioles.
   b. Epinephrine causes bronchoconstriction.
   c. Epinephrine can help relieve the symptoms of asthma.
   d. Epinephrine is released during "fight-or-flight" reactions.
   e. All of these statements regarding epinephrine are true.

___ 29. The disease in which alveolar tissue is destroyed, resulting in fewer but larger alveoli and collapse of the bronchioles, is known as
   a. emphysema
   b. asthma
   c. respiratory distress syndrome (RDS)
   d. pulmonary fibrosis
   e. coal miner's disease

B. True or False/Edit

___ 30. The elastic properties of the rib cage structure, associated cartilages, and of the lungs themselves, operate to oppose inspiratory movements and to facilitate expiratory movements.
___ 31. Unforced or quiet inspiration is a passive process.
___ 32. Contraction of the internal intercostal muscles and the abdominal muscles is seen in forced inspiration.
___ 33. In *restrictive* disorders, such as pulmonary fibrosis, the vital capacity is reduced below normal.
___ 34. *Forced expiratory volume* (FEV) is a diagnostic test for *obstructive* disorders, such as asthma, during which the rate of expiration is measured.
___ 35. *Dyspnea* is term describing the subjective, yet uncomfortable feeling of "shortness of breath".

C. Sequencer — One Normal Ventilation Cycle

36. Number the following events 1-9 as they would occur during one normal inspiration and expiration cycle. *Note*: The last one (9) has been done for you.
   ___ Alveolar pressure falls below atmospheric pressure.
   ___ Intrapulmonary pressure rises above atmospheric pressure.
   ___ Neurons stop firing, intercostal and diaphragm muscles relax.
   ___ Air flows from high to low pressure into the lungs.
   ___ Intercostal and diaphragm muscles contract when stimulated.
   ___ Air volume in the lung alveoli increases.
   ___ Elastic structures of rib cage and lungs passively recoil.

___ Intrapleural pressure falls below atmospheric pressure.
_9_ Air volume in the lung alveoli decreases.

Good work! Now practice this sequence verbally on someone nearby (brother, sister, parent, or friend) until this concept becomes easy for you to recall. (This is a favorite essay question!)

D. Label the Figure — Spirogram Lung Volumes and Capacities

Study the sample spirogram in Figure 16.2. Complete the figure by writing the names of the following lung volumes and capacities on the correct answer lines: Expiratory reserve, Inspiratory reserve, Vital, Residual, Functional residual, Total lung, and Tidal. If you need help, study figure 16.17 in the text. Good luck!

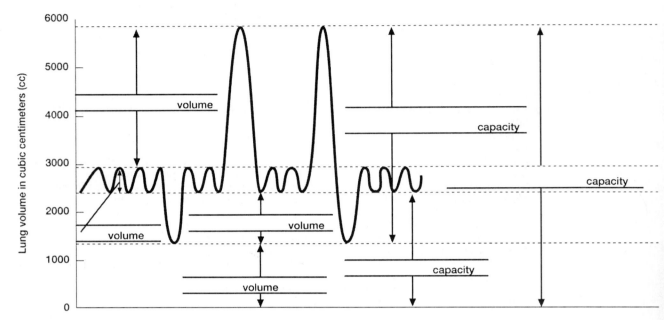

Figure 16.2 A spirogram showing lung volumes and capacities.

IV. GAS EXCHANGE IN THE LUNGS

Gas exchange between the alveolar air and the blood in pulmonary capillaries results in an increased oxygen concentration and a decreased carbon dioxide concentration in the blood leaving the lungs. This blood enters the systemic arteries, where blood gas measurements are taken to assess the effectiveness of lung function.

A. Multiple Choice

___ 37. The *total* pressure exerted by the atmosphere around us at sea level, is
   a. 760 mmHg
   b. 760 torr
   c. one atmosphere
   d. All of these pressures are correct.

___ 38. About 99% of the total atmospheric pressure at sea level is exerted by which *two* gases?
   a. CO_2 and O_2
   b. CO_2 and N_2
   c. N_2 and O_2
   d. O_2 and H_2O

___ 39. Which factor does *not* contribute to the rapid exchange of gases that takes place between the alveoli and the blood capillaries?
   a. a very large surface area present in the alveoli
   b. a very steep temperature gradient between the outside atmosphere and the alveoli
   c. a very short distance required for gases to diffuse
   d. a very extensive supply of capillary blood

___ 40. The P_{O_2} of the blood is
   a. equal to the total oxygen content minus the hemoglobin-bound oxygen
   b. not affected by breathing pure oxygen
   c. a value greater than the P_{O_2} measured in the atmosphere
   d. higher in venous blood and lower in arterial blood

____ 41. In the adult, the rate of blood flow through the *pulmonary* circulation is _____ the rate of blood flow through the *systemic* circulation.
  a. greater than
  b. equal to
  c. less than
  d. not related to

____ 42. The *ventilation* (air flow) to *perfusion* (blood flow) ratio, written as the V/P ratio
  a. results in a ratio with a higher number at the base of the lung than that measured at the apex
  b. usually indicates that blood flow at the base of the lung is greater than that at the apex
  c. is not affected by body position, such as standing or lying down
  d. can never be a number equal to one (1.0)
  e. usually indicates that ventilation at the base of the lung is greater than that at the apex

____ 43. The gas responsible for decompression sickness or the bends (in deep-sea divers) is
  a. oxygen
  b. carbon dioxide
  c. nitrogen
  d. helium

B. True or False/Edit

____ 44. At higher altitudes the partial pressures (P) of the individual gases decrease which result in a corresponding decrease in the total atmospheric pressure.

____ 45. Although water vapor is considered a gas, it does not exert a partial pressure and therefore does not contribute to the total atmospheric pressure.

____ 46. **Henry's law** states that the concentration of a gas in the body that is dissolved in blood plasma is dependent directly on its partial pressure found in the alveolar gas mixture.

____ 47. When using the oxygen electrode to measure partial pressure of oxygen dissolved in the plasma, only the free or unbound oxygen molecules exert measurable pressure.

____ 48. Almost all the oxygen gas in blood is dissolved in the plasma, while only a small "reserve" of oxygen is found inside the red blood cells.

____ 49. Clinically, the only blood gas values of importance are those taken from venous blood rather than from arterial blood.

____ 50. In the pulmonary circulation the resistance to blood flow and its average pressure is lower than the resistance and average pressure found in the systemic circulation.

____ 51. The smooth muscle of the pulmonary arterioles constricts when the P_{O_2} in the alveolus is low, thus sending blood away from these alveoli that are poorly ventilated.

____ 52. Oxygen toxicity following hyperbaric oxygen treatment can result in the oxidation of normal enzymes in the nervous system — causing damage to the retina of the eye and blindness (as demonstrated in retrolental fibroplasia.)

V. REGULATION OF BREATHING

The motor neurons that stimulate the respiratory muscles are controlled by two major descending pathways: one that controls voluntary breathing, and one that controls involuntary breathing. The unconscious, rhythmic control of breathing is influenced by sensory feedback from receptors sensitive to the P_{CO_2}, pH, and P_{O_2} of arterial blood.

A. Multiple Choice

____ 53. Which statement about the *rhythmicity center* of the brain stem is *false*?
  a. It is an aggregation of neurons located in the reticular formation of the medulla oblongata.
  b. It controls breathing involuntarily, such as when we are asleep.
  c. It has interacting collections of both inspiratory neurons and expiratory neurons.
  d. Using spinal motor neurons it controls both the diaphragm and the intercostal respiratory muscles.
  e. All of these statements about the rhythmicity center of the brain stem are true.

____ 54. The **pons**
  a. area called the *apneustic center* continuously stimulates I neurons of the medulla oblongata
  b. area called the *pneumotaxic center* inhibits inspiration by antagonizing the apneustic center
  c. assists the medulla oblongata in the automatic, rhythmic control of breathing
  d. has no direct effect on the muscles of respiration
  e. All of these statements about the pons are correct.

____ 55. Which statement about the *chemoreceptors* of the respiratory system is *false*?
  a. Peripheral chemoreceptors are located in the carotid and aortic sinuses.
  b. Chemoreceptors input to the brain stem modifies both the rate and the depth of breathing.
  c. Central chemoreceptors can be found locally in the medulla oblongata region of the brainstem.
  d. Chemoreceptors are sensitive to blood P_{CO_2}, pH, and P_{O_2}.

___ 56. The partial pressure of carbon dioxide (P_{CO_2})
   a. rises during hyperventilation
   b. when elevated, will cause a decrease in the pH (become more acidic)
   c. has very little effect on the control over the rate and depth of ventilation
   d. is normally about 100 mmHg in arterial blood

___ 57. Which statement about the *central* chemoreceptor neurons located in the medulla oblongata is *false*?
   a. Central chemoreceptors communicate *directly* with the neurons of the respiratory control center in the medulla.
   b. Central chemoreceptors are stimulated *indirectly* by the rise in arterial blood CO_2 concentration.
   c. When properly stimulated, central chemoreceptors are responsible for 70% to 80% of the increased ventilation response.
   d. Central chemoreceptors are stimulated directly by a rise in the pH (fall in H^+ concentration) of the cerebrospinal fluid.
   e. The ventilation response to these chemoreceptors takes several minutes, while that from peripheral chemoreceptors is almost immediate.

___ 58. The Hering-Breuer reflex
   a. involves irritant receptors that stimulate reflex constriction of the bronchioles
   b. is responsible for the sneezing, sniffling, and coughing response when exposed to noxious substances
   c. is stimulated by pulmonary stretch receptors during inspiration that serve to inhibit further inspiration
   d. plays an important role in the regulation of resting tidal volumes in the normal adult during quiet breathing

B. True or False/Edit

___ 59. The motor neurons that leave the spinal cord to control the skeletal muscles of respiration are known as somatic motor neurons.

___ 60. The aortic and carotid artery bodies refer to the same structures as the aortic and carotid artery sinuses.

___ 61. Sensory information about blood chemistry from the aortic bodies travels up the *vagus* nerve to the medulla, while that from the carotid bodies travels along the *glossopharyngeal* nerve.

___ 62. Carbon dioxide can combine with bicarbonate ion in the blood to form carbonic acid, that, in turn, lowers the pH.

___ 63. During *hyperventilation*, the oxygen content of the arterial blood does not increase significantly because most of the O_2 (97%) in the blood is bound to hemoglobin molecules inside the red blood cells.

___ 64. Hyperventilation results in *hypocapnia*.

___ 65. When stimulated, the peripheral chemoreceptors can produce an immediate increase in ventilation, while the medullary chemoreceptor response is slower, taking minutes.

___ 66. Peripheral chemoreceptors in the aortic and carotid bodies are *most* sensitive to a fall in the oxygen content of the arterial blood.

___ 67. The rise in CO_2 during hypoventilation stimulates the medullary chemoreceptors through a lowering of cerebrospinal fluid pH; and stimulates the peripheral chemoreceptors through a lowering of blood pH.

VI. HEMOGLOBIN AND OXYGEN TRANSPORT

Hemoglobin without oxygen, or deoxyhemoglobin, can bond with oxygen to form oxyhemoglobin. This "loading" reaction occurs in the capillaries of the lungs. The dissociation of oxyhemoglobin, or "unloading" reaction, occurs in the tissue capillaries. The bond strength between hemoglobin and oxygen, and thus the extent of the unloading reaction, is adjusted by various factors to ensure an adequate delivery of oxygen to the tissues.

A. Multiple Choice

___ 68. If the lungs are functioning properly, the
   a. P_{O_2} of systemic arterial blood is about 100 mmHg
   b. plasma oxygen concentration is about 0.3 ml per 100 ml of blood
   c. total oxygen concentration is calculated to be about 20 ml of O_2 per 100 ml of blood
   d. hemoglobin molecules bind to and transport most of the oxygen inside the red blood cells
   e. All of these statements are correct.

___ 69. The central atom of each heme group that combines with one molecule of oxygen (O_2) is
   a. Ca^{2+}
   b. Fe^{2+}
   c. Mg^{2+}
   d. Al^{3+}
   e. Zn^{2+}

___ 70. The *unloading* reaction
   a. describes the combination of deoxyhemoglobin and oxygen
   b. occurs in the lung capillaries
   c. results in the formation of oxyhemoglobin
   d. results in the release of free O_2 molecules to the tissues
   e. All of these statements about the unloading reaction are correct.

___ 71. Which of the following statements about combined oxygen-hemoglobin is *false*?
   a. Hemoglobin in the systemic arterial blood is about 97% saturated with oxygen molecules.
   b. About 22% of hemoglobin-bound O_2 will unload as blood flows through the tissues.
   c. Aerobic respiration consumes O_2, lowering the venous blood P_{O_2} to about 40 mmHg and the percent oxygen saturation to 75%.
   d. Almost all of the bound oxygen dissociates from hemoglobin as blood flows past oxygen-depleted tissues with a P_{O_2} of 40 mmHg.

___ 72. The **Bohr effect** describes the specific interaction between oxygen and hemoglobin, whereby hemoglobin molecules
   a. unload more O_2 molecules in the tissues where the pH is lower (more acidic) than normal
   b. load more oxygen in the lungs when the body temperature rises
   c. load more oxygen as the red blood cell levels of 2,3-DPG levels fall
   d. unload more O_2 when exposed to high oxygen levels

___ 73. The **oxyhemoglobin dissociation curve** shifts to the *right* (resulting in greater unloading of O_2) when hemoglobin molecules experience a
   a. fall in the blood pH (becomes more acidic)
   b. rise in blood P_{CO_2}
   c. rise in body temperature
   d. rise in 2,3-diphosphoglyceric acid (2,3-DPG) concentration in the red blood cells
   e. All of these conditions will shift the curve to the right.

___ 74. Which statement about the *hemoglobin S* molecules characteristic of sickle-cell anemia is *false*?
   a. The amino acid valine is substituted for glutamic acid in the synthesis of its protein chains.
   b. It is due to a single base change in the region of DNA that codes for the beta chains.
   c. It comes out of solution when the P_{O_2} is high, causing the shape of red blood cells to become more flexible.
   d. It inhibits the reproduction of the malaria parasite in the red blood cell and thus provides the carriers of sickle-cell anemia with a resistance to this disease.
   e. It can be inherited in the homozygous condition (SS) or in the heterozygous condition (AS).

B. True or False/Edit

___ 75. The four heme portions of a single hemoglobin molecule are composed of nitrogen-containing, disc-shaped organic pigment molecules.

___ 76. Oxidized hemoglobin is known as *methemoglobin* in which the iron loses an electron (is oxidized to Fe^{3+}) and cannot bind or transport oxygen.

___ 77. *Carboxyhemoglobin* is another abnormal form of hemoglobin that binds firmly to carbon dioxide rather than oxygen, thus reducing the transport of oxygen to the tissues.

___ 78. **Erythropoietin** is a hormone produced mainly by the liver to stimulate the production of red blood cells in response to higher than normal oxygen levels in the blood.

___ 79. At rest, as blood passes through the capillaries of the tissues, only about 22% of the oxygen bound to hemoglobin is released or unloaded to the cells.

___ 80. During heavier exercise, the venous blood P_{O_2} can drop from a normal of 40 mmHg to 20mm Hg or less, as more oxygen dissociates from hemoglobin to serve the exercising muscles.

___ 81. A shift in the oxyhemoglobin dissociation curve to the left indicates that more oxygen is unloading from the hemoglobin molecules.

___ 82. Mature red blood cells (RBCs) do not have mitochondria nor do they have a nucleus.

___ 83. Mature red blood cells do not use oxygen for metabolism; instead they obtain their energy from glucose anaerobically, forming 2,3-DPG molecules in a "side reaction."

___ 84. In patients with anemia, when the total hemoglobin concentration is low, more 2,3-DPG molecules are synthesized by RBCs, which promotes a greater dissociation (unloading) of oxygen from hemoglobin.

___ 85. Fetal hemoglobin (*hemoglobin F*) differs from adult hemoglobin (*hemoglobin A*) in that hemoglobin F has two beta protein chains in place of the two gamma chain proteins in adult hemoglobin.

___ 86. **Thalassemia** is a family of diseases that results in the impaired synthesis of either the alpha or the beta protein chain in hemoglobin; thus reducing the ability of such hemoglobin to carry O_2.

___ 87. *Myoglobin*, with only one heme iron, can bind only one oxygen molecule but has a greater affinity for that molecule — releasing it only when muscle oxygen concentrations are very low.

VII. CARBON DIOXIDE TRANSPORT AND ACID-BASE BALANCE

Carbon dioxide is transported in the blood primarily in the form of bicarbonate (HCO_3^-), which is released when carbonic acid dissociates. Bicarbonate can buffer H^+, and thus helps to maintain a normal arterial pH. Hypoventilation raises, and hyperventilation lowers, the carbonic acid concentration of the blood.

A. Multiple Choice

___ 88. In which of these forms is CO_2 *not* carried in plasma?
   a. dissolved directly in the water of the blood (plasma)
   b. as carboxyhemoglobin
   c. bound to an amino acid on hemoglobin (carbaminohemoglobin)
   d. as bicarbonate ion dissolved in the plasma
   e. Carbon dioxide is carried in all these forms.

___ 89. Which statement about the important enzyme, **carbonic anhydrase**, is *false*?
   a. Carbonic anhydrase catalyzes the combination of carbon dioxide and water.
   b. Carbonic anhydrase is found primarily in the plasma.
   c. Carbonic anhydrase catalyzes the formation of carbonic acid in the red blood cells.
   d. Carbonic anhydrase can ultimately result in lowering the blood pH (that is, blood becomes more acidic).
   e. All of these statements regarding carbonic anhydrase are true.

___ 90. Which statement about *ventilation* and *acid-base balance* is *false*?
   a. In *hyperventilation*, the rate of ventilation is greater than the rate of CO_2 production.
   b. In *hyperventilation*, the P_{CO_2} in the arteries would decrease, causing less formation of carbonic acid and a subsequent rise in the pH.
   c. In *hypoventilation*, the ventilation is not sufficient to "blow off" carbon dioxide, causing the carbonic acid production to rise.
   d. In *hypoventilation*, inadequate ventilation leads to a rise in the plasma pH.

___ 91. In **respiratory acidosis**, the
   a. carbon dioxide concentration of the blood would be abnormally high
   b. production of CO_2 exceeds CO_2 loss through ventilation
   c. cause is usually an abnormally low rate and depth of respiration (hypoventilation)
   d. synthesis of carbonic acid is excessively high
   e. All of these statements about respiratory acidosis are true.

___ 92. In **metabolic acidosis**,
   a. the blood pH falls below 7.35
   b. partial compensation results in an abnormal increase in respirations (hyperventilation)
   c. the aortic and carotid bodies are stimulated by the acidosis
   d. abnormally high levels of H^+ (acid) are formed as a result of increased metabolism
   e. All of these statements about metabolic acidosis are true.

B. True or False/Edit

___ 93. The hydrogen ions (H^+) released by the dissociation of carbonic acid (H_2CO_3) can combine with deoxyhemoglobin, that is acting here as a buffer within the red blood cells.

___ 94. The *chloride shift* in the tissue capillaries describes the diffusion of chloride ions out of the red blood cell cytoplasm as bicarbonate ions diffuse into the red blood cells.

___ 95. The *reverse* chloride shift operates in pulmonary capillaries; and ultimately facilitates the conversion of carbonic acid (H_2CO_3) to CO_2 gas (for expiration) and water as products.

___ 96. Ventilation is normally adjusted to keep up with changes in the metabolic rate, and thus keep up with the tissue production of carbon dioxide gas.

___ 97. Through its control over the excretion of hydrogen ion (H^+) and bicarbonate ion (HCO_3^-) in the urine, the kidney is the organ most responsive to metabolic acidosis and alkalosis.

C. Label the Figure — Carbon Dioxide Transport

Figure 16.40 in the text is a terrific summary of CO_2 movement out of a typical living tissue cell and into a nearby capillary red blood cell. Upon entry the CO_2 molecules enter into a remarkable series of chemical reactions, ultimately forming products that play an important role in acid-base balance. In figure 16.3, fill in the blank spaces provided with the correct ion or chemical that will complete the process. As always, try this before resorting to the answers in the text. Good luck!

VIII. EFFECT OF EXERCISE AND HIGH ALTITUDE ON RESPIRATORY FUNCTION

The arterial blood gases and pH do not significantly change during moderate exercise because ventilation increases to keep pace with increased metabolism. This increased ventilation requires neural feedback from the exercising muscles and chemoreceptor stimulation. Adjustments are made at high altitude in both the control of ventilation and the oxygen transport ability of the blood to permit adequate delivery of oxygen to the tissues.

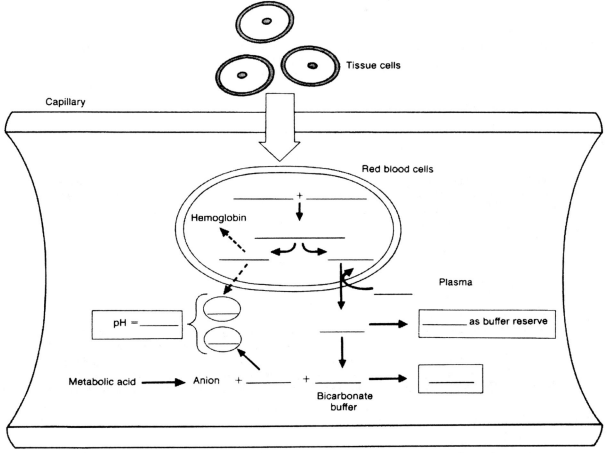

Figure 16.3 Bicarbonate released into the plasma from red blood cells functions to buffer H⁺ produced by the ionization of metabolic acids (lactic acid, fatty acids, ketone bodies, and others). Binding of H⁺ to hemoglobin also promotes the unloading of O_2.

A. Multiple Choice

____ 98. Which statement about *hyperpnea* is *false*?
   a. Hyperpnea is an increase in ventilation rate and/or depth above the usual.
   b. Hyperpnea can occur during exercise.
   c. Hyperpnea causes a decrease in blood P_{CO_2} levels.
   d. Hyperpnea may be caused by chemical factors in the blood (humoral) or by nerve activities (neurogenic), or by both of these means.
   e. All of these statements about hyperpnea are true.

____ 99. Which statement about continued moderate to heavy exercise is *false*?
   a. It may cause muscles to reach a "lactate threshold."
   b. It usually results in increased lactic acid production as muscle respire anaerobically.
   c. It results in a dramatic fall in the arterial oxygen hemoglobin saturation (normally at 97% saturation.)
   d. An increase in the number of mitochondria and respiratory enzymes results in an increase in the muscle's aerobic efficiency.
   e. The "lactate threshold" occurs when 50% to 70% of the person's maximal oxygen uptake has been reached.

___ 100. Which adjustment would *not* occur during acclimatization to high altitude — such as at an altitude of 7,500 feet?
   a. Ventilation is increased due to decreased arterial P_{O_2} (known as the hypoxic ventilatory response).
   b. The percent oxyhemoglobin saturation is reduced below 97%.
   c. Oxygen unloading at the tissues is increased due to an overall decrease in the affinity of oxygen for hemoglobin.
   d. The secretion of the hormone erythropoietin from the kidneys is decreased.
   e. The red blood cell count can rise, resulting in an increase in the hematocrit (to as high as 55% to 60%).

B. True or False/Edit

___ 101. Especially in well-trained athletes, the arterial blood P_{O_2}, P_{CO_2}, and pH remain surprisingly constant during exercise due to the complex action of various homeostatic mechanisms.

___ 102. Early in exercise, a "stitch" may develop in your side as a result of inadequate oxygen delivery to the tissues (hypoxia) and anaerobic respiration in particular muscles (including the diaphragm).

___ 103. The major effect of endurance training is to increase skeletal muscle myoglobin, mitochondria, and metabolic enzymes so that the overall aerobic efficiency of the muscles is improved.

___ 104. Erythropoietin release from kidneys is stimulated by low oxygen delivery — and results in stimulating bone marrow to increase its production of hemoglobin and red blood cells.

IX. CHAPTER REVIEW

A. Match 'n' Spell — Respiratory Volumes and Terms

For each of the following numbered statement below, select the correct term from the column on the right. Place the corresponding letter to the left of the applicable number. Then, write out the term in the larger remaining space between the two columns — be sure to spell the terms correctly!

___ 105. "shortness of breath" feeling _____
___ 106. maximum volume inspired after normal inspiration _____
___ 107. reduced vital capacity (as in pulmonary fibrosis) _____
___ 108. tidal volume X (times) breaths per minute _____
___ 109. maximum inspiration to maximum expiration _____
___ 110. maximum volume expired after normal expiration _____
___ 111. normal, comfortable breathing at rest _____
___ 112. unforced normal volume inspired or expired _____
___ 113. reduced $FEV_{1.0}$ (as in asthma) _____
___ 114. remaining lung volume after maximum expiration _____
___ 115. complete cessation of breathing _____
___ 116. total chest volume after maximum inspiration _____
___ 117. percent of vital capacity expired in 1 second _____

a. tidal volume (TV)
b. vital capacity (VC)
c. total lung capacity (TLC)
d. inspiratory reserve volume (IRV)
e. expiratory reserve volume (ERV)
f. residual volume (RV)
g. total minute volume
h. forced expiratory volume (FEV)
i. restrictive disorder
j. obstructive disorder
k. dyspnea
l. apnea
m. eupnea

B. Acid-Base Balance Brain Teaser

Complete the important acid-base reaction sequence below by supplying the missing chemicals. When finished, use this reaction and the text as references to answer the questions that follow.

_____ + H_2O ↔ _____ ↔ _____ + _____

118. What is the full name of the enzyme that catalyzes this reaction? (*Hint:* 2 words) _____
119. Where is this enzyme typically located in the body? (*Hint:* Where is it most needed?) _____
120. Which chemical in these reactions is considered a major plasma *buffer* (remember, a buffer stabilizes pH by opposing drastic swings in pH)? _____
121. Which chemical is counted directly when pH is measured? _____ ; Can you name the instrument used to measure the pH of solutions? _____

122. Which half of the above reactions is altered primarily by **respiratory** events such as breathing, resulting in a respiratory acidosis or alkalosis? The _____ (right/left) half. Why?
123. Which half of the reaction is altered primarily by metabolic events such as exercise, resulting in **metabolic** acidosis or alkalosis? The _____ (right/left) half Why?

Convince yourself that these reactions are balanced like a teeter-totter and that the momentum can swing in either direction driven by the **law of mass action** (from greater mass to lesser mass). Also, this reaction can be used to **compensate** (correct) for an acidosis or alkalosis condition that is already present. Committing this reaction to memory now will provide you with the best crib note available to answer most acid-base questions and to further your understanding of acidosis and alkalosis in future study.

C. Crossword Puzzle — Respiratory Physiology

Across
1. Equipment used in baseball
3. Blood gas — major stimulant of the carotid inspiration
8. Number of heme subgroups in a molecule of hemoglobin
9. Ease with which the lungs expand under pressure; distensibility
14. Spirometry is used to measure pulmonary _____
15. Female sheep
16. Respiratory control centers alter both the _____ and depth of ventilation
17. Ion most responsible for acid-base measurements and pH
19. What happens to old fruit
20. Secretion from the type II alveolar cells
23. Another name for the pelvis
24. The unloading of oxygen from hemoglobin can be graphed in the shape of a _____
26. Most important oxygen-carrying molecule in the body
32. Storage container
34. Common exclamation when a mistake is made
35. Government security group like the FBI
36. Egyptian snake
38. Oxygen-binding atom in the center of each heme group
39. Small portable bed
40. Method of measuring pulmonary function—aids in the diagnosis of pulmonary disorders
42. Factor that reduces the partial pressure of oxygen in the blood
43. Hemoglobin has two of these polypeptide chains in each subgroup—missing in fetal hemoglobin
45. One location for chemoreceptor bodies sensitive to blood gas and pH
46. Law stating that air pressure is inversely related to volume
48. The branching of the bronchioles is often compared to that of a _____
49. Ventilation of air and perfusion of blood are often expressed in the form of a _____
50. The rib cage is also known as the chest _____

Down
2. One factor that affects the oxygen-hemoglobin dissociation curve
3. Movement of this ion balances the movement of bicarbonate ion across the RBC membrane
4. To forbid by law; prohibit
5. Device for rowing a boat
6. Security group within most cities
7. Airways leading to the alveoli
9. Neural receptors found in the carotid sinus and the aortic arch
10. Obstructive disease characterized by inflammation of the airway
11. Obstructive disease characterized by the destruction of the alveoli
12. The visceral pleura covers this organ
13. Blood cells that contain hemoglobin
18. Abbreviation for a professional basketball organization
21. Slang term for a taxi
22. Cavity that encloses the lungs
25. Salt or fresh water fish shaped like a snake
27. Physical form of oxygen or carbon dioxide in the atmosphere
28. The rhythmicity center that regulates breathing is located in the medulla _____
29. Result of contraction of the diaphragm and intercostal muscles
30. In the absence of oxygen
31. Law separating atmospheric pressure into partial pressures
32. An alkalosis may indicate the presence of too much _____
33. Bone moved by an intercostal muscle
37. The tension of water applied to the law of LaPlace in the description of lung mechanics
41. Membrane covering the lung or lining the chest wall
42. Cessation of breathing
44. The effect of pH on the affinity of hemoglobin for oxygen
47. Like blood flow, air always flows from high pressure to _____ pressure

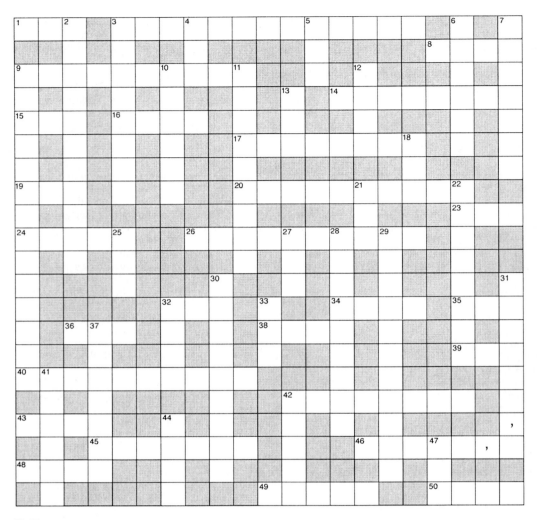

D. Essay

Essay Tutorial

This essay tutorial will answer the first essay question found in the "**Review Activities**" section of your *Human Physiology* textbook. Please look for *Essay Question* 1. at the end of chapter 16, read it carefully, and let me guide you through one possible answer. Watch for key terms in bold-face type, helpful tips and general suggestions on writing the essay or short-answer questions. Enjoy!

124. Using a **flow diagram** to show *cause* and *effect*, explain how contraction of the diaphragm produces *inspiration*.

Note: By careful analysis of the question, we must restrict our answer to the diaphragm muscle and to inspiration only. The flow diagram should focus on both the cause and the effect of stimulating the diaphragm on inspiration. Use arrows to direct the flow of events and to illustrate the proper sequence.

Answer. Contraction of the dome-shaped diaphragm downward (cause); → increase in thoracic volume vertically; → intrapleural pressure is decreased below atmospheric (Boyle's law); → transpulmonary pressure is decreased below atmospheric pressure; → alveolar pressure is decreased below atmospheric; →

air flows into the respiratory passageways to the alveoli from higher to lower pressure, and thus fills the alveoli with inspired air (effect).

Terrific! Now relax, take a deep breath (this is a good chapter to appreciate this, right?) and try these questions.

125. Define the terms compliance and elasticity and demonstrate the differences between these terms during inspiration and expiration.

126. Describe how the alveoli have lowered the high surface tension of water to permit ventilation, incorporating in your answer the law of LaPlace and hyaline membrane disease.

127. From memory, if possible, write the reaction between carbon dioxide and water and the enzyme involved. Define respiratory acidosis and metabolic acidosis, use examples of each, and explain how the body may compensate for each acidosis following this reaction. [*Hint:* Review the acid-base brain teaser, part B.]

128. Describe the structure and function of a single molecule of *hemoglobin*. Now explain why the presence of hemoglobin **S** (substituting valine for glutamic acid) cannot be detected in fetal or neonatal blood.

129. Draw your own oxyhemoglobin dissociation curve on a graph of percent hemoglobin saturation versus partial pressure of O_2 in mmHg. Explain the changes surrounding hemoglobin that cause the O_2 to dissociate from hemoglobin, both at rest and during extensive exercise.

Answers — Chapter 16

I. The Respiratory System
   A. 1. d, 2. a, 3. e, 4. e, 5. b
   B. 6. F—Replace "Respiration" with "Ventilation," 7. T, 8. F—Gas exchanges occur only in the respiratory bronchioles and alveoli, 9. T, 10. T
   C. Label the Figure — The Thoracic Cavity; See figure 16.8 in the text.

II. Physical Aspects of Ventilation
   A. 11. a, 12. c, 13. b, 14. d, 15. d, 16. a, 17. c
   B. 18. T, 19. F—Replace "Inspiration" with "Expiration," 20. F—a better word for compliance is "distensibility" or "stretchable," or how easy is it for the lungs to inflate!, 21. T, 22. T, 23. F—Replace "raise" with "lower"

III. Mechanics of Breathing
   A. 24. d, 25. a, 26. d, 27. c, 28. b, 29. a
   B. 30. T, 31. F—Replace "inspiration'" with "expiration," 32. F—Replace "inspiration" with "expiration," 33. T, 34. T, 35. T
   C. 36. 3, 8, 6, 4, 1, 5, 7, 2, 9
   D. Label the Figure — Lung Volumes and Capacities; See figure 16.17 in the text

IV. Gas Exchange in the Lungs
   A. 37. d, 38. c, 39. b, 40. a, 41. b, 42. b, 43. c
   B. 44. T, 45. F—Water vapor does not exert partial pressure that must be included here, 46. T, 47. T, 48. F—Most (99%) of the O_2 is bound to hemoglobin, 49. F—Switch "venous" and "arterial," 50. T, 51. T, 52. T

V. Regulation of Breathing
   A. 53. e, 54. e, 55. a, 56. b, 57. d, 58. c
   B. 59. T, 60. F—Sinuses sense pressure (baroreceptors), 61. T, 62. F—Replace "bicarbonate ion" with "water," 63. T, 64. T, 65. T, 66. F—Replace "oxygen content" with "pH" 67. T

VI. Hemoglobin and Oxygen Transport
   A. 68. e, 69. b, 70. d, 71. d, 72. a, 73. e, 74. c
   B. 75. T, 76. T, 77. F—Replace "dioxide" with "monoxide," 78. F—Replace "liver" with "kidney" and "higher" with "lower," 79. T, 80. T, 81. F—Replace "left" with "right," 82. T, 83. T, 84. T, 85. F— Switch "gamma" and "beta," 86. T, 87. T

VII. Carbon Dioxide Transport and Acid-Base Balance
   A. 88. b, 89. b, 90. d, 91. e, 92. e
   B. 93. T, 94. F—Switch "out of" and "into," 95. T, 96. T, 97. T
   C. Label the Figure — Carbon Dioxide Transport; See figure 16.40 in the text

VIII. Effect of Exercise and High Altitude on Respiratory Function
   A. 98. c, 99. c, 100. d
   B. 101. T, 102. T, 103. T, 104. T

Chapter Review
   A. 105. k, 106. d, 107. i, 108. g, 109. b, 110. e, 111. m, 112. a, 113. j, 114. f, 115. l, 116. c, 117. h
   B. 118. carbonic anhydrase, 119. inside the red blood cells (RBCs), 120. bicarbonate ion (HCO_3^-), 121. the hydrogen ion (H^+), 122. left half, 123. right half

C. Crossword Puzzle

	1:B	2:A	T		3:C	4:A	R	B	O	N	D	I	5:O	X	I	D	E		6:P		7:B
		E			H		A						A					8:F	O	U	R
9:C	O	M	P	10:L	I	A	N	11:C	E				R		12:L				L		O
H		P		O		S		M		13:R		14:F	U	N	C	T	I	O	N
15:E	W	E		16:R	A	T	E		P		E			N				C		C
M		R		I		H		17:H	Y	D	R	O	G	E	N		18:E		H
O		A		D		M		Y						B					I
19:R	O	T		E		A			20:S	U	R	F	A	21:C	T	A	N	22:T		
E		U							E				A				23:H	I	P
24:C	U	R	V	25:E		26:H	E	M	O	27:G	L	O	28:B	I	N		O		
E		E		E					A		A		B		N			R		
P				L			30:A			S		L		S			A		31:D
T					32:B	I	N		33:R		34:O	O	P	S		35:C	I	A
O	36:A	37:S	P		A		A		38:I	R	O	N		I			I		L
R		U			S		E		B		G		R			39:C	O	T
40:S	41:P	I	R	O	M	E	T	R	Y			A		A				O		N
	L		F				O		42:A	L	T	I	T	U	D	E		N	
43:B	E	T	A		44:B		B		P		A		I							'
	U	45:C	A	R	O	T	I	D		N		46:B	O	Y	47:L	E	'	S
48:T	R	E	E		H		C			E		N			O			
		A			R			49:R	A	T	I	O		50:W	A	L	L

CHAPTER 17
PHYSIOLOGY OF THE KIDNEYS

CHAPTER SCOPE

Imagine yourself at home attaching a plastic tube that protrudes from an opening in the skin over your abdomen to a portable machine. Turning on the machine, several liters of sterile salt solution is pumped into your abdominal cavity between the skin and the internal organs. As time passes, blood wastes are filtered by the thin membrane (*peritoneum*) which covers these organs. Out of your capillary blood, these wastes diffuse into your fluid-filled abdominal cavity, and are drained with this fluid out through the same plastic tube and discarded. This ordeal describes home *peritoneal dialysis* for people whose kidneys do not function properly. Repeated several times each day, this procedure consumes many hours and disrupts the person's daily routine.

Filtration of the blood is only part of the work normally done by healthy kidneys. Much of the work of the kidneys is spent in the return of filtered substance to the blood — a process called **reabsorption**. Requiring an enormous amount of energy, reabsorption rescues many filtered, but important solutes such as *sodium ion (Na$^+$), potassium ion (K$^+$), bicarbonate ion (HCO$_3^-$), glucose, amino acids*; and gas such as *carbon dioxide (CO$_2$)*; and, of course, the solvent, *water*. Meanwhile, those substances that are filtered but *not* reabsorbed remain in the **nephron tubules** to join additional substances that have been added to the nephron by way of the third major function of the kidney, **secretion**. Secretion provides the kidney with an alternate mechanism for ridding the body of specific molecules (in addition to filtration), by moving substances that were not filtered out of the blood and into the nephron tubules at a site downstream from the glomerulus. Together, with a minimum amount of obligatory water, these wastes are excreted as **urine**. Through these three functions — filtration, reabsorption, and secretion — the kidneys are able to eliminate potentially toxic atoms of *nitrogen* (as **urea**) from the metabolism of proteins (chapters 2, 5), to retrieve small electrolytes like *Na$^+$, K$^+$,* and *H$^+$* which have slipped through the glomerular filter, to regulate the overall body pH, and to adjust the circulating water volume in the body. Notice the important role of the kidneys in the manipulation of hydrogen ions (H$^+$) and bicarbonate ions (HCO$_3^-$) to maintain the body's **acid-base balance** (see chapter 16 for discussion of the equally important respiratory influence on acid-base balance).

The kidneys are also intimately involved in regulating the total volume of water in the body. During conditions of dehydration when the total water volume is too low, osmoreceptors located in the hypothalamus are activated and **antidiuretic hormone (ADH)** is secreted from storage vesicles in the posterior pituitary. Through its action on the walls of the nephron tubules, ADH promotes the reabsorption of water from the nephron tubules to restore the body fluid levels. In contrast, when body water is too high such as in hypertension or in patients with excess water in the tissues (edema), different types of *diuretic drugs* may be prescribed that act on specific regions of the nephron tubule to inhibit water reabsorption. Such diuretics promote the loss of extra water in the urine. Other hormones that act on the kidney include **aldosterone** secreted by the adrenal cortex primarily to reabsorb sodium, and the **atrial natriuretic hormone (ANH)** that opposes aldosterone by promoting the excretion of sodium in the urine.

I. STRUCTURE AND FUNCTION OF THE KIDNEYS

Each kidney contains many tiny tubules that empty into a cavity drained by the ureter. Each of the tubules receives a blood filtrate from a capillary bed called the glomerulus. The filtrate is similar to tissue fluid, but is modified as it passes through different regions of the tubule and is thereby changed into urine. The tubules and associated blood vessels thus form the functioning units of the kidneys, which are known as nephrons.

A. Multiple Choice

    1. Which of the following activities is *not* regulated by the kidneys?
        a. the volume of blood plasma, and thus, blood pressure
        b. waste product concentrations in the blood
        c. certain electrolyte concentrations in the blood
        d. the acid-base balance (pH) of the blood plasma
        e. All of these activities are regulated by the kidneys.

    2. The structure of the kidney reveals that the
        a. medulla is in contact with the outer capsule
        b. medulla is divided into eight to fifteen conical renal pyramids
        c. cortex drains into the minor calyces
        d. urethra transports urine to the urinary bladder
        e. female urethra is longer than the male urethra

3. Which statement about the *micturition* process is *false*?
   a. It is controlled by a reflex center located in the sacral levels of the spinal cord.
   b. Stretch receptors in the bladder initiate this reflex when the bladder volume of urine reaches a critical minimum.
   c. Firing of the reflex centers results in simultaneous contraction of the detrusor muscle and relaxation of the internal urethral sphincter, pressuring urine into the urethra.
   d. The urge to urinate, reflexly stimulates the autonomic nerves to contract the external sphincter so that urine is not accidentally released.
   e. All of these statements regarding micturition are true.
4. The vessel delivering blood *directly* to the glomerulus is the
   a. renal artery
   b. interlobar artery
   c. arcuate artery
   d. interlobular artery
   e. afferent arteriole
5. Which statement about the kidney vasculature is *false*?
   a. The kidney has two capillary beds that arranged such that the glomerular capillary bed is drained by an arteriole rather than a venule.
   b. All blood entering the kidney is completely filtered in the glomerulus and forms filtrate that is later returned to the veins by reabsorption.
   c. Peritubular capillaries are the kidney's "real" capillaries since they function in the exchange of gases and nutrients for wastes.
   d. The efferent arteriole contains blood that has been filtered and is leaving the glomerulus.
   e. All of these statements regarding kidney vasculature are true.
6. The section of the nephron consisting of a single layer of cuboidal cells with microvilli to increase the surface area for reabsorption, is known as the
   a. glomerular capsule
   b. proximal tubule
   c. loop of Henle
   d. distal tubule
   e. collecting duct

B. True or False/Edit

7. The *primary* function of the kidney is the regulation of the intracellular fluid environment in the body.
8. The *internal* urethral sphincter (the upper sphincter) is composed of smooth muscle, whereas the *external* urethral sphincter (the lower sphincter) is composed of skeletal muscle and thus its voluntary control is learned early in life.
9. The functional unit of the kidney that is responsible for the formation of urine is called the *renal pyramid*.
10. The *glomerulus* is the structure that is thought of as the "filter" of the kidney since it forms a unique fluid called filtrate from blood.
11. The glomerulus, the glomerular capsule, and the proximal convoluted tubule are all located within the *medulla* region of the kidney.
12. There are two types of nephrons, which are classified according to their position and the lengths of their loops of Henle.
13. The kidney filtrate becomes urine only when is passes through the distal tubules and enters the collecting ducts.

II. GLOMERULAR FILTRATION

The glomerular capillaries have large pores, and the layer of Bowman's capsule in contact with the glomerulus has filtration slits. Water, together with dissolved solutes (but not proteins) can thus pass from the blood plasma to the inside of the capsule and the lumina of the nephron tubules. The volume of this filtrate produced per minute by both kidneys is called the glomerular filtration rate (GFR).

A. Multiple Choice

14. Which substance is filtered by the glomerulus and thus is found in the nephron ultrafiltrate?
    a. red blood cells
    b. platelets
    c. proteins
    d. white blood cells
    e. electrolytes
15. The *net* filtration pressure at the glomerulus that results in the formation of ultrafiltrate is
    a. about equal to arterial blood pressure at 100 mmHg
    b. partially due to the very low colloid osmotic pressure of plasma

c. opposed by the high osmotic pressure of ultrafiltrate
d. estimated to be approximately 10 mmHg

____ 16. Which statement about the *glomerular filtration rate* (GFR) is *false*?
a. GFR averages approximately 180 L (about 45 gallons) per day.
b. GFR will increase during fight-or-flight situations due to the vasodilation of afferent arterioles.
c. A decrease in GFR results in a decrease in the total urine output.
d. Renal autoregulation maintains the GFR at a relatively constant rate despite fluctuations in the mean arterial blood pressure.

B. True or False/Edit

____ 17. Proteins can pass through the glomerular capillary pores yet do not appear in the filtrate mainly because they are too large to pass through the basement membrane outside the capillary wall and are repelled by membrane's negative charges.

____ 18. Our total urine production each day is greater than our daily glomerular filtration rate (GFR).

____ 19. A fall in systemic arterial blood pressure toward 70 mmHg releases locally produced chemicals that dilate the *afferent arterioles*, thus keeping the GFR relatively constant (renal *autoregulation*).

____ 20. When blood pressure falls, sympathetic (fight-or-flight) nerve activity *vasoconstricts* afferent arterioles while renal autoregulation (local) *vasodilates* afferent arterioles.

____ 21. The *tubuloglomerular feedback* process describes how specialized cells of the *macula densa* portion of nephron tubule sense any increased flow of filtrate and signal the incoming afferent arteriole to constrict; thus lowering the GFR and reducing the flow of filtrate (a form of negative feedback)

III. REABSORPTION OF SALT AND WATER

Most of the salt and water filtered from the blood is reabsorbed across the wall of the proximal tubule. The reabsorption of water occurs by osmosis, in which water follows the active extrusion of NaCl from the tubule and into the surrounding peritubular capillaries. Most of the remaining water in the filtrate is reabsorbed across the wall of the collecting duct in the renal medulla. This occurs as a result of the high osmotic pressure of the surrounding tissue fluid, which is produced by transport processes in the loop of Henle.

A. Multiple Choice

____ 22. The *return* of filtered molecules from the tubules to the blood is called
a. filtration
b. reabsorption
c. secretion
d. excretion
e. None of these terms is correct.

____ 23. Which event does *not* occur in the *proximal* tubule section of the kidney nephron?
a. Na^+ is actively pumped across the basal membranes and out of the epithelial cells.
b. From a higher concentration in the filtrate, Na^+ diffuses passively toward a lower concentration in the epithelial cells.
c. Cl^- follows Na^+ passively from the filtrate and into the epithelial cells.
d. Reabsorption of dissolved solutes leaves the remaining filtrate entering the loop of Henle very hypotonic.
e. All of these events occur in the proximal tubule.

____ 24. Which of these statements about the *proximal* tubule is *false*?
a. Sixty-five percent of the original glomerular ultrafiltrate is reabsorbed here and returned to the blood.
b. Reabsorption here is *not* regulated by hormones.
c. Although ATP is consumed, the overall energy expenditure here is small.
d. The tubular fluid entering the loop of Henle remains isosmotic with blood at about 300 mOsm.

____ 25. Which event does *not* occur in the *ascending* portion of the loop of Henle?
a. Na^+, K^+, and Cl^- are all actively pumped from the filtrate into the ascending limb cells.
b. Na^+ is actively pumped across the basolateral membranes of the epithelial cells to the tissue fluid.
c. By passive electrical attraction, Cl^- follows the Na^+.
d. K^+ passively diffuses back into the filtrate or out the basolateral membrane.
e. Water diffuses passively (osmosis) and is reabsorbed, following the ions across the walls of the ascending limb.

____ 26. Which statement regarding the *countercurrent multiplier system* is *false*?
a. The descending limb of the loop of Henle is seemingly permeable to salt and other dissolved solutes, forming a *hypertonic* filtrate.

  b. Interaction between ascending and descending tubular flow in the loop of Henle is an excellent example of negative feedback.
  c. Salt becomes recirculated and trapped in the medullary tissue fluid, increasing in "saltiness" as it accumulates toward the lower tip of the pyramids.
  d. Water is removed from the medulla by the higher colloid osmotic pressure of the blood in the vasa recta capillaries.
  e. Urea is recycled by passively diffusing out of the collecting duct specific urea transporters, through the medullary tissue, and into the ascending limb.
____ 27. When the concentration of *antidiuretic hormone* (ADH) rises in the blood
  a. the walls of the collecting ducts become less permeable to dissolved solutes and water
  b. water channels appear along the collecting duct epithelial cells as vesicles containing proteins called aquaporins arise from the Golgi apparatus and fuse to the epithelial cell membranes
  c. the ultrafiltrate flowing through the collecting duct becomes more hypotonic
  d. a greater volume of dilute urine is excreted
  e. None of these statements regarding ADH is correct.
____ 28. Antidiuretic hormone (ADH)
  a. is synthesized by neurons of the hypothalamus and released from the posterior pituitary gland
  b. binds to receptors on the collecting ducts cells and activates a cAMP second messenger system
  c. is released during body dehydration conditions to place aquaporin proteins (water channels) along the collecting duct, promoting water retention
  d. is released when osmoreceptors in the hypothalamus sense an increase in the blood osmotic pressure (osmolality)
  e. All of these statements regarding ADH are correct.

B. True or False/Edit

____ 29. Only 400 ml of urine per day (known as the *obligatory* water loss) is required to excrete the metabolic wastes produced by the body.
____ 30. *Reabsorption* is the movement of filtered water and molecules from the nephron tubules, through the tubular epithelial cells and eventually into the blood.
____ 31. The osmolality of the filtrate is essentially the same as that of plasma at 300 mOsm/L and is thus *isosmotic* with the plasma.
____ 32. In the *proximal* tubule, the Na^+/K^+ pumps are located along both the apical and basal sides of the epithelial cell membranes.
____ 33. Nearly two-thirds of salt and water in the original ultrafiltrate is reabsorbed from the proximal tubule and returned to the blood.
____ 34. The total metabolic cost for reabsorption in the proximal tubule and the loop of Henle is very high — about 6% of the total calories required by the average adult every day.
____ 35. For water reabsorption (osmosis) to occur from the filtrate, the tissue fluid flowing outside the nephron between the interstitial cells of the renal medulla must be hypotonic.
____ 36. Tubular fluid leaving the loop of Henle and entering the distal tubule in the kidney cortex is hypotonic (about 100 mOsm/L) whereas the tissue fluid in the medulla is made hypertonic.
____ 37. Because proteins (colloids) are present in the blood but not in the medullary fluid, water flows from the medulla into the peritubular (vasa recta) capillaries, thus removing water from the renal medulla.
____ 38. Normally, 99.2% of the 180 L of glomerular ultrafiltrate is reabsorbed in the nephrons so that only 1.5 L of urine is excreted per day.

C. Label the Figure -- Urea and Sodium Flow in the Countercurrent Multiplier System

Figure 17.18 in the text is a summary of some very complex solute and fluid movements into and out of the loop of Henle and collecting tubule portions of the kidney nephron. Starting with the cortex region in the upper left corner of figure 17.1, fill in the proper term(s) or chemical symbol(s) in the blank spaces provided. Think of the properties each portion of the nephron epithelium must possess to cause the net movements you are labeling. This will be a valuable visual aid to help your review of the countercurrent multiplier system when studying for an exam. Check your work against the figure in the text. Good luck!

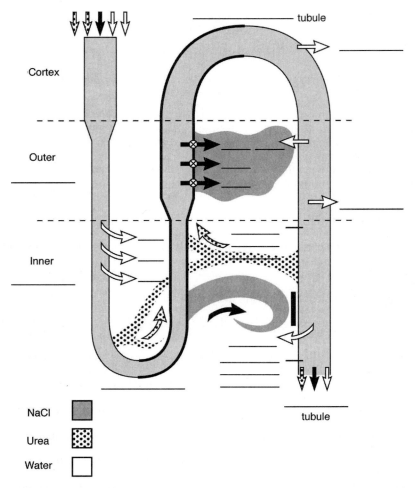

Figure 17.1 Urea diffuses out of the collecting duct and contributes significantly to the concentration of the interstitial fluid fluid in the renal medulla. The active transport of Na⁺ out of the thick segments of the ascending limbs also contributes to the hypertonicity of the medulla so that water is reabsorbed by osmosis from the collecting ducts.

IV. RENAL PLASMA CLEARANCE

As blood passes through the kidneys, some of the constituents of the plasma are removed and excreted in the urine. The blood is thus "cleared," to one degree or another, of particular solutes in the process of urine formation. These solutes may be removed from the blood by filtration through the glomerular capillaries or by secretion by the tubular cells into the filtrate. At the same time, certain molecules in the tubular fluid can be reabsorbed back into the blood.

A. Multiple Choice

___ 39. Which statement about **inulin** is *false*?
  a. Inulin is a polymer of fructose, a simple sugar.
  b. Inulin is easily filtered by the glomerulus of the nephron.
  c. Inulin is not reabsorbed by the walls of the nephron.
  d. Inulin is not secreted by walls of the nephron.
  e. All of these statements about inulin are true.

___ 40. Which plasma molecule is filtered and then completely (100%) reabsorbed by the nephron?
  a. protein
  b. inulin
  c. urea
  d. glucose
  e. creatinine

41. Which plasma molecule is both filtered and secreted by the nephron? [hint: used to measure the renal blood flow]
    a. potassium ion (K⁺)
    b. inulin
    c. urea
    d. glucose
    e. para-aminohippuric acid (PAH)
42. Which plasma substance is filtered, reabsorbed, and secreted by the nephron?
    a. potassium ion (K⁺)
    b. inulin
    c. urea
    d. glucose
    e. para-aminohippuric acid (PAH)
43. Which statement about the movements of glucose and amino acids within the kidney nephron is *false*?
    a. They are easily filtered by the glomeruli into the renal tubules of the nephrons.
    b. They are normally not found in the urine.
    c. They are reabsorbed into the nephron tubule cells by primary rather than secondary active transport.
    d. They are reabsorbed completely until their concentrations exceed their transport maximum (T_m).
    e. They are able to saturate their membrane carriers and appear in the urine if their renal plasma thresholds are exceeded.

B. True or False/Edit

44. *Secretion* is the movement of solutes in a direction opposite to that of reabsorption.
45. The amount of inulin passing into the urine and excreted each minute is exactly equal to the glomerular filtration rate (GFR).
46. Renal plasma clearance is the volume of plasma from which a substance is completely removed or "cleared" in one minute by excretion in the urine.
47. If a substance is secreted into the nephron, its plasma clearance rate is less than the glomerular filtration rate (GFR).
48. Urea, formed in the liver from amino acids during protein metabolism, is filtered at the glomerulus and partially reabsorbed along the nephron.
49. Blood entering the kidneys through the renal artery will be completely free of wastes when it exits the kidneys through the renal vein.
50. The plasma clearance of para-aminohippuric acid (PAH) can be used to measure the total renal blood flow in ml per minute.
51. Roughly 80% of the total renal plasma flow is filtered at the glomerulus; while the remaining 20% passes on to the efferent arterioles.
52. The appearance of glucose in the urine (*glycosuria*) occurs only when the plasma concentration of glucose is abnormally high (*hyperglycemia*), exceeding its renal plasma threshold.
53. **Diabetes mellitus** is a disease characterized by the inadequate secretion or action of insulin resulting in hypoglycemia (measured after fasting) and glycosuria.
54. **Diabetes insipidus** and diabetes mellitus are similar diseases, differing only in severity of their symptoms.

V. RENAL CONTROL OF ELECTROLYTE AND ACID-BASE BALANCE

The kidneys regulate the blood concentration of Na⁺, K⁺, HCO₃⁻, and H⁺. Aldosterone stimulates the reabsorption of Na⁺ in exchange for K⁺ in the distal tubule. Aldosterone thus promotes the renal retention of Na⁺ and the excretion of K⁺. Secretion of aldosterone from the adrenal cortex is stimulated directly by a high blood K⁺ concentration, and indirectly by a low Na⁺ concentration via the renin-angiotensin system.

A. Multiple Choice

55. Which electrolyte is *not* regulated mainly by the action of the kidneys on the blood?
    a. sodium
    b. potassium
    c. iron
    d. bicarbonate
    e. phosphate
56. Which statement about *aldosterone* is *false*?
    a. Aldosterone is a major steroid (*mineralocorticoid*) hormone secreted by the kidney.
    b. Aldosterone promotes the reabsorption of Na⁺ in the late distal tubule and the cortical region of the collecting duct.
    c. Aldosterone stimulates the secretion of K⁺ from the peritubular blood into the distal tubule.

d. Without aldosterone, no K⁺ is ever excreted in the urine.
e. The combined action of aldosterone on the kidney can lead to an increased blood volume and blood pressure.

____ 57. Which statement about the *juxtaglomerular apparatus* (JGA) of the kidney is *false*?
a. The JGA is a location in each nephron where the afferent arteriole and the distal convoluted tubule contact each other.
b. The role of the JGA macula densa region of the distal tubule is to secrete the enzyme *renin*.
c. The JGA granular cells within the afferent arteriole are sensitive to renal blood flow (acting as baroreceptors?).
d. High Na⁺ concentrations in the filtrate can inhibit the secretion of renin from the JGA.
e. All of these statements regarding the JGA are true.

____ 58. Which homeostatic response to a *high* blood volume would *not* likely occur?
a. a decrease in renin secretion
b. a decrease in aldosterone secretion
c. a decrease in atrial natriuretic peptide (ANP) secretion
d. an increase in Na⁺ excretion in the urine
e. an decrease in antidiuretic hormone (ADH) secretion.

____ 59. Which statement about the role of the kidneys the regulation of normal blood pH is *false*?
a. The kidneys work to excrete bicarbonate ion in the urine and to reabsorb hydrogen ion.
b. Hydrogen ion (H⁺) can enter the filtrate in two ways: by filtration through the glomerulus and by tubular secretion.
c. Most of the hydrogen ion (H⁺) secretion occurs across the wall of the proximal tubule in exchange for the reabsorption of sodium ion (Na⁺).
d. Buffers, like bicarbonate ion, can bind and release free H⁺ when necessary, thus stabilizing pH.
e. Normal urine has little bicarbonate and is slightly acidic, with a pH range between 5 and 7.

____ 60. Which statement about the reabsorption of *bicarbonate* in the proximal tubule is *false*?
a. The apical membranes of the tubule cells are impermeable (do not allow diffusion) to bicarbonate.
b. Bicarbonate in the filtrate is converted to carbon dioxide and water by the action of the enzyme, carbonic anhydrase.
c. The enzyme, carbonic anhydrase, is located both in the apical cell membrane and in the tubule cell cytoplasm.
d. During alkalosis, less bicarbonate is reabsorbed and more bicarbonate is excreted to help stabilize the pH.
e. All of these statements regarding bicarbonate reabsorption in the proximal tubule are true.

____ 61. The two organs most responsible for acid-base balance are the
a. heart and kidneys
b. liver and lungs
c. kidneys and lungs
d. lungs and heart
e. liver and heart

____ 62. Which statement about acid-base regulation in the kidneys is *false*?
a. The kidneys can filter and secrete H⁺ into the filtrate.
b. The kidneys normally reabsorb all bicarbonate ion filtered at the glomerulus.
c. Normally some H⁺ is excreted each day in the urine, thus lowering the urine pH value below 7.
d. Filtered bicarbonate present in the filtrate is reabsorbed into the blood indirectly as CO_2 gas.
e. All of these statements about acid-base regulation in the kidneys are true.

B. True or False/Edit

____ 63. Approximately 90% of the filtered Na⁺ and K⁺ is reabsorbed without the influence of hormones in the early part of the nephron, closer to the glomerulus.

____ 64. In the absence of aldosterone, an impressive 2% of the filtered Na⁺ (roughly 30 g) will be excreted with the urine each day.

____ 65. Aldosterone works to reabsorb sodium primarily in the proximal convoluted tubule and in the cortical region of the collecting duct.

____ 66. The action of aldosterone on the nephron is the only means by which the body can get rid of any *excess* plasma potassium (K⁺).

____ 67. Cardiac arrhythmias, and even death, can occur when plasma K⁺ concentrations are either abnormally high or abnormally low.

____ 68. A rise in plasma Na⁺ concentration directly stimulates the secretion of aldosterone from the adrenal cortex.

____ 69. Renin and angiotensin converting enzyme (ACE) are the only two *enzymes* in the renin-angiotensin-aldosterone system.

___ 70. The *macula densa* cells of the juxtaglomerular apparatus (JGA) act to inhibit renin and aldosterone secretion when the blood and filtrate Na⁺ concentrations are raised.
___ 71. During severe acidosis an increase in H⁺ secretion into the distal tubule will take the place of K⁺ as Na⁺ is reabsorbed, leading to a rise in blood K⁺ levels (hyperkalemia).
___ 72. Bicarbonate ion (HCO₃⁻) is a buffer to which free H⁺ can bind, thus causing the H⁺ concentration to fall and the pH to rise.
___ 73. In the regulation of whole body pH, the lungs are primarily responsible for the control of bicarbonate ions whereas the kidneys are primarily responsible for the control of carbon dioxide levels in the blood.
___ 74. Given a normal level of bicarbonate ion in the blood (21-26 mEq/L), a rise in PCO₂ levels greater than 45 mmHg results in a *respiratory alkalosis*.
___ 75. A blood pH lower than 7.35 due to high PCO₂ is called a *respiratory acidosis*.
___ 76. The enzyme, carbonic anhydrase, is located on the apical membrane and in the cytoplasm of proximal tubule cells.
___ 77. In order for bicarbonate ion to be reabsorbed from the filtrate and returned into the blood, it must first combine with carbon dioxide gas.
___ 78. Most of the H⁺ that is excreted in the urine is first combined (and buffered) to either phosphates (HPO₄⁻²) or ammonia (NH₃) molecules.

C. Label the Figure - Plasma Sodium Homeostasis

The maintenance of **sodium ion** (Na⁺) levels in the blood plasma is a beautiful example of a functioning negative feedback system (homeostasis). In figure 17.25 in the text, the fall in blood sodium levels due to a low sodium dietary intake is sensed by receptors in the hypothalamus, and specific pathways are activated to restore sodium levels by promoting the reabsorption of Na⁺ from the kidney filtrate. The last leg of this pathway involves the *renin-angiotensin-aldosterone* mechanism originating in the nephron of the kidney. Test your understanding of this important series of events by completing the flowchart in figure 17.2. Remember, most homeostatic mechanisms in the body can be demonstrated using a similar flowchart format; some simpler and others more complex. Notice that if you start with a *high* Na⁺ intake, you can follow the same flowchart; however, the arrows must be reversed along the way. Try it!

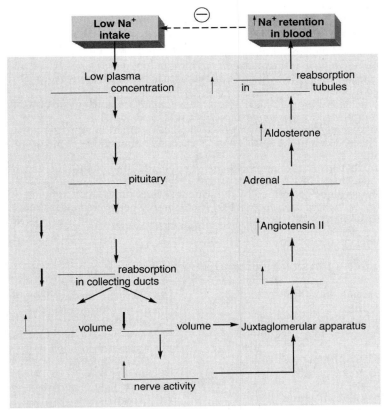

Figure 17.2 The sequence of events by which a low sodium (salt) intake leads to increased sodium reabsorption by the kidneys. The dashed arrow and negative sign show the completion of the negative feedback loop.

VI. CLINICAL APPLICATIONS

Different types of diuretic drugs act on specific segments of the nephron tubule to indirectly inhibit the reabsorption of water and thus promote the lowering of blood volume. A knowledge of the mechanism of action of diuretics thus promotes better understanding of the physiology of the nephron. Clinical analysis of the urine, similarly, is meaningful only when the mechanisms that produce normal urine composition are understood.

A. Multiple Choice

___ 79. The purpose for taking *diuretic drugs* as medication is to
   a. lower blood volume
   b. lower blood pressure
   c. treat congestive heart failure
   d. reduce edema
   e. All of these conditions can benefit from diuretic drug medication.

___ 80. The most powerful diuretics, inhibiting salt and water reabsorption by as much as 25%, are the
   a. carbonic anhydrase inhibitors
   b. loop diuretics
   c. thiazides
   d. potassium-sparing diuretics

___ 81. Diuretics that competitively block the aldosterone-induced stimulation of Na^+ reabsorption and K^+ secretion in the distal tubule, are the
   a. carbonic anhydrase inhibitors
   b. loop diuretics
   c. thiazides
   d. potassium-sparing diuretics

___ 82. The major kidney function that can *not* be performed by artificial dialysis membranes is to
   a. separate molecules on the basis of size
   b. prevent the diffusion of plasma proteins
   c. reabsorb Na^+, K^+, glucose, and other molecules
   d. allow the free movement of water (solvent)
   e. Dialysis membranes perform all of these functions.

B. True or False/Edit

___ 83. Clinically, one of the most important kidney functions involves the ability of the kidneys to regulate blood volume in the management of high blood pressure.

___ 84. That part of the nephron where most diuretic drugs act to promote water loss is the *proximal convoluted tubule*.

___ 85. The carbonic anhydrase inhibitors like *acetazolamide* are much more powerful diuretics than the loop diuretics like *furosemide* and *ethacrynic acid*.

___ 86. *Potassium-sparing diuretics* may be used in place of other diuretics when there is a risk of excess K^+ secretion into the filtrate and its excessive elimination in the urine; resulting in hypokalemia.

___ 87. *Glomerulonephritis* is currently believed to be an autoimmune disease which involves the person's own antibodies.

___ 88. Hemodialysis can be performed by the patient several times a day at home, whereas *continuous ambulatory peritoneal dialysis* (CAPD) is commonly performed three times a week for several hours each session.

CHAPTER REVIEW

A. Crossword Puzzle — Physiology of the Kidneys

Across

2. proximal tubule membrane surface with Na^+ active transport pumps
4. all nephrons originate here
6. drug used to measure the total renal blood flow
7. approximately 65% of filtrate, salt, and water reabsorbed in this portion of the nephron
9. the "filter" of the kidney nephron
12. reabsorption of water occurs by this process
14. abbreviation of the enzyme that combines carbon dioxide and water; helps acid-base balance
16. *abbreviation* describing the point at which all reabsorption carrier molecules are saturated
17. hypothalamic hormone responsible for water reabsorption in the collecting duct of the nephron
18. another name for an electrolyte
19. the kidney medulla is divided into wedges known as _____
21. the working functional unit of the kidney is called the _____
22. proximal tubule carriers reabsorb all glucose and _____ acids from the ultrafiltrate

23. _____ recta capillaries in the medulla help establish the countercurrent multiplier system
24. adrenal cortex hormone that promotes Na$^+$ reabsorption and K$^+$ secretion in the distal tubule
25. the loop of _____ has descending and ascending limbs
26. another term for urination

Down
1. the three functions of the kidney are filtration, reabsorption, and _____
3. the opposite of secretion
5. salt form of solutes most responsible for the hypertonic fluid in the medulla
8. Na$^+$, Cl$^-$, K$^+$, and H$^+$ are all known as _____

10. fluid forced out of the blood in the glomerulus is called _____
11. polymer of fructose used to measure the GFR
13. proximal tubule membrane surface with carriers for glucose and amino acid cotransport with sodium diffusion
14. positive feedback multiplication of solutes within the medulla to promote water reabsorption
15. ultrafiltrate buffer which is completely reabsorbed such that none is present in normal urine, normally
19. cytoplasmic extensions of podocytes found in the glomerular capsule
20. amino acids and _____ are both reabsorbed in the proximal tubule by cotransport carriers

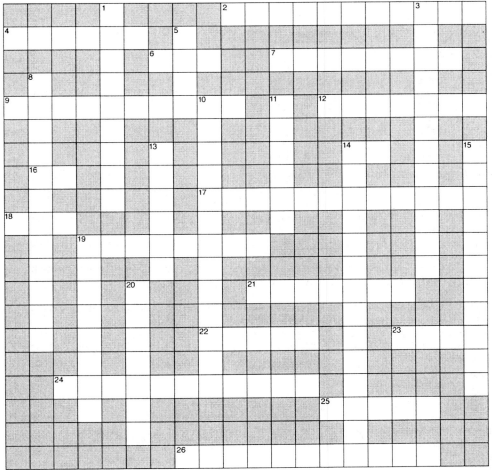

B. Essay

Essay Tutorial

This essay tutorial will answer the first essay question found in the "**Review Activities**" section of your *Human Physiology* textbook. Please look for *Essay Question* 1. at the end of chapter 17, read it carefully, and let me guide you through one possible answer. Watch for key terms in bold-face type, helpful tips and general suggestions on writing the essay or short-answer questions. Enjoy!

89. Explain **how** *glomerular ultrafiltrate* is produced and **why** it has a low **protein** concentration.

Answer. Glomerular ultrafiltrate is produced by the hydrostatic pressure of the blood, forcing fluid out of the blood and into the glomerular capsule. This ultrafiltrate does not contain cells (too large) and very few proteins. Plasma proteins are often too large for filtration or are repelled by the negatively-charged glycoproteins in the glomerular basement membranes. The hydrostatic pressure of the blood is opposed by two forces: (1) the hydrostatic pressure of the capsule pushing back against the fluid being filtered; and (2) the higher osmotic (oncotic) pressure of proteins left behind in the filtered blood leaving the glomerulus. The higher oncotic pressure in the efferent blood attracts water away from the glomerular filtration capillaries. The blood pressure force is greater, however, such that the *net* filtration pressure at the glomerulus is approximately 10 mmHg, favoring the formation of filtrate.

I hope you understand glomerular filtration a little better after wrestling with this one. Now try a few more if time permits.

90. Explain how the *glomerular filtration rate* GFR is maintained fairly constant both by **extrinsic** (from outside) neural control and by **intrinsic** (local) autoregulation mechanisms.

91. Explain how 65% of filtered salt and water can be reabsorbed across the *proximal* convoluted tubule membranes without the influence of hormones.

92. *Draw* and *label* a complete nephron of the kidney. Describe three major functions of the kidney and highlight your drawing with examples of each function in action along the nephron.

93. Using your drawing from the previous question, describe the location of aldosterone receptors along the nephron and the effects of aldosterone on Na^+, K^+, and H^+ concentrations in the body.

94. Explain the mechanisms that result in the formation of excess tissue fluid (edema) in patients with glomerulonephritis.

Answers — Chapter 17

I. Structure and Function of the Kidneys
   A. 1. e, 2. b, 3. d, 4. e, 5. b, 6. b
   B. 7. F—Replace "intra-" with "extra-," 8. T, 9. F--Replace "pyramid" with "nephron," 10. T, 11. F—Replace "medulla" with "cortex," 12. T, 13. F—Filtrate forms urine in the renal pelvis

II. Glomerular Filtrationc
   A. 14. e, 15. d, 16. b
   B. 17. T, 18. F—GFR = 180 L/day, 19. T, 20. T, 21. T

III. Reabsorption of Salt and Water
   A. 22. b, 23. d, 24. c, 25. a, 26. b, 27. b, 28. e
   B. 29. T, 30. T, 31. T, 32. F—Replace "apical" with "lateral," 33. T, 34. T, 35. F—Replace "hypo-" with "hyper-", 36. T, 37. T, 38. T
   C. Label the Figure —Urea and Sodium Flow in the Countercurrent Multiplier System; See figure 17.18 in the text

IV. Renal Plasma Clearance
   A. 39. e, 40. d, 41. e, 42.a, 43. c
   B. 44. T, 45. T, 46. T, 47. F—Replace "less" with "greater", 48. T, 49. F—Only 20% of renal plasma flow is filtered, 50. T, 51. F—Switch 80% and 20%, 52. T, 53. F—Replace "hypoglycemia" with "hyperglycemia,"
   54. F—D. insipidus is caused by inadequate ADH secretion from the hypothalamus

V. Renal Control of Electrolyte and Acid-Base Balance
   A. 55. c, 56. a, 57. b, 58. c, 59. a, 60. e, 61. c, 62. e
   B. 63. T, 64. T, 65. F—Replace "proximal" with "distal," 66. T, 67 T, 68. F—Replace "Na$^+$" with "K$^+$," 69. T, 70. T, 71. T, 72. T, 73. F—Switch "bicarbonate" and "CO$_2$," 74. F—Replace "alkalosis" with "acidosis," 75. T, 76 T, 77. F—Replace "carbon dioxide" with "H$^+$," 78. T
   C. Label the Figure — Plasma Sodium Homeostasis See figure 17.25 in the text

VI. Clinical Applications
   A. A. 79. e, 80. b, 81. d, 82. c
   B. B. 83. T, 84. F—Replace "proximal" with "distal and loop of Henle," 85. F—Loop diuretics are among the most powerful diuretics, 86. T, 87. T, 88. F—Switch "Hemodialysis" with "continuous ambulatory peritoneal dialysis (CAPD)

Chapter Review

A. Crossword Puzzle

				1 S					2 B	A	S	O	L	A	T	E	3 R	A	L
4 C	O	R	T	E	X		5 N										E		
				C		6 P	A	H			7 P	R	O	X	I	M	A	L	
	8 E			R			C										B		
9 G	L	O	M	E	R	U	L	10 U	S		11 I		12 O	S	M	O	S	I	S
	E			T				L			N						O		
	C			I		13 A		T			U			14 C	A		R		15 B
	16 T	M		O		P		R			L			O			P		I
	R			N		I		17 A	N	T	I	D	I	U	R	E	T	I	C
18 I	O	N				C		F			N			N			I		A
	L		19 P	Y	R	A	M	I	D	S				T			O		R
	Y		E			L		L						E			N		B
	T		D		20 G			T		21 N	E	P	H	R	O	N			O
	E		I		L			R						C					N
	S		C		U			22 A	M	I	N	O		U		23 V	A	S	A
			E		C			T						R					T
		24 A	L	D	O	S	T	E	R	O	N	E		R					E
			S		S								25 H	E	N	L	E		
					E									N					
							26 M	I	C	T	U	R	I	T	I	O	N		

CHAPTER 18
THE DIGESTIVE SYSTEM

CHAPTER SCOPE

Question: Why do we eat? **Answer:** To survive, right? Yet the answer is more complex than simply survival. As we learned in chapters 2-5, we eat primarily for two reasons: 1) to supply our tissue cells with the necessary **carbohydrate, lipid (fat)**, and **protein** nutrients as *fuel* for cell respiration and ATP production; and 2) to provide simple, raw materials for the *biosynthesis* of vital structural and functional molecules of the body. Among the functional molecules are the neurotransmitter substances, described in the nervous system (chapters 7 through 10), all of the hormones described in chapter 11, and the digestive enzymes to be discussed in this chapter. All of these chemicals, and indeed most of your body molecules, are assembled from the basic raw materials which have been digested and absorbed from the foods we eat.

In the nervous system, and the kidney (chapter 17), energy (ATP) from fuel foods was used by membrane pumps to establish the membrane potential, making action potentials and reabsorption along the nephron possible. The energy that hormones demand from their target tissues also is derived from fuel foods. Skeletal muscles (chapter 12), smooth and cardiac muscles (chapters 13 and 14), also have a great demand for metabolic energy as we move bones of the skeleton and pump blood around the body. Similarly, our respiratory system (chapter 15) expends energy drafting O_2 gas into the body and blowing CO_2 wastes out into the atmosphere. This ventilation effort enables metabolic processes to occur in all cells.

This chapter introduces the digestive system tissues through which carbohydrates, lipids, and protein fuel foods are **digested** by enzymes and **absorbed** into the bloodstream. Notice that we have come a full circle in the book — with enzyme *hydrolysis* reactions that are the reverse of the *dehydration synthesis* steps we traced earlier in chapter 2. Digestion and absorption is controlled by the **nervous system** (especially the *parasympathetic* division) and the **endocrine system**. The next chapter will expand on the topics that are concerned with the regulation of metabolic processes in the body and their regulation by hormones, most of which are very familiar to us.

I. INTRODUCTION TO THE DIGESTIVE SYSTEM

Within the lumen of the gastrointestinal tract, large food molecules are hydrolyzed into their monomers (subunits). These monomers pass through the inner layer, or mucosa, of the small intestine to enter the blood or lymph in a process called absorption. Digestion and absorption are aided by specializations of the mucosa and by characteristic movements caused by contractions of the muscle layers of the gastrointestinal tract.

A. Multiple Choice

____ 1. Which statement about the *digestive system* is *false*?
   a. Fully active digestive enzymes are limited in their location to the lumen (cavity).
   b. Indigestible materials never actually enter the body.
   c. Wavelike muscle contractions and sphincter muscles regulate movement throughout the system.
   d. Transport is normally in one direction only.
   e. All of these statements about the *digestive system* are true.

____ 2. Which term best describes the process of swallowing food?
   a. ingestion
   b. mastication
   c. deglutition
   d. absorption
   e. defecation

____ 3. Which is *not* an accessory organ of the digestive system?
   a. stomach
   b. salivary glands
   c. liver
   d. tongue
   e. pancreas

____ 4. Which is *not* a layer (*tunic*) found along the gastrointestinal (GI) tract?
   a. mucosa
   b. submucosa
   c. capsule
   d muscularis
   e. serosa

___ 5. Which GI layer (*tunic*) features blood vessels, glands, and nerves?
   a. mucosa
   b. submucosa
   c. capsule
   d. muscularis
   e. serosa

___ 6. The myenteric (*Auerbach's*) plexus is a major nerve supply that innervates which layer of the gastrointestinal (GI) tract?
   a. mucosa
   b. submucosa
   c. capsule
   d. muscularis
   e. serosa

___ 7. Which statement about *parasympathetic* nerves of the gastrointestinal (GI) tract is *false*?
   a. The vagus nerve stimulates an increase in motility (smooth muscle contractions) and secretions of the GI tract.
   b. The lower portion of the large intestine is innervated by spinal nerves emerging from the sacral region.
   c. Preganglionic parasympathetic neurons synapse with postganglionic neurons at the submucosal plexus and myenteric plexus.
   d. Parasympathetic stimulation decreases peristalsis and reduces GI secretions.

B. True or False/Edit

___ 8. The primary functions of the digestive system are digestion and absorption.
___ 9. The digestive system is open to the environment at both ends, and its epithelial lining is considered an outside surface.
___ 10. The esophagus runs along the back wall of the thoracic cavity, behind the lungs, and enters the abdominal cavity at the level of the diaphragm.
___ 11. The *submucosa* layer is both an absorptive and major secretory layer composed of simple columnar epithelium and an underlying lamina propria.
___ 12. Sympathetic nerve fibers act antagonistically to the effects of parasympathetic fibers, reducing peristalsis and secretions and stimulating the contraction of sphincter muscles.

II. ESOPHAGUS AND STOMACH

Swallowed food is passed through the esophagus to the stomach by wavelike contractions known as peristalsis. The mucosa of the stomach secretes hydrochloric acid and pepsinogen. Upon entering the lumen of the stomach, pepsinogen is activated to become the protein-digesting enzyme known as pepsin. The stomach partially digests proteins and functions to store its contents, called chyme, for later processing by the small intestine.

A. Multiple Choice

___ 13. The *pyloric* sphincter is located at the end of the
   a. esophagus leading into the stomach
   b. stomach leading into the small intestine
   c. pancreatic duct leading into the small intestine
   d. common bile duct leading into the small intestine

___ 14. Which statement about the *esophagus* is *false*?
   a. The esophagus passes through the thoracic cavity and through the diaphragm.
   b. The esophagus is lined with nonkeratinized stratified squamous epithelium.
   c. The upper one-third contains smooth muscle and the bottom one-third contains skeletal muscle.
   d. Constriction of the lower esophageal (gastroesophageal) sphincter normally prevents stomach contents from regurgitating into the esophagus.
   e. All of these statements regarding the esophagus are true.

___ 15. The *antrum* region of the stomach is most associated with which other region of the stomach?
   a. cardiac
   b. undus
   c. body
   d. pyloric
   e. None of these terms is associated with the antrum.

___ 16. Which of the following is a true *endocrine* cell within the gastric glands of the stomach?
   a. goblet cell
   b. G cell
   c. parietal cell
   d. chief cell
   e. enterochromaffin-like cell (ECL)

___ 17. Which function is *not* served by the presence of *hydrochloric acid* in the stomach (gastric) juices?
  a. Hydrochloric acid denatures the tertiary structure of ingested proteins making them more digestible.
  b. Hydrochloric acid alters the structure of pepsinogen, resulting in activation of the enzyme, pepsin.
  c. Hydrochloric acid partially digests carbohydrate and fat molecules as well as protein molecules in chyme.
  d. Hydrochloric acid is the ideal (optimum) pH for maximum pepsin activity.
  e. All of these functions are served by the acidic gastric juice.

___ 18. Which mechanism does *not* explain how the *stomach mucosa* resists self-digestion and ulcer formation?
  a. The gastric mucosa is lined by a thin layer of alkaline mucus that contains bicarbonate buffer.
  b. The gastric mucosa cells are very impermeable to the acid in the stomach lumen.
  c. The entire epithelial lining is replaced every three days.
  d. Buffers are released from Brunner's glands and the pancreas to neutralize the stomach acids.
  e. All of these mechanisms help resist self-digestion and ulcer formation in the stomach.

B. True or False/Edit

___ 19. Peristaltic contractions are wavelike, due first to the squeezing action of circular muscles, followed by the shortening action of longitudinal muscles.
___ 20. The esophagus empties its contents into the *cardiac* region of the stomach.
___ 21. Hydrochloric acid (HCl) present in the stomach does not directly digest protein ingested with foods, but rather facilitates the activation of the enzyme, pepsin.
___ 22. Ingested proteins are completely digested in the stomach by the combined action of the enzyme, pepsin and the presence of HCl.
___ 23. Ingested carbohydrates and fats are not digested in the stomach at all.
___ 24. The only substances absorbed by stomach epithelium are alcohol and aspirin, which are soluble in the lipid component of the membranes.
___ 25. Ulcers of the stomach and duodenum are known collectively as *gastric* ulcers.
___ 26. The *duodenum* is normally protected against gastric acid erosion by the buffering action of bicarbonate found both in alkaline pancreatic juice and in secretions from Brunner's glands.
___ 27. The only function of the stomach that appears to be essential for life is the secretion of the *intrinsic factor*, a molecule necessary for vitamin B_{12} absorption.
___ 28. Antihistamine drugs such as those used to treat cold and allergy symptoms are found to be effective in blocking the secretion of stomach acid.

C. Match 'n' Spell — Secretory Cells of the Stomach Mucosa

Match the letter of the cell type from the stomach mucosa listed on the right with the correct numbered secretion given below. Then practice your spelling by writing the cell types for each secretion in the center space provided.

___ 29. secrete histamine _____   a. D cells
___ 30. secrete pepsinogen (inactive) _____   b. parietal cells
___ 31. secrete somatostatin _____   c. chief (zymogenic) cells
___ 32. secrete intrinsic factor for vitamin B_{12} absorption _____   d. enterochromaffin-like cells
                   e. G cells
___ 33. secrete hydrochloric acid (HCl) _____   f. mucosa (parietal?) cells
___ 34. secrete gastrin _____

D. Label the Figure — The Stomach

Knowledge of the stomach anatomy is crucial to understanding how it works (physiology). Study the figure of the stomach below. Label the structures of the stomach by writing each term on the appropriate line provided. Some terms have been provided to help you. When you are finished check your work with figure 18.5 in the text. Then, erase your work and set aside until its time to review for the next examination!

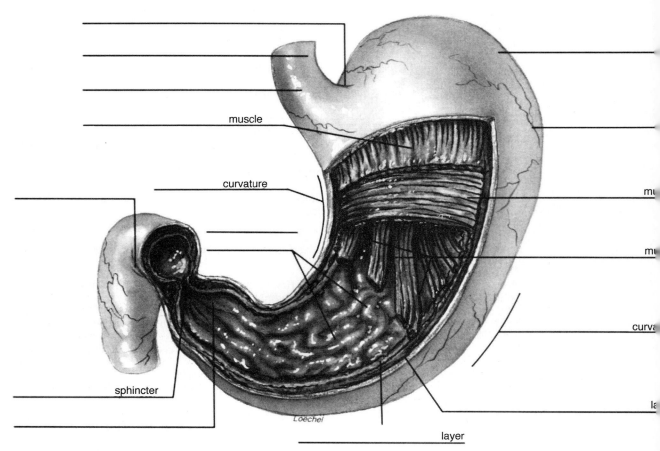

Figure 18.1 The primary regions and structures of the stomach.

III. SMALL INTESTINE

The mucosa of the small intestine is folded into villi that project into the lumen. In addition, the cells that line these villi have foldings of their plasma membrane called microvilli. This arrangement greatly increases the surface area for absorption. It also improves digestion, since the digestive enzymes of the small intestine are embedded within the cell membrane of the microvilli.

A. Multiple Choice

____ 35. The *longest* portion of the small intestine is the
   a. duodenum
   b. ileum
   c. jejunum

____ 36. Bile salts, vitamin B_{12}, water, and electrolytes are absorbed primarily by the
   a. jejunum
   b. ileum
   c. duodenum

____ 37. Which structure does *not* increase the surface area for absorption in the small intestine?
   a. rugae
   b. plicae circularis
   c. villi
   d. microvilli
   e. None of these structures increase the small intestine surface area.

____ 38. Absorbed *fat* enters the unique lymphatic vessels in the lamina propria core of each villus known as
   a. villi capillaries
   b. microvilli
   c. central lacteals
   d. intestinal crypts (of Lieberkühn)
   e. plicae circularis

____ 39. Which statement about *microvilli* is *false*?
   a. They are fingerlike projections formed by the foldings of the epithelial cell membrane itself.

b. In the light microscope, they appear as a vague "brush border" along the luminal border of the columnar epithelial cells of the intestinal mucosa layer.
c. "Fixed" digestive enzymes attached to the membranes of microvilli face the lumen and hydrolyze various substrates in chyme.
d. They may activate pancreatic juice enzymes such as trypsin, that flow into the intestine.
e. All of these statements regarding microvilli are true.

___ 40. Which statement about *smooth muscle* in the small intestine is *false*?
a. They are connected to each other by an electrical synapse known as a nexus.
b. Pacesetter potentials, or *slow waves*, are spontaneous depolarizations that, like excitatory postsynaptic potentials (EPSPs) between neurons, weaken as they travel.
c. Pacesetter potentials, when depolarized to a threshold, can fire action potentials that cause contraction in smooth muscle cells.
d. The frequency and strength of smooth muscle contractions are increased by stimulation of sympathetic nerves.
e. All of these statements regarding small intestine smooth muscle are true.

B. True or False/Edit

___ 41. The absorption of carbohydrates, lipids, amino acids, calcium, and iron occurs primarily in the duodenum and jejunum of the small intestine.
___ 42. Electron microscopic foldings of the apical cell membrane of epithelial cells lining the small intestine are called villi.
___ 43. At the base of each intestinal villus, crypts of Lieberkühn form narrow pouches, producing new epithelial cells to replace those cells that are continuously exfoliated (shed) from the tips.
___ 44. Milk sugar, or lactose is digested by the brush border enzyme, lactase; and whose absence in adults causes the unpleasant symptoms known as lactose intolerance.
___ 45. The small intestine has two major types of smooth muscle contractions: peristalsis and pendular action.
___ 46. Like cardiac muscle, intestinal smooth muscle is capable of spontaneous electrical activity and automatic rhythmic contractions.
___ 47. Stimulation of the vagus (parasympathetic) nerve releases the neurotransmitter, acetylcholine that increases the excitability and contractility of intestinal smooth muscle.
___ 48. The major smooth muscle contractile activity of the small intestine is called peristalsis.

IV. LARGE INTESTINE

The large intestine absorbs water and electrolytes from the chyme it receives from the small intestine and, in a process regulated by the action of sphincter muscles, passes waste products out of the body through the rectum and anal canal.

A. Multiple Choice

___ 49. *Chyme* from the ileum passes into the _____ of the large intestine; leading to an increase in pressure in the final section, or _____ before exiting through the anus.
a. colon; cecum
b. sigmoid colon; cecum
c. cecum; rectum
d. ascending colon; sigmoid colon
e. sigmoid colon; rectum

___ 50. Which statement about the large intestine, or *colon*, is *false*?
a. The colon is covered by columnar epithelium cells interspersed with mucus-secreting goblet cells.
b. Like the small intestine, the epithelium of the large intestine also forms crypts of Lieberkühn.
c. There are no villi present in the large intestine.
d. Bulges or pouches of the outer surface form pouches, called haustra.
e. All of these statements about the colon are true.

___ 51. The *vermiform appendix* is a thin outpouching of the
a. cecum
b. ascending colon
c. transverse colon
d. sigmoid colon
e. rectum

___ 52. The total volume of water excreted in the feces each day is about
a. 200 ml
b. 500 ml
c. 1.0 L
d. 1.5 L
e. 2.0 L

___ 53. Which analogy between the intestine and the kidney is *false*?
   a. Both areas contain tight junctions between adjacent epithelial cells.
   b. Both areas have Na$^+$/K$^+$ active transport pumps in the basolateral membranes.
   c. Both areas can both secrete water into the lumen as well as absorb (or conserve) water.
   d. Both areas have receptors for the hormone *aldosterone*, which stimulates salt and water reabsorption.
   e. Both areas contribute to the loss of water from the body as a way of excreting other waste materials.

___ 54. Which of the following is *not* a direct cause of *diarrhea*?
   a. cholera
   b. celiac sprue
   c. appendicitis
   d. lactose intolerance

B. True or False/Edit

___ 55. A *diverticulum* is a pouch larger than a *haustrum* that forms when the wall of the muscularis externa weakens and stretches lengthwise.

___ 56. The *vermiform appendix* is a short, thin outpouching of the cecum that has no true digestive function.

___ 57. Most of the fluid and electrolytes in the lumen of the gastrointestinal tract are absorbed by the large intestine.

___ 58. Water absorption in the large intestine occurs by osmosis down a water concentration gradient set up by Na$^+$/K$^+$ active transport pumps similar to that found in the kidney nephron.

___ 59. *Aldosterone*, the hormone that stimulates salt and water reabsorption along the renal tubules, also appears to stimulate salt and water absorption from the *ileum* of the small intestine.

___ 60. The defecation reflex is regulated to a large degree by habit.

V. LIVER, GALLBLADDER, AND PANCREAS

The liver regulates the chemical composition of the blood in numerous ways. In addition, the liver produces and secretes bile, which is stored and concentrated in the gallbladder prior to its discharge into the duodenum. The pancreas produces pancreatic juice, an exocrine secretion containing bicarbonate and important digestive enzymes that is passed into the duodenum via the pancreatic duct.

A. Multiple Choice

___ 61. As part of the *reticuloendothelial system*, the *Kupffer cells* in the liver are responsible for the
   a. synthesis and secretion of bile
   b. phagocytosis of blood swirling within the sinusoids
   c. metabolism of carbohydrates and lipids
   d. synthesis of large plasma proteins
   e. torage of particular vitamins.

___ 62. Which statement about the functional unit of the liver, known as the *liver lobules*, is *false*?
   a. A central vein collects mixed blood from the sinusoids to help form the hepatic vein.
   b. Incoming blood from the hepatic artery and from the portal vein mix in the sinusoids.
   c. Bile is made and released into the central vein of each lobule.
   d. Liver lobules are destroyed by diseases such as cirrhosis.
   e. All of these statements regarding liver lobules are true.

___ 63. The *enterohepatic circulation* refers to the specific pathway of many compounds, that are
   a. absorbed from the intestine; and then travel to the liver
   b. carbohydrate and lipid metabolism
   c. synthesis of proteins
   d. synthesis and secretion of bile
   e. All of these are major liver functions.

___ 64. Which of the following is not a major function of the liver?
   a. detoxication of blood
   b. carbohydrate and lipid metabolism
   c. synthesis of proteins
   d. synthesis and secretion of bile
   e. All of these are major liver functions.

___ 65. Which statement about substance called *bilirubin* is *false*?
   a. Bilirubin is a pigment secreted from the liver in bile.
   b. Bilirubin is derived from liver cholesterol molecules.
   c. Bilirubin is bound to albumin in the bloodstream since it is not very water-soluble.
   d. In the intestine, bacteria convert bilirubin into another pigment called urobilinogen.
   e. Bilirubin can be conjugated (combined) with glucuronic acid to change its solubility properties.

___ 66. As part of bile secretions, the bile salts are compounds derived from
   a. sodium and potassium compounds
   b. cholesterol
   c. bilirubin
   d. lecithin
   e. None of these form bile salts.

___ 67. Which statement about *jaundice* is *false*?
   a. Jaundice is due to high levels of either free or conjugated bilirubin in the blood.
   b. Jaundice may be due to the excessive destruction of white blood cells in newborn babies.
   c. Jaundice may be seen in premature infants with inadequate amounts of liver enzymes.
   d. Jaundice may be seen in adults whose bile ducts are blocked by gallstones.
   e. Jaundice is seen in newborn babies who suffer from erythroblastosis fetalis.

___ 68. Which route of elimination is *not* used primarily by the liver?
   a. excretion of compounds in the bile
   b. excretion of compounds in the urine
   c. phagocytosis by Kupffer cells lining the sinusoids
   d. chemical alteration (detoxication) within the hepatocytes
   e. All of these routes are used by the liver.

___ 69. Which detoxication reaction is *not* used by the liver?
   a. Toxic ammonia molecules are converted into less toxic urea molecules.
   b. Toxic porphyrins are converted into the yellow pigment, bilirubin.
   c. Toxic organic acids are converted to pH stabilizing bases.
   d. Toxic steroid hormones and other nonpolar compounds (drugs) are converted to polar (more water-soluble) ones.
   e. All of these reactions occur in the liver.

___ 70. The plasma protein that is most common (70% of all plasma protein) and is responsible for much of the colloid osmotic (oncotic) pressure of blood, is
   a. albumin
   b. K-globulin
   c. fibrinogen
   d. prothrombin
   e. angiotensinogen

___ 71. Which statement about the gallbladder is *false*?
   a. The gallbladder's major function is to store and concentrate bile.
   b. The gallbladder's storage capacity is about 35-100 ml of bile.
   c. Bile accumulates in the gallbladder only when the sphincter of Oddi is closed.
   d. When full, the gallbladder is the shape of a small pear.
   e. Contraction of the muscular gallbladder ejects bile through the common bile duct and into the stomach.

___ 72. Which statement about the digestive enzymes secreted by the acini of the pancreas, is *false*?
   a. These enzymes digest ingested carbohydrates, proteins, and triglycerides.
   b. These enzymes are mostly produced as inactive molecules (zymogens) that become active in the small intestine.
   c. Enterokinase is one of the more important pancreatic enzymes.
   d. Activated trypsin activates many of the other pancreatic zymogens.
   e. All of these statements regarding pancreatic enzymes are true.

B. True or False/Edit

___ 73. The *liver*, located immediately beneath the diaphragm in the abdominal cavity, is the largest internal organ.

___ 74. Liver cells or *hepatocytes* form plates that are one or two cells thick and are separated by highly permeable capillary spaces called *sinusoids*.

___ 75. All digestion products (except fat) that are absorbed into the blood are delivered to the liver first, and then released into the general circulation.

___ 76. The *hepatic portal vein* connects the liver to the inferior vena cava that returns blood to the heart.

___ 77. Blood and bile travel in different vessels and therefore do not mix in the liver lobules.

___ 78. The liver has a wider variety of functions than any other organ in the body.

___ 79. *Bilirubin* is the pigment in the blood that is filtered by the kidney and thus gives urine its yellow color.

___ 80. *Urobilinogen*, formed by bacteria in the intestine, can return to the blood via the *enterohepatic circulation*, where it may be filtered by kidneys, adding yellow color to the urine.

___ 81. The liver *cytochrome P450 enzymes* that metabolize thousands of toxic compounds, such as benzopyrene (a carcinogen from tobacco smoke and charbroiled meat) and dioxin, are not related to the cytochromes of cell respiration fame located in the mitochondrion.

___ 82. After a carbohydrate-rich meal, the liver removes blood glucose and converts this glucose into glycogen (*glycogenesis*) and triglycerides (*lipogenesis*).

___ 83. During fasting (or starvation), stored liver glycogen molecules are broken down into free glucose molecules (*gluconeogenesis*), that are subsequently released into the blood.

___ 84. When the small intestine is empty of food, the sphincter of Oddi at the end of the common bile duct closes so that bile backs up and fills the gallbladder.

___ 85. After the gallbladder has been surgically removed, bile will continue to flow into the intestine since it is continuously produced by the liver.

___ 86. The *endocrine* cells of the pancreas are in secretory units known as *acini*.

___ 87. The complete digestion of food molecules in the small intestine requires the activity of both pancreatic enzymes and fixed brush border intestinal enzymes.

VI. NEURAL AND ENDOCRINE REGULATION OF THE DIGESTIVE SYSTEM

The activities of different regions of the GI tract are coordinated by the actions of the vagus nerve and various hormones. The stomach begins to increase its secretion in anticipation of a meal, and further increases its activities in response to the arrival of chyme. The entry of chyme into the duodenum stimulates the secretion of hormones that promote contractions of the gallbladder, secretion of pancreatic juice, and inhibition of gastric activity.

A. Multiple Choice

___ 88. During the *cephalic* phase of gastric regulation
   a. the brain exerts its reflex control via the vagus nerve
   b. HCl is secreted from chief cells
   c. pepsinogen is secreted from parietal cells
   d. gastrin is secreted from enterochromaffin-like cells

___ 89. Which statement about the *gastric* phase is *false*?
   a. The gastric phase exhibits both positive and negative feedback mechanisms that occur as protein arrives in the stomach.
   b. The presence of fat in the stomach chyme, but not glucose, stimulates gastric acid secretion.
   c. As the pH of the gastric juice drops (acid levels rise), the secretion of gastrin hormones also drops, correspondingly.
   d. The amount of HCl and pepsinogen secreted by the stomach is directly proportional to the amount of short polypeptides and amino acids present in the chyme.
   e. The amount of acid secreted by the parietal cells of the stomach is closely matched to the amount of protein ingested.

___ 90. Which statement about the *intestinal* phase is *false*?
   a. The increased osmolality of chyme in the duodenum may inhibit gastric activity and secretion via nerve reflexes.
   b. Stretch (distension) caused by chyme entering the duodenum may inhibit gastric activity.
   c. The presence of protein polypeptides in intestinal chyme may stimulate the release of a hormone (enterogastrone) that inhibits gastric function.
   d. Somatostatin, cholecystokinin (CCK) and glucagon-like peptide-1 (GLP-1) are polypeptide hormones that collectively serve to inhibit gastric activity.
   e. The presence of glucose in the intestinal chyme may cause GIP release, which, in turn stimulates the secretion of insulin from the islets of Langerhans.

___ 91. The arrival of chyme causes the reflex secretion of pancreatic juice and bile during the
   a. cephalic phase
   b. gastric phase
   c. intestinal phase
   d. progress through all of these phases

___ 92. The presence of _____ in chyme stimulates *secretin* release, while the presence of _____ in chyme stimulates *cholecystokinin (CCK)* release.
   a. acid; alkaline
   b. acid; fat and protein
   c. fat; protein and glucose
   d protein and fat; acid
   e. alkaline; protein and glucose

___ 93. As chyme enters the duodenum, bile secretion is enhanced by
   a. secretin secretion
   b. enterogastrone secretion
   c. CCK secretion
   d. both a and b
   e. both a and c

B. True or False/Edit
___ 94. Autonomic nerve activity and various hormones modify the existing gastric motility and glandular secretions due to the presence of food.
___ 95. *Gastrin* is a hormone secreted by G cells that promotes HCl secretion from the parietal cells and pepsinogen secretion from the chief cells.
___ 96. Distension of the stomach by the arrival of a large amount of chyme will reduce gastric secretions.
___ 97. The amino acids *tryptophan* and *phenylalanine* have been shown to be potent stimulators of both *pepsinogen* secretion from chief cells and *gastrin* secretion from G cells of the stomach.
___ 98. A breakfast of pancakes and syrup takes longer to digest and pass through the stomach than a breakfast of bacon and eggs, due partly to the inhibitory action of *enterogastrone*.
___ 99. *Secretin* promotes the synthesis and release of bicarbonate by the pancreas while *cholecystokinin* (CCK) increases the digestive enzyme content of pancreatic juice.
___ 100. In the acinar cells of the pancreas, the cytoplasmic second messenger responding to the hormone, secretin is Ca^{2+}, whereas the second messenger for CCK is cyclic AMP.
___ 101. Since nerve reflexes can regulate digestion, it seems the role of GI hormones may be primarily *trophic*, or supportive.
___ 102. The structure of the gastric mucosa is dependent upon the supportive, or *trophic*, effects of the hormone, *secretin*.
___ 103. The structure of the acinar (exocrine) cells of the pancreas is dependent upon the *trophic* effects of *cholecystokinin* (CCK).

VII. DIGESTION AND ABSORPTION OF CARBOHYDRATES, LIPIDS, AND PROTEINS

Polysaccharides and polypeptides are hydrolyzed into their subunits. These subunits enter the epithelial cells of the intestinal villi and are secreted into blood capillaries. Fat is emulsified by the action of bile salts, hydrolyzed into fatty acids and monoglycerides, and absorbed into the intestinal epithelial cells. Once in the cells, triglycerides are resynthesized and combined with proteins to form particles that are secreted into the lymphatic fluid.

A. Multiple Choice
___ 104. The nutrients in foods that serve predominantly as "fuel food," providing energy for metabolism are
   a. vitamins, minerals, and carbohydrates
   b. carbohydrates, lipids (fats), and vitamins
   c. protein, lipids (fats), and water
   d. carbohydrates, proteins, and lipids (fats)
   e. protein, vitamins, and carbohydrates
___ 105. Which statement about the digestion of *protein* in ingested food is *false*?
   a. Protein digestion begins in the mouth with enzymes in saliva.
   b. The stomach enzyme, pepsin, only partially digests proteins.
   c. Most protein digestion occurs in the duodenum and jejunum.
   d. Peptide bonds between amino acids are broken by both endopeptidases and exopeptidases, depending upon their location along the protein chain.
   e. Microvilli brush border peptidase enzymes are also involved in protein digestion.
___ 106. Which statement about the digestion of *lipid* in ingested food is *false*?
   a. Lipid digestion begins in the duodenum with the digestion of large lipid globules into smaller globules.
   b. The emulsification process requires the mixture of lipids with bile.
   c. Emulsification digests lipids, forming free fatty acids and glycerol.
   d. Pancreatic enzymes, lipase and colipase, aid the hydrolysis of lipids.
   e. Mixed micelles of digested lipids are absorbed primarily by diffusion.
___ 107. Which statement about the intestinal absorption or the transport of lipids in the blood is *false*?
   a. Chylomicrons are lipid-protein particles formed within the intestinal epithelial cells during lipid absorption.
   b. Chylomicrons enter the lacteal of the intestinal villus for transport through lymphatic vessels.
   c. Absorbed lipids do not travel through the hepatic portal vein.
   d. Chylomicrons enter and blend with the general blood circulation via the thoracic duct.
   e. All of these statements regarding the intestinal absorption or the transport of lipids in the blood are true.

B. True or False/Edit
___ 108. The enzyme *amylase*, or ptyalin, is secreted with the saliva and is responsible for most of the digestion of starch molecules into maltose, maltriose, and oligosaccharides.

___ 109. The digestive enzymes "fixed" to the brush border of epithelial cells in the duodenum complete the digestion of starch, forming monosaccharides for absorption.
___ 110. Absorption of digested carbohydrates such as glucose or fructose in the intestine occurs by coupled transport (cotransport, or secondary active transport coupled to Na⁺ diffusion).
___ 111. Like glucose absorption, the absorption of free amino acid from the intestine requires coupled transport (cotransport, or secondary active transport coupled to Na⁺ diffusion).
___ 112. Bile emulsification of fat is the process by which droplets of fat are formed with less surface area for the hydrolytic action of *lipase* and *colipase* enzymes.
___ 113. Once inside the epithelial cells, digested free fatty acids and monoglycerides are reassembled to form triglycerides and phospholipids.
___ 114. *Lipoprotein lipase* enzymes are attached to the endothelium of blood vessels, hydrolyzing triglycerides and releasing fatty acids and glycerol for use by the tissues.

CHAPTER REVIEW

A. Sequencer — The Cheeseburger

115. Lipid digestion, absorption, and transport in the blood follow a particularly intricate sequence of events. After consuming a large high-fat cheeseburger, start with the movement of lipid-loaded chyme out of the stomach and into the intestine. From one through fourteen, number the events below in their proper order — the last one has been done for you. As always, use your text to redirect your thinking if you go astray!

___ Mixed micelles of bile salts, lecithin, and cholesterol are secreted from the liver into the duodenum.
___ Triglycerides and phospholipids are reassembled in the intestinal epithelial cells.
___ Cholecystokinin (CCK) hormones are released into the blood in response to the presence of fat in the intestinal chyme.
___ Remnant particles (mostly cholesterol) are removed from the blood by receptor-mediated endocytosis in the liver.
___ Fat hydrolysis occurs due to the presence of pancreatic lipase, colipase, and phospholipase A enzymes.
_14_ Lipoproteins secreted by the liver provide tissue cells with triglycerides, forming low-density lipoproteins (LDL), which transport cholesterol to various organs, including blood vessels.
___ Lipoprotein lipase enzymes attached to the endothelium of blood vessels release free fatty acids and glycerol from chylomicrons for use by tissue cells.
___ Large fat globules flow into the duodenum.
___ Chylomicrons are transported through the lymphatic system and enter the venous blood by way of the thoracic duct.
___ Mixed micelles of bile salts, digested lipids and lecithin move to the brush border of the intestinal epithelium for absorption.
___ Cholecystokinin (CCK) stimulates bile secretion from the liver and contraction of the gallbladder.
___ Liver repackages cholesterol and triglyceride with apoproteins, forming very-low-density lipoproteins (VLDL).
___ Inside the epithelial cells cholesterol and protein are packaged with triglycerides and phospholipids, forming chylomicrons, that migrate into the lymphatic lacteals of the villi.
___ Emulsification results in the formation of tiny droplets of triglycerides in the duodenum.

B. Match 'n' Spell — Digestive Enzymes and Hormones

The large number of digestive enzymes and gastrointestinal tract hormones, with funny-sounding names, often confuses students. Prove me wrong by selecting the correct enzyme or hormone from the list on the right for each of the numbered descriptive statements on the left, below. Write the corresponding letter in the space provided. Of course, you should try to spell these hand-cramping words in the center space. Good luck!

___ 116. liberates intestinal free fatty acids and glycerol _____ a. enterokinase
___ 117. duodenal hormone inhibiting gastric function _____ b. CCK
___ 118. carbohydrate-digesting enzyme inactivated by HCl _____ c. salivary amylase
___ 119. cleaves interior peptide bonds of polypeptides _____ d. pancreatic amylase
___ 120. hormone stimulated by fat and protein in chyme _____ e. gastrin
___ 121. microvilli brush border enzyme (trypsin activator) _____ f. lipoprotein lipase
___ 122. blood vessel enzyme releasing free fatty acids _____ g. lipase and colipase
___ 123. duodenum starch-digesting enzyme _____ h. endopeptidase
___ 124. the first hormone discovered in 1902 _____ i. exopeptidase
___ 125. carboxypeptidase and aminopeptidase are examples _____ j. enterogastrone
___ 126. hormone stimulating gastric secretion and motility _____ k. maltase and sucrase
___ 127. digests disaccharides into monosaccharides _____ l. secretin

C. Essay

Essay Tutorial

This essay tutorial will answer the first essay question found in the "**Review Activities**" section of your *Human Physiology* textbook. Please look for *Essay Question* 1. at the end of chapter 18, read it carefully, and let me guide you through one possible answer. Watch for key terms in bold-face type, helpful tips and general suggestions on writing the essay or short-answer questions. Enjoy!

128. Explain how the gastric secretion of **HCl** and **pepsin** is regulated during the cephalic, gastric, and intestinal phases.

Answer. We have two ways to answer this question. (1) Start with HCl, and follow HCl regulation through these three extrinsic phases; then, in a similar fashion, follow the control of pepsin secretion. (2) First, discuss the three phases of gastric control in their proper sequence, and then compare the control of HCl and pepsin secretion that occurs in each phase.

Let's use the latter method.

Cephalic phase — refers to control by the brain as the vagus nerve carries impulses to the *chief* cells, stimulating *pepsinogen* secretion, and indirectly stimulates the *parietal* cells to secrete HCl. Simultaneously, the vagus nerve directly stimulates *G cells* in the antrum to secrete *gastrin* and the *ECL cells* to secrete *histamine*. The gastrin is circulated back to the stomach, where it also stimulates the ECL cells to release histamine. Histamine, in turn, activates H_2 receptors on the parietal cells to stimulate acid secretion.

Gastric phase — in the stomach, both the distension of the stomach and the presence of polypeptides in chyme increase gastrin release, increasing pepsinogen and HCl secretion as described above. The activity of pepsin and HCl makes more polypeptides, leading to more secretions — a *positive* feedback mechanism. However, by *negative* feedback, too much acid (lower pH) reduces the secretion of gastrin so that stomach pH is related somewhat to the amount of ingested protein. This inhibition of gastrin secretion from G cells may be mediated by the hormone *somatostatin*, secreted by the *D cells* of the stomach.

Intestinal phase — the presence of chyme in the small intestine inhibits both HCl and pepsinogen secretion from the stomach by two mechanisms: (1) the bulk and osmolality of chyme, together with other stimuli, seem to activate neural reflexes which inhibit gastric motility and secretion, and (2) fat in the chyme stimulates the release of the hormone, *enterogastrone*, (and perhaps others such as gastric inhibitory peptide (GIP), CCK, somatostatin, and glucagon-like peptide-1 (GLP-1)) that inhibits the release of HCl and pepsinogen and gastric activity ceases.

Note: An answer in table form (see table 18.7 in the text) is also acceptable, and may be more easily read by your instructor, perhaps leading to a better grade! Now, got time for a couple more?

129. Describe the *digestion*, *absorption*, and *transport* of fats from the intestine to the liver for processing. (*Hint:* see the sequencer, part A.)

130. From the lumen to the outside, list the four layers of the GI wall. Include all smooth muscle layers and nerve networks (plexuses) that innervate these muscles.

131. Draw and label one intestinal *villus*--include the four layers of the intestine, crypts of Lieberkühn, central lacteal, and brush border (simple columnar epithelium). You can check your drawing against figures 18.3 and 18.13 in the text. State the function of each anatomical feature.

132. Describe the structure and function of the *large* intestine. Include a description of the defecation reflex.

133. Describe the unique architecture of the *liver lobule* and the inflow of blood from both the hepatic portal vein and the hepatic artery. How is bile formed in the lobule and where does it go for elimination from the body?

Let's try something new! Here is a comprehensive essay question that is perhaps typical of an essay question on a large examination. I would like you to answer the following "grand essay question."

134. You have just consumed a large, cold, frothy glass of whole milk containing milk sugar (lactose), milk protein, and milk fat. From the mouth, trace the pathway of each nutrient as it is (1) digested, (2) absorbed, (3) transported in the blood, and finally, (4) processed by the tissue cells for energy.

Answers — Chapter 18

I. Introduction to the Digestive System
   A. 1. e, 2. c, 3. a, 4. c, 5. b, 6. d, 7. d
   B. 8. T, 9. T, 10. T, 11 F—Replace "submucosa" with "mucosa," 12. T
II. Esophagus and Stomach
   A. 13. b, 14. c, 15. d, 16. b, 17. c, 18. d
   B. 19. T, 20. T, 21. T, 22. F— Replace "completely" with "partially," 23. T, 24. T, 25. F—Replace "gastric" with "peptic," 26. T, 27. T, 28. F—Antihistamines taken to block gastric acid secretion block H_2 histamine receptors; antihistamines for colds block H_1 histamine receptors
   C. 29. d, 30. c, 31. a, 32. f, 33. b, 34. e

D. Label the Figure — The Stomach; See figure 18.5 in the text.
III. Small Intestine
   A. 35. b, 36. b, 37. a, 38. c, 39. e, 40. d
   B. 41. T, 42. F—Replace "villi" with "microvilli," 43. T, 44. T, 45. F—Replace "pendular action" with "segmentation," 46. T, 47. T, 48. F—Replace "peristalsis" with "segmentation"
IV. Large Intestine
   A. 49. c, 50. e, 51. a, 52 a, 53. c, 54. c
   B. 55. T, 56. T, 57. F—Replace "large" with "small," 58. T, 59. T, 60. T
V. Liver, Gallbladder, and Pancreas
   A. 61 b, 62. c, 63. b, 64. e, 65. b, 66. b, 67. b, 68. b, 69. c, 70. a, 71. e, 72. c
   B. 73. T, 74. T, 75. T, 76. F—Delete "portal," 77. T, 78. T, 79. F—Replace "Bilirubin" with "Urobilinogen," 80. T, 81. T, 82. T, 83. F—Replace "gluconeogenesis" with "glycogenolysis," 84. T, 85. T, 86. F—Replace "endocrine" with "exocrine," 87. T
VI. Neural and Endocrine Regulation of the Digestive System
   A. 88 a, 89. b, 90. c, 91. c, 92 b, 93 e
   B. 94. T, 95. T, 96. F—Replace "reduces" with "increases," 97. T, 98. F—Replace "longer" with "shorter," 99. T, 100. F—Switch "Ca^{2+}" and "cyclic AMP," 101. T, 102. F—Replace "secretin" with "gastrin," 103. T
VII. Digestion and Absorption of Carbohydrates, Lipids, and Proteins
   A. 104. d, 105. a, 106. c, 107. e
   B. 108. F—Replace "Salivary amylase, or ptyalin" with "Pancreatic amylase," 109. T, 110. T, 111. T, 112. F—Replace "less" with "greater," 113. T, 114. T

Chapter Review
   A. 115. 4, 8, 2, 12, 6, 14, 11, 1, 10, 7, 3, 13, 9, 5
   B. 116. g, 117. j, 118. c, 119. h, 120. b, 121. a, 122. f, 123. d, 124. l, 125. i, 126. e, 127.

CHAPTER 19
REGULATION OF METABOLISM

CHAPTER SCOPE

Why do we eat? This simple question, posed in our last chapter scope, actually has a two-part Answer. In the digestive system chapter, we learned that the larger fuel food polymers are digested by specific enzyme reactions into smaller molecules that are absorbed into the blood and distributed to all cells of the body. The second part of the answer is provided in this chapter on the regulation of metabolism. We eat to provide all body cells with absorbed fuel foods, such as *carbohydrates*, *lipids*, and *proteins*, that release energy when combusted along specific **metabolic pathways**. This energy is transferred to make molecules of **ATP**, used immediately by the cell for various functions such as active transport, or is stored for future use as glycogen or fat. Energy that is not directly applied is lost as *heat*. Still more of these absorbed raw materials are required for the synthesis of new molecules to replace those that routinely wear out or are broken down.

These carbohydrate, lipid, and protein fuel molecules are continuously built up (**anabolism**) or broken down (**catabolism**) by tissue cells. **Metabolism** refers to both of these processes occurring simultaneously throughout all body tissues. In chapter 2, anabolic processes were discussed in which these fuel molecules were assembled by *dehydration synthesis*. The catabolic, or hydrolytic, processes were covered later in chapter 5. Here, (1) carbohydrates were combusted during glycolysis, the Krebs cycle, and oxidative phosphorylation reactions; (2) lipids were dismantled during beta-oxidation to acetyl-CoA; and (3) proteins were disassembled during transamination and oxidative deamination reactions. If your memory of these pathways is hazy it should be, because these complicated reactions were discussed very early in the text. If you have the time, this would be an ideal opportunity to review these pages.

Most of this chapter is devoted to the **endocrine** and **neural** control over these metabolic pathways and the problems that can develop when these control systems malfunction, such as in **diabetes mellitus**. The organs and hormones featured will include the (1) *pancreas*, that releases insulin (beta cells) and glucagon (alpha cells); (2) the *adrenal glands*, that release epinephrine (from the medulla) and glucocorticoids (from the cortex); (3) the *anterior pituitary gland*, that releases growth hormone; (4) the *thyroid gland*, that releases throxine (follicle cells) and calcitonin (parafollicular cells); and (5) the *parathyroid glands*, that release parathyroid hormone (PTH) from chief cells. (Please review chapter 11, for further descriptions of these endocrine glands, the general properties of their hormones, and the operation of their second messenger systems.)

I. NUTRITIONAL REQUIREMENTS

The body's requirements must be met by the caloric value of food to prevent catabolism of the body's own fat, carbohydrates, and protein. Additionally, food molecules — particularly the essential amino acids and fatty acids — are needed for replacement of molecules in the body that are continuously degraded. Vitamins and elements do not directly provide energy but instead are required for diverse enzymatic reactions.

A. Multiple Choice

____ 1. Which statement about the total rate of body metabolism, or metabolic rate, is *false*?
    a. The metabolic rate can be measured by the amount of heat generated by the body.
    b. The metabolic rate can be measured by the amount of oxygen consumed by the body per minute.
    c. The metabolic rate is increased both by eating and by physical exercise.
    d. The metabolic rate is decreased when the ambient temperature is lowered (as in hypothermia).
    e. All of these statements regarding the metabolic rate are true.

____ 2. Which factor is *not* involved in the *direct* determination of the *basal metabolic rate* (BMR)?
    a. male or female gender
    b. age
    c. level of thyroid hormone secretions
    d. body frame size
    e. body surface area

____ 3. Which of the following molecules is *not* either an essential fatty acid or an essential amino acid?
    a. riboflavin
    b. methionine
    c. linolenic acid

        d. tryptophan
        e. inoleic acid
___ 4. Which of the following is *not* a *fat-soluble* vitamin?
        a. vitamin A
        b. vitamin D
        c. vitamin C
        d. vitamin E
        e. vitamin K
___ 5. The vitamin that is converted into a hormone with the help of the sun, serving to regulate calcium levels in the blood, is
        a. vitamin D.
        b. vitamin K.
        c. vitamin C.
        d. thiamine.
        e. pyridoxine.
___ 6. Of the following elements, which one is needed in relatively *large* amounts to function as a cofactor for specific enzymes, and therefore, is not a trace element?
        a. fluorine
        b. zinc
        c. magnesium
        d. iron
        e. selenium

B. True or False/Edit

___ 7. A *kilocalorie* is equal to 1,000 calories and can also be written as 1 kCal, or 1 C.
___ 8. A person with *hyperthyroidism* would be expected to have an abnormally high BMR, and a person with *hypothyroidism* to have an abnormally low BMR.
___ 9. A higher than normal BMR in certain obese people may be due to genetic factors which have been inherited.
___ 10. When the intake of carbohydrates, protein, or fat exceeds the energy output, the excess calories are stored in the body primarily as fat.
___ 11. Weight loss can be achieved by dieting alone or in combination with an exercise program to raise the metabolic rate.
___ 12. *Anabolism* (the assembly of polymers) and *catabolism* (the breakdown of polymers) are processes that normally occur simultaneously within cells of the body.
___ 13. Since fat can be made from excess carbohydrates, only a small amount of fat is necessary in the diet to supply the body with the essential fatty acids and adequate quantities of fat-soluble vitamins.
___ 14. There are more essential fatty acids required by the body than there are essential amino acids required by the body.
___ 15. Derivatives of the waterc-soluble vitamins primarily serve as cofactors for specific enzymes involved in the metabolism of carbohydrates, lipids, and proteins.

II. REGULATION OF ENERGY METABOLISM

The blood plasma contains circulating glucose, fatty acids, amino acids, and other molecules that can be used by the body tissues for cell respiration. These circulating molecules may be derived from food or from the breakdown of the body's own glycogen, fat, and protein. The building of the body's energy reserves following a meal, and the utilization of these reserves between meals, is regulated by the action of a number of hormones that act to promote either anabolism or catabolism.

A. Multiple Choice

___ 16. Which of the following is *not* a *circulating energy substrate*?
        a. vitamins
        b. fatty acids
        c. glucose
        d. amino acids
        e. ketone bodies
___ 17. Which statement about *eating behavior* is *false*?
        a. The ventromedial and the lateral areas of the hypothalamus may regulate the feeding and the satiety responses, respectively.
        b. Chemical neurotransmitters such as endorphins may increase eating activity.
        c. The neurotransmitters norepinephrine (stimulates) and serotonin (inhibits) seem to have opposing actions on eating behavior.
        d. The intestinal hormone cholecystokinin (CCK) may act as a neurotransmitter to stop eating activity and promote satiety.
        e. All of these statements regarding eating behavior are true.

____ 18. Which statement about *adipose cells* (*adipocytes*) is *false*?
   a. Adipocytes store fat in large vacuoles, releasing primarily free fatty acids during times of fasting.
   b. Adipocytes are very active cells, and may themselves secrete hormones that play a pivotal role in the regulation of metabolism.
   c. A rise in circulating fatty acid levels promotes the conversion of preadipocytes (derived from fibroblasts) into new adipocytes.
   d. Mostly in children, the prostaglandin, 15d-PGJ$_2$, produced by adipocytes and some other tissues appears to stimulate the formation of new adipocytes.
   e. All of these statements regarding adipocytes are true.

____ 19. The molecule (cytokine) secreted by adipose cells (and other cell types) of obese people that may contribute to the increase in *insulin resistance* (decrease in insulin sensitivity), is called
   a. leptin
   b. 15d-PGJ$_2$ (prostaglandin)
   c. TNFI (Tumor Necrosis Factor, alpha)
   d. CCK (cholecystokinin)
   e. neuropeptide Y

____ 20. The hormone, or *satiety factor* that is coded for by the obese gene, *ob*, and secreted by adipose tissue to decrease appetite, is
   a. leptin
   b. 15d-PGJ$_2$ (prostaglandin)
   c. TNFI (Tumor Necrosis Factor, alpha)
   d. CCK (cholecystokinin)
   e. neuropeptide Y

____ 21. Which of the following substances is a neurotransmitter in the hypothalamus region of the brain with a potent effect of stimulating appetite?
   a. neuropeptide Y
   b. leptin
   c. TNFI (Tumor Necrosis Factor, alpha)
   d. 15d-PGJ$_2$ (prostaglandin)
   e. melanocyte stimulating hormone

____ 22. In which of the following conditions is *obesity not* considered a risk factor?
   a. some malignancies (especially endometrial and breast cancer)
   b. gallbladder disease
   c. diabetes mellitus
   d. Parkinson's disease
   e. cardiovascular diseases

____ 23. Which two hormones have *both* anabolic and catabolic effects? [Hint: see table 19.5]
   a. insulin and glucagon
   b. epinephrine and glucocorticoids
   c. growth hormone and thyroxine
   d. glucagon and thyroxine

B. True or False/Edit

____ 24. Protein is combusted as a secondary, or an emergency, energy source only after glycogen and fat primary *energy reserves* have been utilized.

____ 25. Resting skeletal muscles have an almost absolute requirement for blood glucose as its primary energy source.

____ 26. The *satiety factor* hormone known as *leptin* appears to counterbalance the action of neuropeptide Y, a neurotransmitter and potent stimulator of appetite.

____ 27. When weight is gained, a reduced secretion of leptin from the adipocytes may result in increased production of neuropeptide Y, thus reducing hunger and food intake.

____ 28. Obesity in childhood is due to an increase in both adipocyte size and number; whereas weight gain in adults is due mainly to an increase in adipocyte size.

____ 29. The "pear shape" distribution of body fat places more intra-abdominal fat in the mesenteries and greater omentum, and thus, is a better predictor of cardiovascular disease than is an increase in subcutaneous fat seen in the "apple shape"

____ 30. Obesity is often diagnosed using a measurement derived from body weight (in kilograms) and height (in meters, squared) called the *body mass index* (BMI).

____ 31. The *postabsorptive* state starts about 4 hours after a meal and continues until the next meal; and is generally referred to as the fasting state.

____ 32. Glucagon, growth hormone, glucocorticoids, and epinephrine are all catabolic hormones that break down larger lipid energy reserves into simpler circulating free fatty acid substrates (lipolysis). [*Hint:* see table 19.5]

C. Label the Figure — Hormones That Balance Metabolism

Study figure 19.1 carefully. In the spaces provided, write the proper *metabolic process, fuel molecule,* or the *name of the hormone* that is involved in the balanced regulation of anabolism (buildup) and catabolism (breakdown) of carbohydrates, lipids, and protein. Notice the direction of the arrows. Can you name the two hormones that are active in *both* anabolism and catabolism? If you get stuck, sneak a peak at figure 19.2 in your text.

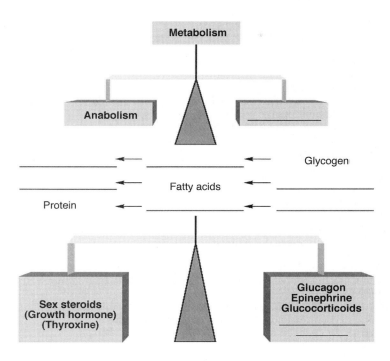

Figure 19.1   The balance of metabolism can be tilted toward anabolism (synthesis of energy reserves) or catabolism (utilization of energy reserves) by the combined actions of various hormones. Growth hormone and thyroxine have both anabolic and catabolic effects.

III. ENERGY REGULATION BY THE ISLETS OF LANGERHANS

Insulin secretion is stimulated by a rise in blood glucose concentration, and insulin promotes the entry of blood glucose into tissue cells. Insulin thus increases the storage of glycogen and fat while causing the blood glucose concentration to fall. Glucagon secretion is stimulated by a fall in blood glucose, and glucagon acts to raise the blood glucose concentration by promoting glycogenolysis in the liver.

A. Multiple Choice

___ 33. The hormone secreted by the delta cells of the islets of Langerhans, that is identical to that produced by the hypothalamus and the intestine, is
   a. insulin
   b. glucagon
   c. somatostatin

___ 34. The most numerous cells of the islets of Langerhans are the _____ cells that secrete the hormone _____.
   a. alpha; insulin
   b. beta; insulin
   c. delta; glucagon
   d. beta; glucagon
   e. delta; insulin

___ 35. Which statement about the regulation of insulin and glucagon from the islets of Langerhans is *false*?
   a. Alpha and beta cells respond to changes in both the glucose and the amino acid concentrations in the plasma.
   b. Homeostasis regulates insulin and glucagon levels by negative feedback loops.
   c. Alpha and beta cells act both as sensors and effectors in regulation of their secretion of hormones.

        d. After a meal, the rise in plasma glucose levels stimulates the release of insulin.
        e. All of these statements about the regulation of insulin and glucagon from the islets of Langerhans are true.

____ 36. Which response to stimulation of the autonomic nervous system is *not* correct?
        a. Both sympathetic and parasympathetic nerves innervate the islets of Langerhans.
        b. Parasympathetic stimulation decreases insulin secretion.
        c. Sympathetic stimulation increases glucagon secretion.
        d. Together with epinephrine, glucagon is involved in "stress hyperglycemia," when the sympathetic nerves are stimulated.
        e. During meals, parasympathetic nerve activity stimulates gastrointestinal motility and secretion.

____ 37. Which of the following effects is *not* promoted by insulin?
        a. Increase in cellular uptake of plasma glucose.
        b. Synthesis of glycogen in liver and muscle cells (glycogenesis).
        c. Synthesis of triglycerides (fat) in adipose cells (lipogenesis).
        d. Increase in cellular uptake of plasma fatty acids.
        e. Increase in cellular uptake of plasma amino acids.

____ 38. Which statement about the *postabsorptive*, or fasting state, is *false*?
        a. Glucagon secretion is high and insulin secretion is low.
        b. Glucose-6-phosphatase enzymes in the liver stimulate hydrolysis of liver glycogen to free glucose molecules (glycogenolysis).
        c. Muscle glycogen stores can only be used by the muscle cells for energy.
        d. Liver glycogen stores can only be used by the liver cells for energy.
        e. Hormones promote the formation of glucose from noncarbohydrate molecules (gluconeogenesis).

____ 39. The enzyme, hormone-sensitive lipase
        a. is found only in liver cells.
        b. is sensitive to, and activated by, the hormone insulin.
        c. promotes the hydrolysis of stored triglycerides, releasing free fatty acids and glycerol into the blood.
        d. converts triglycerides into ketone bodies as an alternative energy source.
        e. is most active immediately following ingestion of a meal.

B. True or False/Edit

____ 40. In the islets of Langerhans of the pancreas, the alpha and beta cells act as both the sensors and effectors in the negative feedback regulation (homeostasis) of plasma glucose levels.

____ 41. During the absorption of a carbohydrate meal, stimulation of the alpha cells causes the secretion of *glucagon* which acts to lower blood glucose levels by promoting its uptake by the tissues.

____ 42. A fall in plasma glucose will stimulate the alpha cells to secrete glucagon and inhibit the release of insulin from beta cells.

____ 43. One effect of glucagon is to lower the concentration of glucose in the blood by promoting the synthesis of glucose by the liver (gluconeogenesis).

____ 44. The *oral glucose tolerance test* is a clinical procedure in which a high glucose solution is drunk that challenges the ability of the beta cells to secrete insulin and lower the subsequent rise in blood glucose levels.

____ 45. Meals rich in protein and low in carbohydrates can stimulate the secretion of both insulin and glucagon from the pancreas — promoting amino acid entry into tissue cells and a rise in blood glucose.

____ 46. Relaxed eating environments will encourage parasympathetic stimulation of the pancreas and the subsequent increase in insulin secretion.

____ 47. *Gastric inhibitory peptide (GIP)* is also known as *glucose-dependent insulinotropic peptide* since it is released by the presence of glucose in the intestinal chyme to stimulate insulin secretion from the pancreas, even before plasma glucose levels begin to rise.

____ 48. The overall effect of glucagon is to lower blood *glucose* and *amino acid* levels by promoting their cellular uptake and incorporation into glycogen and proteins, respectively.

____ 49. One anabolic effect of insulin is the synthesis of triglycerides (lipogenesis) from glucose transported into adipose cells following a meal.

____ 50. There is a maximum of about 100 g of stored glycogen in the skeletal muscles, whereas the liver can store approximately 375-400 g of glycogen.

____ 51. Glycogen stores in liver and skeletal muscle have a maximum, in that once these stores are filled, continued ingestion of excess calories will increase the production of fat.

____ 52. During fasting, *gluconeogenesis* promotes the synthesis of new glucose molecules from noncarbohydrate substrates such as certain amino acids and pyruvic acid molecules derived from muscle tissue.

___ 53. During fasting or starvation, several organs in the body can use *ketone bodies* derived from fatty acid metabolism as an alternative energy source; and thus spare glucose for use by the brain.

___ 54. Insulin is active primarily after eating (absorption), whereas glucagon is most active between meals (fasting).

C. Label the Figure — Insulin and Glucagon Effects on Glucose Metabolism

Study figure 19.2 carefully. In the spaces provided, write the name of the hormone (*insulin* or *glucagon*) or the terms *cellular uptake*, *glycogenolysis*, or *gluconeogenesis*. Notice the upward (increase) and downward (decrease) direction on all arrows. Can you explain why the effects of these hormones are said to be *antagonistic*. If you need help, refer to figure 19.5 in the text.

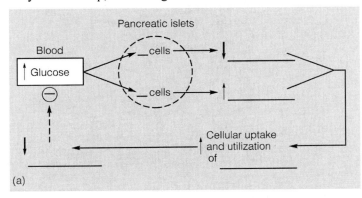

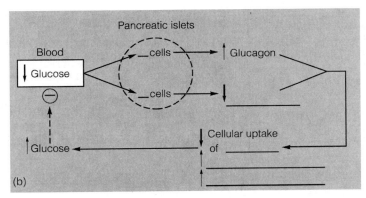

Figure 19.2 The secretion from the β (beta) cells and α (alpha) cells of the pancreatic islets (of Langerhans) is regulated largely by the blood glucose concentration. (a) A high blood glucose concentration stimulates insulin and inhibits glucagon secretion. (b) A low blood glucose concentration stimulates glucagon and inhibits insulin secretion.

IV. DIABETES MELLITUS AND HYPOGLYCEMIA

Inadequate secretion of insulin, or defects in the action of insulin, produce metabolic disturbances that are characteristic of the disease diabetes mellitus. A person with type I diabetes requires injections of insulin; a person with type II diabetes can control this condition by other methods. In both types, hyperglycemia and glycosuria result from the deficiency and/or defective action of insulin. A person with reactive hypoglycemia, by contrast, secretes excessive amounts of insulin, and thus experiences hypoglycemia in response to the stimulus of a carbohydrate meal.

A. Multiple Choice

___ 55. Which general statement about diabetes mellitus is *false*?
  a. Diabetes mellitus is characterized by low blood sugar levels (hyoglycemia).
  b. Diabetes mellitus can result from inadequate insulin release when beta cells are destroyed.
  c. Diabetes mellitus can result from target cells not responding to insulin (increased resistance).
  d. Glucose usually "spills over" into the urine (glycosuria).
  e. There are two basic forms of diabetes mellitus, type I and type II.

___ 56. *Type II diabetes mellitus* is characterized by
  a. the destruction of the beta cells by an autoimmune attack or by viruses, for example.

      b. the absence of the hormone insulin in the plasma.
      c. its occurrence in people over age 40, representing 90% of the people with diabetes mellitus.
      d. diagnosis in people under age 30, and thus, once called *juvenile-onset diabetes*.
      e. abnormally high plasma levels of the hormone, glucagon.

___ 57. In people with *type I diabetes mellitus*,
      a. large amounts of free fatty acids are released from adipose cells (lipolysis).
      b. the liver raises the blood levels of ketone bodies (ketosis).
      c. the pH of the blood may go down (become more acidic) as more acids are made.
      d. osmotic diuresis may cause dehydration and thirst as water follows the excess solute into the urine.
      e. All of these occur in people with type I diabetes mellitus.

___ 58. *Reactive hypoglycemia* is a condition characterized by
      a. inadequate insulin secretion from the beta cells.
      b. being genetically predisposed to type I diabetes (IDDM).
      c. an exaggerated response of beta cells to a rise in blood glucose levels.
      d. diagnosis when the oral glucose tolerance test results in blood glucose levels that rise sharply and stay elevated for 5 hours.
      e. treatment consisting of two or three large, high-carbohydrate meals a day.

B. True or False/Edit

___ 59. *Type I* diabetes is *insulin-dependent diabetes mellitus (IDDM)*, formerly called *juvenile-onset* diabetes, occurring in about 10% of the patients with diabetes in this country.

___ 60. *Type II* diabetes mellitus, also known as *non-insulin-dependent diabetes mellitus (NIDDM)* usually occurs in adults over thirty years of age (*maturity-onset* diabetes) and is commonly associated with obesity.

___ 61. *Type I* diabetics (IDDM) may actually secrete normal or slightly elevated amounts of the hormone insulin from the beta cells of the islets of Langerhans.

___ 62. *Obesity* seems to increase the sensitivity of target cells to insulin, increasing the efficiency of glucose uptake by tissue cells.

___ 63. People with *NIDDM* have an abnormally high tissue sensitivity to insulin, or a lowered *insulin resistance*.

___ 64. People with *NIDDM* do not usually develop ketoacidosis; but are at risk of blindness, kidney failure, and amputation of the lower extremities due to prolonged exposure to high blood glucose levels.

___ 65. *Hypoglycemia*, and possibly a coma, can result in patients with type I diabetes (IDDM) who inject themselves with an overdose of insulin to prevent hyperglycemia and ketoacidosis.

V. METABOLIC REGULATION BY ADRENAL HORMONES, THYROXINE, AND GROWTH HORMONE

Epinephrine, the glucocorticoids, thyroxine, and growth hormone stimulate the catabolism of carbohydrates and lipids. These hormones are thus antagonistic to insulin in their regulation of carbohydrate and lipid metabolism. Thyroxine and growth hormone, however, stimulate protein synthesis and are needed for body growth and proper development of the central nervous system. These hormones thus have an anabolic effect on protein synthesis, which is complementary to that of insulin.

A. Multiple Choice

___ 66. Which statement about the *adrenal gland* is *false*?
      a. The adrenal *medulla* secretes the catecholamine hormones, epinephrine, and norepinephrine.
      b. The adrenal *cortex* secretes mineralocorticoids, such as aldosterone, and glucocorticoids, such as cortisol.
      c. The adrenal medulla responds to sympathetic nerve activity.
      d. The adrenal cortex secretes adrenocorticotropic hormone (ACTH).
      e. The adrenal cortex and medulla have different embryonic origins.

___ 67. Which statement about the hormone, *thyroxine* is *false*?
      a. Thyroxine is also called tetraiodothyronine, or T_4.
      b. Thyroxine is released from the thyroid follicles when stimulated by TSH from the anterior pituitary.
      c. Thyroxine has target cells in almost every organ of the body.
      d. Thyroxine is a prehormone that must first be converted to T_3 within the target cells to be active.
      e. All of these statements about thyroxine are true.

___ 68. Which action of *thyroxine* is *false*?
      a. Thyroxine stimulates the rate of cell respiration in almost all cells of the body.
      b. Thyroxine reduces the concentration of ATP in target cells.
      c. Thyroxine reduces body heat production during cold adaptation.

  d. Thyroxine concentration is directly related to the basal metabolic rate (BMR).
  e. All of these statements about thyroxine are true.
___ 69. Cretinism
  a. is due to an overactive thyroid (hyperthyroidism).
  b. results in severe mental retardation.
  c. results from a lack of growth hormone.
  d. s a permanent condition and cannot be treated.
  e. usually occurs after puberty.
___ 70. Symptoms of *hyperthyroidism* include
  a. decreased activity, lethargy, and increased sleep.
  b. irritability and an intolerance to heat.
  c. myxedema, accumulation of subcutaneous mucoproteins and fluid.
  d. constipation, decreased appetite, and weight gain.
  e. psychological depression and apathy.
___ 71. Which statement about *growth hormone* (GH) is *false*?
  a. GH is secreted in adults as well as in children.
  b. GH is also known as *somatotropic* hormone.
  c. GH is inhibited by *somatostatin* from the hypothalamus.
  d. GH is synthesized and released by the posterior pituitary.
  e. GH secretion follows a *circadian* rhythm, rising during sleep.
___ 72. Which statement about *growth hormone* (GH) is *false*?
  a. GH secretion increases after absorbing a high protein meal.
  b. GH secretion falls during prolonged fasting.
  c. GH secretion rises when plasma glucose levels fall.
  d. GH stimulates the catabolism of fat and release of fatty acids from adipose tissue.
  e. GH has both anabolic (protein) and catabolic (fat) effects.
___ 73. In adults, the oversecretion of *growth hormone* (GH) causes
  a. gigantism.
  b. Graves' disease.
  c. acromegaly.
  d. dwarfism.
  e. cretinism.

B. True or False/Edit

___ 74. The metabolic effects of epinephrine on its target cells are similar to those of the hormone, insulin.
___ 75. Both glucagon and epinephrine stimulate glycogenolysis, with release of glucose from the liver; and lipolysis, with release of fatty acids from adipose cells.
___ 76. Epinephrine and glucagon hormones have similar mechanisms of action that are both mediated by *cyclic AMP second messengers* in their target cells.
___ 77. Prolonged fasting or exercise stimulates the release of *ACTH* from the anterior pituitary, which, in turn, stimulates an increase in the secretion of *glucocorticoid* hormones from the adrenal cortex.
___ 78. Stress-induced release of *glucocorticoids* such as hydrocortisone (cortisol), results in the release of amino acids, glucose, fatty acids, and ketone bodies into the blood to help compensate for the state of stress.
___ 79. Thyroxine inhibits the rate of cell respiration in almost all cells in the body.
___ 80. Thyroxine is also considered an *anabolic* hormone since it is necessary for normal growth of the skeleton and for proper development of the central nervous system (CNS).
___ 81. *Graves' disease* is a disorder in which autoantibodies are produced that have TSH-like effects, stimulating the thyroid gland and forming a goiter.
___ 82. Blood levels of growth hormone fluctuate each day (circadian), with highest levels reached when awake (daytime).
___ 83. Growth hormone has both *anabolic* (protein synthesis) and *catabolic* (fat breakdown) effects on various target cells.
___ 84. The skeleton growth-promoting effects of growth hormone seem to be mediated by the *somatomedins*, IGF-1 and IGF-2 proteins, which stimulate the chondrocytes (cartilage cells) to divide and secrete more matrix and exhibit insulin-like actions.
___ 85. An inadequate secretion of growth hormone during the growing years results in *dwarfism*.

VI. REGULATION OF CALCIUM AND PHOSPHATE BALANCE

A normal blood Ca^{2+} concentration is critically important for contraction of muscles and maintenance of proper membrane permeability. Parathyroid hormone promotes an elevation in blood Ca^{2+} by stimulating *resorption of the calcium phosphate crystals from bone and renal excretion of phosphate. A derivative of vitamin D produced in the body, 1,25-dihydroxyvitamin D₃, promotes the intestinal absorption of calcium and phosphate.*

A. Multiple Choice

___ 86. Which statement about *bone* is *false*?
    a. Bone serves as a large store of calcium and carbonate
    b. Calcium is stored as *calcium phosphate* in the form of hydroxyapatite crystals in bone.
    c. *Osteoblasts* (bone-forming cells), secrete an organic matrix of collagen protein that becomes hardened by deposits of hydroxyapatite.
    d. *Osteoclast* cells routinely dissolve hydroxyapatite crystals, a process called *resorption*.
    e. Bone formation and resorption rates are determined by hormones.

___ 87. Which effect is *not* mediated by calcium ion (Ca^{2+})?
    a. excitation-contraction coupling in muscles
    b. as the second messenger in the action of certain hormones
    c. oxygen-binding ion within heme groups of hemoglobin
    d. maintain proper membrane permeability to Na^+ and to other ions
    e. combines with phosphate to harden bone

___ 88. Which bone disorder is due to excessive secretion of *parathyroid hormone* (PTH)?
    a. rickets
    b. osteomalacia
    c. osteoporosis
    d. steitis fibrosa cystica

___ 89. Which statement about *parathyroid hormone* (PTH) is *false*?
    a. PTH is released when blood Ca^{2+} levels fall.
    b. PTH stimulates the resorption of bone by osteoclasts.
    c. PTH increases Ca^{2+} (but not phosphate) reabsorption from the glomerular filtrate of the kidney nephrons.
    d. PTH promotes the formation of *1,25-dihydroxyvitamin D₃* in the kidneys.
    e. All of these statements about PTH are true.

___ 90. The synthesis of 1,25-dihydroxyvitamin D₃
    a. begins when sunlight strikes the skin.
    b. requires activity of hydroxylation enzymes made in liver cells.
    c. requires activity of hydroxylation enzymes made in the kidneys.
    d. is promoted by parathyroid hormone (PTH) stimulating the enzymes involved synthesis of the vitamin.
    e. All of these statements about the synthesis of *1,25-dihydroxyvitamin D₃* are true.

___ 91. In a normal diet, *1,25-dihydroxyvitamin D₃* stimulates the
    a. intestinal absorption of calcium and phosphate.
    b. deposition of calcium and phosphate into bone.
    c. body's loss of calcium and phosphate in the urine.
    d. fall in both calcium and phosphate levels in the blood.
    e. distribution of the pigment, *melanin*, in the skin following sun exposure (a tan).

___ 92. Which statement about *calcitonin* is *false*?
    a. Calcitonin is secreted by the *parafollicular* cells, or *C cells* of the thyroid gland.
    b. Calcitonin acts to lower blood Ca^{2+} levels by inhibiting the activity of *osteoclasts*, thus reducing bone resorption.
    c. Calcitonin inhibits the reabsorption of calcium and phosphate in the kidney nephrons, thus increasing their urinary excretion.
    d. Calcitonin's action is clearly antagonistic to that of parathyroid hormone and is, therefore, required to maintain calcium homeostasis.
    e. Very large doses (pharmacological doses) of calcitonin are clinically useful in the treatment of Paget's disease of the bone.

B. True or False/Edit

___ 93. Continuously throughout life the bone-forming cells, or *osteoclasts*, serve to construct bone while simultaneously, the bone-dissolving cells, or *osteoblasts* work to resorb bone.

___ 94. By the age of fifty or sixty, the rate of bone resorption often exceeds the rate of bone deposition.

___ 95. The three hormones most involved in the endocrine regulation of calcium and phosphate balance are *parathyroid hormone* (PTH), *1,25-hydroxyvitamin D₃*, and *calcitonin*.

___ 96. Osteoporosis is most common in postmenopausal women, where the reduction in the secretion of estrogen from the ovaries may be related to inadequate osteoblast activity.

___ 97. *Parathyroid hormone* (PTH) is released when the plasma Ca^{2+} levels rise, stimulating the activity of osteoblast cells in bone.

___ 98. Surgical removal of the parathyroid glands results in a rise in calcium levels in the plasma (*hypercalcemia*).
___ 99. *Vitamin D₃* functions as a prehormone which must be chemically changed in order to become biologically active.
___ 100. The primary function of *1,25-dihydroxyvitamin D₃* is to raise the blood levels of calcium and phosphate, by promoting their absorption in the intestine from food.
___ 101. Low blood calcium levles can be raised by the combined actions of parathyroid hormone (PTH) and 1,25-dihydroxyvitamin D₃.

VII. CHAPTER REVIEW

A. Completion

102. Your metabolic rate is influenced by a number of factors, including _____, _____, and _____ _____; and is often measured as the rate of _____ consumption. 103. Chemical energy, or potential energy, in food we eat is measured in units of hear caled _____. Excess energy from carbohydrates, protein, and fat that is not comusted will be stored primarily as _____. 104. The fat-soluble vitamins are _____, _____, _____, and _____, with the remaining vitamins soluble in the solvent _____.

105. In the body, the three main energy reserves (stores) available for use by the tissues are _____, _____, and _____, which are broken down into simpler energy substrates for combustion in cell respiration. 106. Eating behavior seems to be controlled by the _____ region of the brain, stimulating overeating (hyperphagia) or undereating _____. Four neurotransmitters (neurohormones?) have also been associated with eating behavior, including _____, _____, _____, and _____.

107. Hormones also regulate the distribution of energy through specific actions on metabolism. The islets of _____ in the _____ secrete two important hormones: _____ from the alpha cells and insulin from the _____ cells. 108. A rise in plasma glucose concentration stimulates the secretion of _____ and inhibits the secretion of _____ from the islets; whereas a rise in plasma amino acids _____ (stimulates/inhibits) secretion of both insulin and glucagon. Both parasympathetic stimulation and enterogastrone or gastric inhibitory peptide (GIP) from the intestine _____ (increase/decrease) the release of insulin, which _____ (raises/lowers) blood glucose levels and _____ (stimulate/inhibits) the synthesis of fat within adipose cells. 109. Fasting _____ (increases/decreases) glucagon secretion, which stimulates the breakdown _____ (anabolism/catabolism) of stored _____ and _____, thus increasing blood glucose levels.

110. Type I, or _____ (IDDM/NIDDM) diabetes mellitus results when pancreatic _____ (alpha/beta) cells are destroyed such that plasma insulin levels _____ (rise/fall) and plasma glucagon levels _____ (rise/fall). 111. In Type II, or _____ (IDDM/NIDDM), diabetes, the target cells are _____ (more/less) responsive to the insulin present and is associated with _____ (obesity/leanness). Type _____ diabetes mellitus is the more common form.

112. Epinephrine from the adrenal _____ (cortex/medulla) has effects that are similar to those of the hormone _____ from the pancreas, whereas _____ is a glucocorticoid from the adrenal _____ (cortex/medulla) that promotes muscle protein _____ (anabolism/catabolism) and conversion of amino acids to _____ (gluconeogenesis) in the liver. 113. The basal metabolic rate (BMR) is set by the hormone _____, which _____ (increases/decreases) the rate of cell respiration in most body cells. Thyroxine is especially important in synthesis of _____ during normal growth and development of the _____ nervous system. 114. Growth hormone (GH) is synthesized by the _____ _____ (2 words) gland, where it is released and inhibited by hormones from the _____. Growth hormone is secreted following a high-_____ meal and when blood glucose levels _____ during fasting. The promotion of body growth by growth hormone occurs indirectly through polypeptides such as IGF-1 and IGF-2, known as _____.

115. Hydroxyapatite crystals in bone contain the minerals _____ and _____. Bone formation is performed by _____ (osteoblasts/osteoclasts), whereas bone resorption is done by _____. 116. Parathyroid hormone (PTH) is released when plasma Ca^{2+} levels are _____ (high/low), thus stimulating bone _____ (deposition/resorption) and _____ (increasing/decreasing) reabsorption of Ca^{2+} from the kidney. PTH also activates a kidney hydroxylation enzyme, which adds a hydroxyl group (OH) to the number 25 carbon of vitamin _____, forming _____. 117. This vitamin _____ (increases/decreases) the intestinal absorption of calcium and phosphate, _____ (increases/decreases) bone resorption, and _____ (increases/decreases) the reabsorption of phosphate from the kidney tubules. This overall effect results in a rise in both Ca^{2+} and phosphate

levels when Ca²⁺ concentrations in the blood fall. 118. Calcitonin is a hormone secreted by the _____ cells of the _____ gland when plasma Ca²⁺ levels are too _____ (high/low). Calcitonin _____ (raises/lowers) blood Ca²⁺ by inhibiting bone _____ (resorption/deposition) and _____ (increasing/decreasing) urinary excretion of calcium and phosphate.

B. Crossword Puzzle — Regulation of Metabolism

Across
1. most available source of energy, especially for brain tissue
2. islet of Langerhans cells that secrete *glucagon*
3. _____ism: glandular condition that results in an increase in BMR
6. coenzyme derived from the vitamin, *niacin* (B₃)
8. circulating energy substrate that can be stored in large quantity-known as a(an) _____ acid
10. the sum total of catabolism and anabolism
12. measure of energy provided in foods — unit of heat
14. person who suffered from hypothyroidism during the prenatal or early infant growth periods
15. hormone secreted by the intestine to stimulate insulin secretion
18. the process of hydrolysis and other chemical reactions that break down larger molecules
20. a property common to vitamins A, D, E, and K
21. islet of Langerhans cells that secrete *insulin*
23. a festive occasion; celebration
26. when not idle, you are _____
27. an abnormal blood glucose condition that may develop following excessive insulin injection by a diabetic
28. circulating energy substrate, other than carbohydrate or fat
30. hormones from the *adrenal cortex*, such as hydrocortisone
31. endocrine gland with a distinct cortex and medulla that secrete various hormones for regulating metabolism
33. hormone that stimulates the rate of cell respiration in almost all cells of the body
35. a period of time characterized by not eating
36. physical property common to vitamin C and other vitamins involved in cell respiration
37. an essential trace element, needed to assemble hemoglobin molecules
38. common expression when departing
39. disfiguring bone disease of children due to a lack of *1,25-dihydroxyvitamin D₃*
41. hormone most responsible for the uptake of blood glucose into tissue cells
42. a primary target tissue for *growth hormone*
44. abnormally high levels of glucose in the blood
46. part of the brain somewhat involved in regulating eating behavior
52. one component of hydroxyapatite crystals
53. insulin stimulates the uptake of glucose into the _____
54. another component of hydroxyapatite crystals
55. vitamin that, if deficient, causes *pellagra*

Down
1. storage form of carbohydrate in liver and muscle tissue
2. another name for fat cells
4. molecules that the body cannot make and therefore must be eaten as part of the diet
5. what happens to blood calcium levels in the presence of *parathyroid hormone* (PTH)
7. destination for excess calories that are not expended by activity
8. a *coenzyme* derived from the vitamin, riboflavin (B₂)
9. pancreatic hormone that raises blood glucose levels during periods of fasting
11. main "fight-or-flight" hormone released from the *adrenal medulla*
13. food that is not properly cared for or preserved will _____
16. hired enforcer at the door to your favorite dance hall
17. thyroid hormone secreted when blood calcium levels rise above normal
19. the buildup or assembly of larger molecules from smaller molecules
22. gland that secretes a hormone that stimulates bone *resorption* and kidney calcium *reabsorption*
24. glandular condition, _____ism: with symptoms including *myxedema* and *goiter*
25. essential compounds that serve primarily as *coenzymes* to assist metabolic enzymes
29. disease often described as type I or type II
32. an important *trace element* and enzyme *cofactor*
34. inappropriately high body weight; a risk factor in many disorders such as cardiovascular disease
40. the general name for any atom found in the periodic table
43. portion of the adrenal gland that secretes epinephrine and norepinephrine
45. hormone regulated by both releasing and inhibiting hormones from the *hypothalamus*
47. bone-softening disease caused by increased osteoclast activity
48. one important metabolic organ that hydroxylates vitamin D
49. the assemblage of food and drink consumed while eating
50. Mrs. _____, a former U.S. president's wife with Graves' disease
51. measured by oxygen consumption 12-14 hours after eating and comfortable

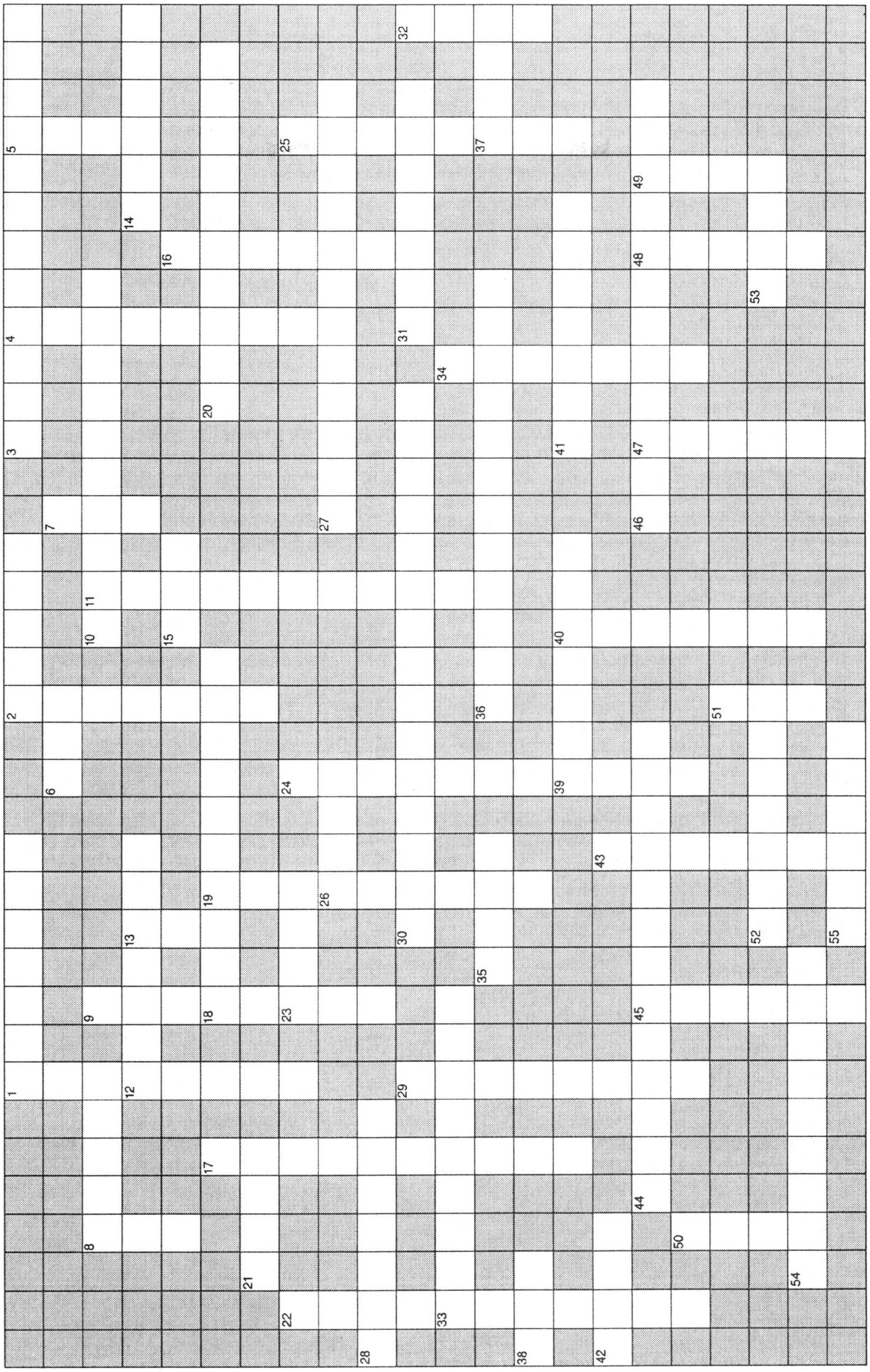

C. Essay

Essay Tutorial

This essay tutorial will answer the first essay question found in the "**Review Activities**" section of your *Human Physiology* textbook. Please look for *Essay Question* 1. at the end of chapter 19, read it carefully, and let me guide you through one possible answer. Watch for key terms in bold-face type, helpful tips and general suggestions on writing the essay or short-answer questions. Enjoy!

119. Compare the metabolic effects of **fasting** to the state of uncontrolled *insulin-dependent diabetes mellitus*. Explain the hormonal *similarities* of these conditions.

Answer. Fasting results in lowered blood glucose concentrations as glucose is expended as fuel in cell respiration. In response, *glucagon* hormones are released from the alpha cells of the pancreas. Glucagon stimulates the hydrolysis of glycogen reserves (glycogenolysis) mainly in the liver, the breakdown of fat (lipolysis) from adipose tissue, the synthesis of glucose from amino acids (gluconeogenesis) in the liver, and the formation of ketone bodies (ketosis) — all in the effort to provide circulating *energy substrates* for use by the starving cells. Since plasma glucose and amino acid levels are low, insulin secretion is also low.

Type I diabetes mellitus (*IDDM*) is uncontrolled when insulin is not being provided (usually by injection) in response to a rise in blood sugar levels. Hormone levels during fasting conditions are similar to those during this type of uncontrolled diabetes in that the blood concentrations of glucagon are high and insulin concentrations are low. Without insulin yet with increased amounts of glucagon, type I diabetics have high blood glucose concentrations (hyperglycemia) in addition to an increased release of fatty acids from adipose cells. In the liver, newly releasaed fatty acids are converted to ketone bodies causing blood levels of ketones to rise (ketosis). When the blood buffers such as bicarbonate are limited, *ketoacidosis* results, just as it does in fasting conditions. Therefore, both fasting and type I diabetic individuals are similar in that each is unable to utilize glucose molecules as a source of fuel, so that cells must depend on other circulating energy substrates such as fatty acids and ketone bodies (ketoacids) liberated by the actions of primarily glucagon for meeting metabolic demands.

Whew! This was a tough question. Again, don't be disappointed if your answer differs from mine. Your efforts will give you valuable practice in answering essay-formatted questions and help you understand concepts in physiology. Now, let's work on a few more.

120. Define the term **Calorie.** Describe how this unit of heat is used as a measure of the energy *content* of fuel food — such as carbohydrate, fat, and protein — and as a measure of energy *output* during physical activity.

121. Discuss the possible roles played by the *sex hormones*, *growth hormone*, and *somatomedins* (IGF-1 and IGF-2) in the growth and development that occur during puberty.

122. Distinguish between the target cell actions of *parathyroid hormone* (PTH), *1,25-dihydroxyvitamin D₃*, and *calcitonin* in the effort to maintain blood levels of calcium and phosphate constant (homeostasis).

123. Describe how a state of prolonged fasting or exercise can be partially compensated by synthesis of *corticosteroids* (e.g., hydrocortisone). Explain how these effects are similar to those of *glucagon*.

Answers — Chapter 19

I. Nutritional Requirements
   A. 1.e 2.d 3.a 4.c 5.a 6.c
   B. 7.T 8.T 9.F—Replace "higher" with "lower" 10.T 11.T 12.T 13.T 14.F—Switch "fatty" and "amino" 15.F—Replace "cofactors" with "coenzymes"

II. Regulation of Energy Metabolism
   A. 16.a 17.e 18.e 19.c 20.a 21.a 22.c 23.c
   B. 24.T 25.F—Replace "Skeletal muscle" with "The brain" 26.T 27.F—Switch "reduced" with "increased" 28.T 29.F—Switch "pear" with "apple" 30. T 31.T 32.T
   C. Label the Figure — Hormones That Balance Metabolism; See figure 19.2 in the text.

III. Energy Regulation by the Islets of Langerhans
   A. 33.c 34.b 35.e 36.b 37.d 38.d 39.c
   B. 40.T 41.F—Replace "alpha" with "beta," "glucagon" with "insulin" 42.T 43.F—Replace "gluconeogenesis" with "glycogenolysis" 44.T 45.T 46.T 47.T 48.F—Replace "glucagon" with "insulin" 49.T 50.F—Switch "liver" and "skeletal muscles" 51.T 52.T 53.T 54.T
   C. Label the Figure — Insulin and Glucagon Effects on Glucose Metabolism.
   See figure 19.5 in the text.

IV. Diabetes Mellitus and Hypoglycemia
   A. 55.a 56.c 57.e 58.c
   B. 59.T 60.T 61.F—Replace "I (NIDDM)" with "II (IDDM)" 62.F—Replace "obesity" with "exercise" 63.F-Replace "high" with "low," "lowered" with "raised" 64.T 65.T

V. Metabolic Regulation by Adrenal Hormones, Thyroxine, and Growth Hormone
   A. 66.d 67.e 68.c 69.b 70.b 71.d 72.b 73.c
   B. 74.F—Replace "insulin" with "glucagon" 75.T 76.T 77.T 78.T 79.F—Replace "inhibits" with "stimulates" 80.T 81.T 82.F—Replace "awake (daytime)" with "asleep (nighttime)" 83.T 84.T 85.T

VI. Regulation of Calcium and Phosphate Balance
   A. 86.a 87.c 88.d 89.e 90.e 91.a 92.d
   B. 93.F—Switch "osteoclasts" and "osteoblasts" 94.T 95.T 96.T 97.F—Replace "rise" with "fall;" "osteoblast" with "osteoclast", 98.F—Replace "rise" with "fall;" "hypercalcemia" with "hypocalcemia" 99.T 100.T 101.T

VII. Chapter Review
   A. 102.temperature, eating, physical activity, oxygen 103.kilocalories; fat; coenzymes, cofactors, 104.A, D, E, K, water, 105.glycogen, fat, protein, 106.hypothalamus, hypophagia; endorphins, norepinephrine, serotonin, CCK, 107.Langerhans, pancreas, glucagon, beta, 108.insulin, glucagon, stimulates; increase, lowers, stimulates, 109.increases, catabolism, glycogen, fat, 110.IDDM, beta, fall, rise, 111.NIDDM, less, obesity; II. 112.medulla, glucagon, cortisol, cortex, anabolism, glucose, 113.thyroxine, increases; proteins, central, 114.anterior pituitary, hypothalamus; protein, fall; somatomedins, 115.calcium, phosphate; osteoblasts, osteoclasts, 116.low, resorption, increasing; D₃, 1,25-dihydroxyvitamin D₃, 117.increases, increases, increases, 118.parafollicular, thyroid, high; lowers, resorption, increasing.

B. Crossword Puzzle

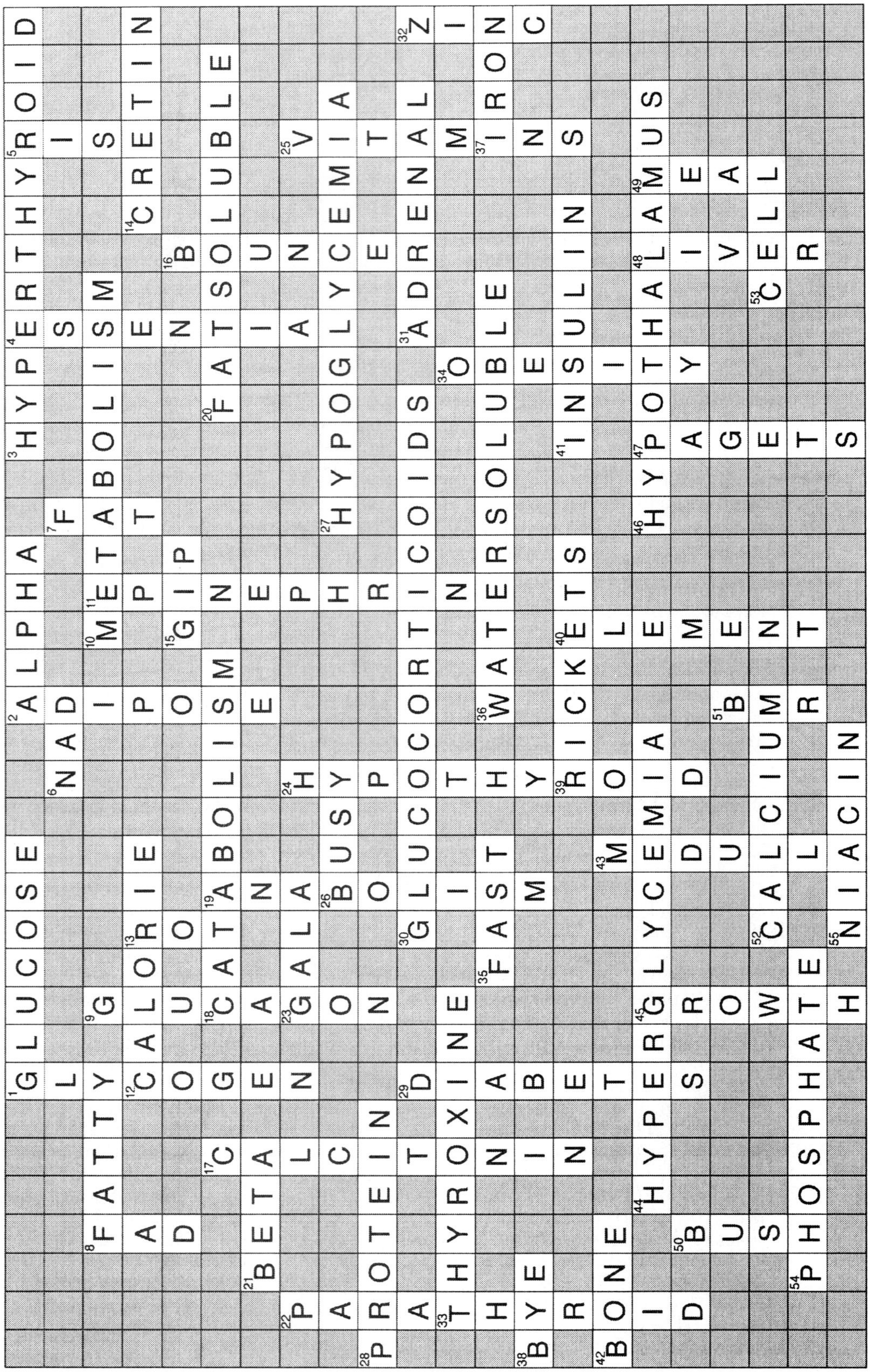

CHAPTER 20
REPRODUCTION

CHAPTER SCOPE

This is the final chapter of the textbook. Odd as it may seem to present this topic on *human reproduction* last, there are many practical reasons to support this format. First, sexual reproduction is a subject of enduring popularity to college students and is directly applicable to the their lives. Second, the student finishes with the miraculous development of a multicellular organism from a single cell and is left, hopefully, with a sense of awe and inspiration for further study. Finally, reproduction is an exceedingly complex subject. Your successful comprehension of the structural and functional developments that occur from the moment of organism conception to death is dependent upon your understanding of the many complex hormonal and neural control systems that were introduced in previous chapter discussions.

Chapter 1 introduced the concept of *homeostasis*, using an example of the secretion of sex steroid hormones and their control involving negative feedback mechanisms. Much of this hormonal regulation involves the hypothalamus and pituitary gland tissues that ultimately regulate the synthesis and release of hormones from the gonads. This regulation is influenced by the *central nervous system* (chapter 8). The *nervous system* also plays a role in reproductive performance, providing the delivery of sensory neuron (chapters 7 and 9) action potentials to the brain for interpretation and the relay of autonomic motor (chapter 10) signals back to the gonads and accessory organs. In chapter 3, during the description of the cell cycle and cell division (**mitosis**), the process of **meiosis** was introduced as a preview of male sperm and female ova formation. This chapter will challenge your memory of meiosis during the discussions of sperm production (**spermatogenesis**) and ovum development (**oogenesis**).

Perhaps a review of *endocrine* physiology (chapter 11) will help you the most in understanding this chapter. The clear descriptions of *steroid* hormone structure and their actions at specific target tissues around the body are especially noteworthy. Also recommended for review is the influence of higher brain centers, the hypothalamic control over the pituitary, and the roles these regions play in the overall endocrine administration of the gonads, the placenta, and the lactating breast.

The remaining concepts in this chapter include the intricate hormonal changes that occur during the female menstrual cycle, and the related concepts of **ovulation, fertilization, implantation** (pregnancy), **parturition** (childbirth), and **lactation** (breastfeeding). All of these processes bring us to the end of this chapter, the end of the text, the end of this study guide, and the beginning of a new living person. *Celebrate!*

I. SEXUAL REPRODUCTION

Early embryonic gonads can become either testes or ovaries. A particular gene on the Y chromosome induces the embryonic gonads to become testes. Females lack a Y chromosome, and the absence of this gene causes the development of ovaries. The embryonic testes secrete testosterone, which induces the development of male accessory sexual organs and external genitalia. The absence of testes (rather than the presence of ovaries) in a female embryo causes the development of the female accessory sexual organs.

A. Multiple Choice

___ 1. In sexual reproduction, the *sperm* and *ova*, known as , are formed within the *testes* and *ovaries*, called , by a process of reduction division known as _____.
   a. gonads; germ cells; meiosis
   b. gametes; gonads; meiosis
   c. zygotes; gametes; mitosis
   d. zygotes; germ cells; mitosis

___ 2. The *total* number of chromosomes found in a zygote is
   a. twenty-one
   b. twenty-three

       c. thirty-eight
       d. forty-two
       e. forty-six

____ 3. The *total* number of *autosomes* found in a zygote is
       a. twenty-one
       b. twenty-six
       c. thirty-eight
       d. forty-four
       e. forty-eight

____ 4. All *ova* must contain one chromosome, whereas each *sperm* must contain one chromosome.
       a. Y; X
       b. X; X
       c. X; Y
       d. Y; X or Y
       e. X; X or Y

____ 5. The genotype in *Klinefelter's syndrome* patients is _____, whereas the genotype in *Turner's syndrome* patients is _____.
       a. XXY; XXX
       b. XXY; XO
       c. XYY; XXY
       d. XYY; XO

____ 6. The hormone, *testosterone*, is synthesized early in the embryo, by the _____ of the testes.
       a. Leydig cells
       b. seminiferous tubules
       c. Sertoli cells
       d. spermatogonia
       e. germinal cells

____ 7. Which statement about the *Müllerian Inhibition Factor (MIF)* is false?
       a. MIF is a polypeptide secreted from the seminiferous tubules of the testes.
       b. MIF causes regression of the Müllerian ducts beginning about the eighth week.
       c. MIF is necessary for normal development of the female embryo.
       d. MIF allows the growth and development of the Wolffian ducts to proceed in the male.
       e. MIF is made by the Sertoli cells of the male.

____ 8. The *homologous* structure of the male penis is the female; while the homologous structure of the male scrotum is the female .
       a. vagina; uterus
       b. ovary; vagina
       c. uterus; labia
       d. clitoris; labia majora
       e. ovary; fallopian tube

____ 9. The *active* form of testosterone in target organs is
       a. testis-determining factor (TDF)
       b. 5α-reductase
       c. Müllerian inhibition factor (MIF)
       d. dihydrotestosterone (DHT)
       e. progesterone.

____ 10. The abnormal condition in which an individual has normal functioning testes but lacks the target cell receptors for testosterone, is called
       a. congenital adrenal hyperplasia
       b. hermaphroditism
       c. testicular feminization syndrome
       d. 5β-reductase deficiency
       e. None of these abnormal conditions is correct.

B. True or False/Edit

___ 11. Each zygote has twenty-three pairs of chromosomes from its mother and twenty-three pairs from its father; and when paired together are known as *homologous* chromosomes.

___ 12. The X and Y sex chromosomes form one homologous pair of chromosomes that look very much alike and contain similar genes.

___ 13. As each pair of homologous chromosomes from the mother and father separate during *meiosis*, the distribution of chromosomes to the haploid gamete is entirely random.

___ 14. The chromosomal sex of the zygote is determined entirely by the sperm.

___ 15. Only one X chromosome of the pair found in the female cells is active; the other chromosome forms a clump of inactive "heterochromatin," called a *polar body*.

___ 16. The gene for sex determination is located on the short arm of the Y chromosome and is presumed to synthesize the *testis-determining factor* (TDF).

___ 17. In the formation of the embryo, the ovarian follicles of the female ovaries appear before the seminiferous tubules of the male testes.

___ 18. The descent of the testes from the abdomen into the scrotum cavity is required since the production of sperm (*spermatogenesis*) requires cooler temperatures.

___ 19. The female sex accessory organs develop due to the absence of testes rather than to the presence of ovaries.

II. ENDOCRINE REGULATION OF REPRODUCTION

The functions of the testes and ovaries are regulated by gonadotropic hormones secreted by the anterior pituitary. The gonadotropic hormones stimulate the gonads to secrete their sex steroid hormones, and these steroid hormones, in turn, have an inhibitory effect on the secretion of the gonadotropic hormones. This interaction between the anterior pituitary and the gonads forms a negative feedback loop.

A. Multiple Choice

___ 20. Which of the following is *not* a *primary* effect of the **gonadotropic hormones** (*FSH* and *LH*) in either males or females?
   a. stimulate the formation of sperm (*spermatogenesis*) or ova (*oogenesis*)
   b. stimulate steroid hormone secretion from the gonads
   c. maintain the structure of the gonad tissue
   d. stimulate the formation of the sexual accessory organs
   e. All of these are primary gonadotropic hormone effects.

___ 21. *Gonadotropin-releasing hormone* (GnRH), also known as *luteinizing hormone-releasing hormone* (LHRH), is secreted by the
   a. hypothalamus
   b. anterior pituitary
   c. posterior pituitary
   d. gonads

___ 22. The polypeptide hormone, *inhibin*, is an important hormone secreted by the
   a. hypothalamus
   b. anterior pituitary
   c. gonads
   d. cerebral cortex
   e. posterior pituitary

___ 23. Which of the following is *not* a secondary sexual characteristic that occurs during puberty in boys?
   a. growth of the testes
   b. growth of the penis
   c. darkening and distribution of pubic hair
   d. growth of the larynx
   e. descent of the testes into the scrotum

___ 24. The hormone derived from the amino acid, tryptophane, and secreted by the *pineal gland* primarily at night, is
   a. melatonin
   b. gonadotropin releasing hormone (GnRH)
   c. inhibin
   d. estradiol
   e. melanin

B. True or False/Edit

___ 25. Unlike the embryonic *testes* that mature early and are active in development, the embryonic *ovaries* do not mature until the third trimester of pregnancy.

___ 26. Testosterone is most active in the third trimester of pregnancy, masculinizing the male embryo's external genitalia and sex accessory organs.

___ 27. In castrated male or female animals, the blood levels of the gonadotropins, FSH and LH, are much lower than those measured in the intact animal.

___ 28. The sex steroid hormones (estrogen, progesterone, and testosterone) have a *negative feedback* effect both on the hypothalamus to inhibit its secretion of GnRH, and on the anterior pituitary to inhibit its responsiveness to GnRH.

___ 29. The polypeptide hormone *inhibin* appears to specifically inhibit the *anterior* pituitary's secretion of LH without affecting the secretion of FSH.

___ 30. The onset of puberty may result from the normal maturation of brain tissue and from the hypothalamus and pituitary tissues becoming less sensitive to the negative feedback effects of the sex steroid hormones.

___ 31. The onset of puberty occurs sooner in children with very high levels of physical activity and lower levels of body fat.

___ 32. In the daytime, as light strikes the retina, the neurons responsible for activating pineal gland secretion are indirectly inhibited and the secretion of *melatonin* from the pineal gland is decreased.

III. MALE REPRODUCTIVE SYSTEM

The Leydig cells in the interstitial tissue of the testes are stimulated by LH to secrete testosterone, a potent androgen that acts to maintain the structure and function of the male accessory sex organs and to promote the development of male secondary sex characteristics. The Sertoli cells in the seminiferous tubules of the testes are stimulated by FSH. Spermatogenesis requires the cooperative actions of both FSH and testosterone.

A. Multiple Choice

___ 33. The cellular receptor proteins for *FSH* are found exclusively on the
   a. Sertoli cells
   b. Leydig cells
   c. prostate gland
   d. spermatogonia cells
   e. interstitial cells

___ 34. Which substance is *not* derived from testosterone within the target cells of the male brain?
   a. estradiol-17β
   b. inhibin
   c. 3α-diol
   d. 3β-diol
   e. dihydrotestosterone (DHT)

___ 35. Which of the following hormones is *not* produced by the interstitial cells of Leydig?
   a. adrenocorticotropic hormone (ACTH)
   b. melanocyte stimulating hormone (MSH)
   c. testosterone
   d. β-endorphin
   e. All of these hormones are produced by Leydig cells.

___ 36. *Spermatogonia* are
   a. stem cells that have migrated from the yolk sac to the testes during early embryonic development
   b. located nearest the lumen of the seminiferous tubules in the adult testes
   c. haploid cells (with twenty-three chromosomes) within the seminiferous tubules of the testes
   d. also known as interstitial cells located between the tubules
   e. produced during the second meiotic division.

___ 37. Which statement about *meiosis* in the testes is *false*?
   a. Primary spermatocytes are diploid.
   b. Secondary spermatocytes are haploid.
   c. During the first meiotic division duplicate chromatids separate as two daughter cells are formed.
   d. The second meiotic division results in the formation of four haploid spermatids.
   e. Meiosis occurs entirely within the walls of the seminiferous tubules.

___ 38. The *Sertoli cells* of the testes
   a. are found in the interstitial spaces of the testes
   b. are the germinal "stem" cells from the embryo that will undergo meiosis
   c. form the blood-testis barrier to the movement of molecules to the germinal cells
   d. are formed during the process of *spermiogenesis*
   e. are responsible for the synthesis of testosterone

___ 39. Which statement about *semen* is *false*?
   a. Most of the semen volume (60%) comes from the two seminal vesicles.
   b. Semen normally contains fructose and clotting proteins.
   c. Semen is produced entirely in the lumen of the seminiferous tubules of the testes.
   d. The prostate gland contributes citric acid, calcium and coagulation proteins to the semen composition.
   e. Semen is carried by two ejaculatory ducts to the single urethra.

B. True or False/Edit

___ 40. The secretion of *testosterone* by the interstitial cells of Leydig is stimulated by the arrival of the hormone FSH but not by LH.

___ 41. *Inhibin* is a protein (and therefore, water-soluble) hormone secreted by the Sertoli cells of the seminiferous tubules.

___ 42. Older males experience an abrupt drop in sex steroid secretions similar to that experienced by females during menopause.

___ 43. Examples of anabolic steroids include the androgens in males and the estrogens in females.

___ 44. There is evidence that in males both the Sertoli cells of the seminiferous tubules and the interstitial Leydig cells can produce small amounts of *estradiol*.

___ 45. FSH acts on the Sertoli cells to secrete *inhibin*, which, in turn, enhances the response of Leydig cells to LH, resulting in an overall increase in *testosterone* secretion.

___ 46. *Spermiogenesis* is the process whereby Sertoli cells eliminate the cytoplasm of spermatids by phagocytosis, thus forming spermatozoa.

___ 47. During puberty both LH and androgens are required to complete the initiation of *spermatogenesis* within the seminiferous tubules.

___ 48. Spermatozoa that enter the "head" of the epididymis are nonmotile, relatively immature, and are therefore, not capable of fertilizing an ovum.

___ 49. Emission and ejaculation refer to the same process.

___ 50. Male sexual function requires the antagonistic action of the parasympathetic and sympathetic nervous systems.

___ 51. Approximately 70% of men with vasectomies develop antibodies to their own sperm, which may reduce the possibility of restoring fertility if desired.

IV. FEMALE REPRODUCTIVE SYSTEM

The ovaries contain a large number of follicles, each of which encloses an ovum. Some of these follicles mature during the ovarian cycle, and the ova they contain progress to the secondary oocyte stage of meiosis. At ovulation, the largest follicle breaks open to extrude a secondary oocyte from the ovary. The empty follicle then becomes a corpus luteum, which ultimately degenerates at the end of a nonfertile cycle.

A. Multiple Choice

____ 52. The *cervix* is considered part of the
   a. vagina
   b. uterus
   c. fallopian tube
   d. ovary
   e. clitoris

____ 53. Like spermatogenesis in the testes of prenatal males, *oogenesis* in the ovary of prenatal females is arrested in _____ of meiosis.
   a. prophase I
   b. metaphase I
   c. anaphase I
   d. prophase II
   e. metaphase II

____ 54. The ring of granulosa cells surrounding the ovum is the
   a. corona radiata
   b. cumulus oophorus
   c. antrum
   d. zona pellucida
   e. theca interna

____ 55. The thin gel-like layer of proteins and polysaccharides just outside the *oocyte* is called the
   a. corona radiata
   b. cumulus oophorus
   c. antrum
   d. zona pellucida
   e. theca interna

____ 56. Within the *graafian follicle* of the ovary, the process of meiosis will be arrested in the *secondary* oocyte at
   a. metaphase I
   b. anaphase I
   c. prophase II
   d. metaphase II
   e. anaphase II

____ 57. The *corpus luteum* is an endocrine structure that is formed from the
   a. enlarged primary oocyte
   b. graafian follicle after ovulation
   c. secondary oocyte after fertilization by sperm
   d. corpus albicans of the ovary

B. True or False/Edit

____ 58. *Fimbriae* extensions of the uterine or fallopian tubes are not directly connected to the ovary; and therefore ova released during ovulation are "swept" along by the ciliated epithelial lining of the tubes.

____ 59. After birth, the number of *primary* oocytes increases steadily, reaching 300,000-400,000 by the time the girl enters puberty.

____ 60. As the ovarian follicles grow, FSH stimulates the *granulosa* cells to convert precursor testosterone molecules into estrogen.

___ 61. Only *after* the secondary oocyte has been ovulated and fertilized by sperm does the oocyte complete its second meiotic division and form a second *polar body*.

___ 62. Unlike the *corpus luteum* that secretes only estrogen, the ovarian *follicles* secrete both estrogen and progesterone.

___ 63. Only one hypothalamic releasing hormone (*GnRH*) controls the release of both FSH and LH, consequently the blood levels of these two hormones rise and fall together.

V. MENSTRUAL CYCLE

Cyclic changes in the secretion of gonadotropic hormones from the anterior pituitary cause the ovarian changes during a monthly cycle. The ovarian cycle is accompanied by cyclic changes in the secretion of estradiol and progesterone, which interact with the hypothalamus and pituitary to regulate gonadotropin secretion. The cyclic changes in ovarian hormone secretion also cause changes in the endometrium of the uterus during a menstrual cycle.

A. Multiple Choice

___ 64. The average duration of the *menstrual cycle* is
   a. fourteen days
   b. twenty-one days
   c. twenty-eight days
   d. thirty-six days
   e. seventy-two days

___ 65. Which of the following is *not* a menstrual phase taking place either in the ovarian follicle or the endometrium of the uterus?
   a. menstrual phase
   b. follicular phase
   c. proliferative phase
   d. luteal phase
   e. lunar phase

___ 66. "Day one" of the menstrual cycle conveniently refers to that particular day when
   a. ovulation of the ovum from the graafian follicle occurs
   b. the loss of endometrial tissue as menstrual flow begins
   c. fertilization of the ovum by sperm occurs
   d. implantation of the fertilized ovum takes place
   e. the secondary oocyte undergoes its second meiotic division

___ 67. The _____ phase of the ovaries spans day one through fourteen, while the _____ phase covers day fourteen through twenty-eight.
   a. menstrual; proliferative
   b. luteal; secretory
   c. proliferative; secretory
   d. follicular; luteal
   e. secretory; proliferative

___ 68. In the uterus, days fourteen through twenty-eight are known as the _____ phase.
   a. menstrual
   b. luteal
   c. secretory
   d. follicular
   e. proliferative

___ 69. The *anterior pituitary* hormone that stimulates the secretion of estradiol (the principal estrogen) from the granulosa cells of the growing follicle before ovulation is
   a. gonadotropin releasing hormone (GnRH)
   b. follicle stimulating hormone (FSH)
   c. luteinizing hormone (LH)
   d. progesterone
   e. adrenocorticotropic hormone (ACTH)

___ 70. The *positive* feedback effect on the pituitary gland and the hypothalamus near the end of the *follicular phase* is primarily caused by the rapid rise in the blood levels of
   a. FSH
   b. LH
   c. estradiol
   d. progesterone
   e. GnRH

___ 71. The hormone whose blood concentration "surges" near day fourteen and is most responsible for triggering the rupture of the graafian follicle, or *ovulation*, is
   a. FSH
   b. LH
   c. estrogen
   d. progesterone
   e. GnRH

___ 72. The hormone that is present in negligible quantities in the first half (follicular phase) of the menstrual cycle but rises rapidly to peak levels during the second half (luteal phase), is
   a. FSH
   b. LH
   c. estrogen
   d. progesterone
   e. GnRH

___ 73. The thin, watery mucus secreted by the cervix close to the time of ovulation is caused by high blood levels of the hormone,
   a. FSH
   b. LH
   c. estradiol
   d. progesterone
   e. GnRH

___ 74. Careful measurement of oral basal body temperature can be used to predict
   a. the day of ovulation
   b. the day of the peak LH "surge"
   c. the amount of estrogen secreted in the blood
   d. whether or not fertilization has occurred
   e. the day of implantation of the zygote

___ 75. As a result of the *birth control pill*, hormone levels are altered so that the menstrual cycle resembles one long phase of the ovary.
   a. proliferative
   b. menstrual
   c. luteal
   d. follicular
   e. secretory

___ 76. *Menopause* is caused primarily by a decrease in the normal activity of the
   a. anterior pituitary
   b. hypothalamus
   c. ovary
   d. uterine endometrium
   e. vagina

B. True or False/Edit

___ 77. *Estrous* in nonprimate female mammals and *menstruation* in most female primates refer to the same basic process.

___ 78. Toward the end of the *follicular* phase of the normal menstrual cycle in the ovary, one follicle in one ovary reaches maturity and becomes the graafian follicle.

___ 79. Although blood levels of FSH stay relatively constant during the early *follicular* phase, estrogen production by the follicles increases as the number of new FSH *receptors* in the granulosa cells increases.

___ 80. During *ovulation* the ovum sheds its *zona pellucida* and *corona radiata*, which remain behind with the follicle as the ovum is released.

___ 81. There is only one *corpus luteum* formed during each menstrual cycle.

___ 82. Estrogen and progesterone levels fall during the nonfertile late *luteal* phase (about day twenty-two) because the corpus luteum regresses and stops functioning.

___ 83. The *proliferative* phase of the endometrium occurs during the same menstrual cycle time period as the *luteal* phase of the ovaries.

___ 84. The appearance of blood during the *menstrual* phase seems to be due to blood loss as newly developed spiral arteries constrict causing necrosis (cell death) and sloughing of the stratum functionale of the endometrium.

___ 85. Birth control pills provide both synthetic estrogen and synthetic progesterone which prevent the process of implantation by suppressing the release of the gonadotropins.

C. Label the Figure — The Menstrual Cycle

Figure 20.36 in the text is an excellent summary of the female menstrual cycle. This cyclical flow diagram roughly in the shape of a clock, outlines the hormonal control over the sequence of events that occur in the ovary (follicle) during one menstrual cycle. These follicular events are correlated with the phases of the uterus (endometrium) that are taking place simultaneously. In figure 20.1 below, identify and write the name of the appropriate hormone in the space provided. Choose the hormones from this list: *estradiol*, *progesterone*, *GnRH*, *FSH*, and *LH*. Notice that each hormone can be used more than once. Be sure to attempt to label the figure *without* using the text, and then check your work. For an extra challenge when you are finished, erase the answers and come back later for another practice session!

VI. FERTILIZATION, PREGNANCY, AND PARTURITION

Once fertilization has occurred, the secondary oocyte completes meiotic division and then undergoes mitosis to form first a ball of cells and then an early embryonic structure called a blastocyst. Cells of the blastocyst secrete a hormone known as human chorionic gonadotropin, that maintains the mother's corpus luteum and its production of estradiol and progesterone. This prevents menstruation, so that the embryo can implant into the endometrium, develop, and form a placenta. Birth is dependent upon strong contractions of the uterus, which are stimulated by oxytocin from the posterior pituitary.

A. Multiple Choice

___ 86. The term *capacitation* refers to the
a. formation of the sperm head, body, and tail
b. process by which sperm become able to fertilize an ovum
c. recognition of the ova by approaching sperm
d. removal of the sperm body and tail after fertilization

___ 87. During the *acrosomal reaction* that occurs when the sperm meets the ovum,
a. hyaluronidase and protein-digesting enzymes are activated
b. sperm tunnels its way through the corona radiata and zona pellucida layers of the ovum
c. a chemical change in the zona pellucida allows the entry of only one sperm
d. the secondary oocyte is about to complete its second meiotic division
e. All of these statements regarding the acrosomal reaction are correct.

___ 88. In the female reproductive tract, the *secondary* oocyte (ovum) lives about day(s); whereas sperm live about day(s).
a. one; two
b. one; three
c. two; one
d. two; three
e. three; one

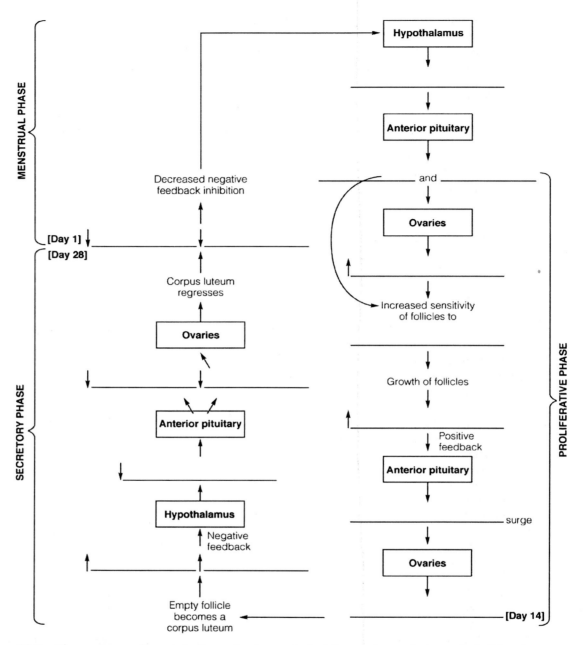

Figure 20.1 The sequence of events in the endocrine control of the ovarian cycle in context of the phases of the endometrium during the menstrual cycle.

___ 89. By about fifty to sixty hours after fertilization a third cleavage occurs, producing a ball of cells called a(an).
  a. two; zygote
  b two; embryo
  c. four; blastocyst
  d. eight; morula
  e. sixteen; trophoblast

___ 90. The term *nidation* refers to the process of
  a. ovulation
  b. fertilization
  c. cleavage

244

    d. implantation
    e. parturition
___ 91. *Human chorionic gonadotropin* (hCG) is an important hormone secreted by the
    a. trophoblast cells of the chorion
    b. inner cell mass (fetus)
    c. endometrium of the uterus
    d. corpus luteum of the ovary
___ 92. The effects of hCG on the corpus luteum of the ovary resemble those of which other hormone?
    a. follicle stimulating hormone (FSH)
    b. luteinizing hormone (LH)
    c. estradiol 17-ϑ
    d. progesterone
    e. oxytocin
___ 93. Which two structures — one from *fetal* tissue and one from *maternal* tissue — together form the functional unit known as the **placenta**?
    a. endoderm and ectoderm
    b. decidua basalis and mesoderm
    c. endoderm and chorion frondosum
    d. ectoderm and mesoderm
    e. decidua basalis and chorion frondosum
___ 94. Which of the following techniques is *not* used to evaluate the status of the growing embryo during pregnancy?
    a. chorionic villus biopsy
    b. amniocentesis
    c. ultrasound imaging
    d. All of these techniques are used to evaluate the growing embryo.
___ 95. The high metabolic activity seen in the placenta including its rapid rate of protein synthesis most resembles that seen in the following organ
    a. kidney
    b. liver
    c. thyroid
    d. pancreas
    e. heart
___ 96. The two placental hormones — *human chorionic gonadotropin* (hCG) and *human chorionic somatomammotropin* (hCS) — duplicate the actions of four hormones that are secreted by the
    a. anterior pituitary gland
    b. posterior pituitary gland
    c. thyroid gland
    d. hypothalamus
    e. ovaries
___ 97. The two agents most responsible for the powerful smooth muscle contractions of the uterus in labor during *parturition* (childbirth), are
    a. LH and progesterone
    b. oxytocin and estrogen
    c. hCG and prostaglandins
    d. oxytocin and prostaglandins
    e. estrogen and progesterone
___ 98. During pregnancy, high estrogen levels in the blood inhibit breast milk production by stimulating the secretion of *prolactin-inhibiting hormone* (PIH, thought to be dopamine) produced by the
    a. anterior pituitary
    b. posterior pituitary
    c. ovary

                d. hypothalamus
                e. placenta
___ 99. Successful *lactation*, including the *milk-ejection reflex* or milk let-down, results from the combined action of these two hormones.
                a. PIH and oxytocin
                b. estrogen and progesterone
                c. prolactin and oxytocin
                d. PIH and prostaglandins
                e. progesterone and PIH

B. True or False/Edit

___ 100. Freshly ejaculated sperm are not capable of immediately fertilizing an ovum.
___ 101. Each ovulation releases a *secondary* oocyte arrested during *prophase* of its second meiotic division.
___ 102. The *second* polar body is formed after fertilization by a sperm as the second meiotic division is completed; and, like the first polar body, ultimately fragments and disintegrates.
___ 103. The ball of cells called a *morula* consists of two parts, an inner cell mass (that later forms the fetus) and a surrounding trophoblast layer or chorion (that later forms the placenta).
___ 104. An important effect of *human chorionic gonadotropin* (hCG) is to prevent menstruation and thus maintain pregnancy by prolonging the secretions of the corpus luteum.
___ 105. The last of three embryonic cell layers to form from the cytotrophoblast portion of the chorion is the *mesoderm* layer.
___ 106. The entire fetus with its umbilical cord are located within the amniotic sac and bathed by amniotic fluid.
___ 107. The umbilical artery carries oxygenated blood from the placenta to the fetus, as the umbilical vein carries deoxygenated blood from the fetus to the placenta.
___ 108. The maternal and fetal blood come close together within the placenta but never mix.
___ 109. During pregnancy the *placenta* becomes a major sex steroid-producing gland secreting increasing amounts of estrogen and progesterone until the end of gestation, when plasma levels of both hormones are significantly higher than normal.
___ 110. Mammary gland development during pregnancy and the subsequent lactation response require complex interactions among many hormones and their regulation by the neuroendocrine system.
___ 111. Before childbirth the low secretion of prolactin from the anterior pituitary gland is controlled by prolactin-inhibiting hormone (PIH), which is believed to be the neurotransmitter, dopamine.
___ 112. Breast-feeding, acting through reflex inhibition of GnRH secretion from the hypothalamus, can ultimately inhibit ovulation and thereby serve as a natural contraceptive mechanism in some mothers with limited caloric intake.

C. Label the Figure — The Control of Mammary Gland Development During Pregnancy and Lactation

Figure 20.52 in the text outlines the complex hormonal control of mammary gland development during gestation (pregnancy) and explains why milk is not produced until after parturition (childbirth). Study figure 20.2 below, identify the correct hormone for each blank answer line, then write the name of that hormone in the space provided. As always, once you have completed the figure, check your work with figure 20.52 in the text.

VII. CHAPTER REVIEW

A. Match 'n' Spell - Hormones and Chemicals of the Reproductive System

The text of this chapter includes the descriptions of many hormones and chemicals involved in the normal development and function of the reproductive system. Some of these names are real tongue-twisters or are often reduced to initials (such as PIH). To help you become more familiar with these terms, study the following list of substances on the right and match the appropriate letter with the numbered statements on the left. Write the proper letter in the space provided. As an extra study aid, try to spell correctly the chosen hormone or chemical on the line that follows each numbered phrase.

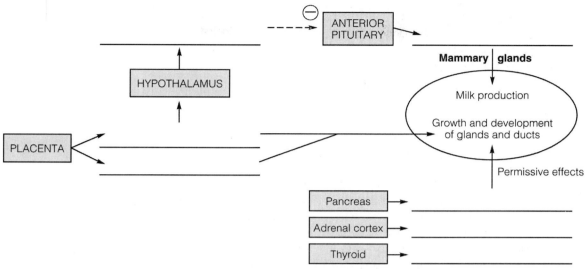

Figure 20.2 The hormonal control of mammary gland development during pregnancy and lactation. Note that milk production is prevented during pregnancy by estrogen inhibition of prolactin secretion. This inhibition is accomplished by the stimulation of PIH (prolactin-inhibiting hormone) secretion from the hypothalamus.

113. produced by a specific gene only on the Y chromosome _____
114. produced by developing seminiferous tubules--causes regression of tissues that would become female sex organs _____
115. active androgen synthesized by 5α-reductase _____
116. hypothalamic hormone stimulating FSH and LH release _____
117. specific inhibitor of FSH secretion in response to GnRH, but does not inhibit LH secretion _____
118. pineal gland hormone responsive to light-dark cycles _____
119. anterior pituitary hormone that stimulates Leydig cells of the testes to secrete androgens _____
120. hypothalamic hormone stimulated by high estrogen during pregnancy — prevents the production of milk _____
121. posterior pituitary hormone released by nipple suckling, initiating the milk-ejection reflex _____
122. after childbirth, this hormone stimulates the production of milk proteins (casein and lactalbumin) _____
123. cyclic fatty acids produced in the uterus that appear involved in uterine contractions during labor _____
124. key chemicals in the head of sperm, responsible for tunneling through the corona radiata and zona pellucida _____
125. placental hormone with growth hormone (GH) and prolactin effects — causes a "diabeticlike" effect in mothers _____
126. ovarian hormone responsible for the *positive* feedback LH "surge" resulting in ovulation on day fourteen _____
127. placental hormone that mimics LH, maintaining the corpus luteum for the first few weeks of pregnancy _____
128. anterior pituitary hormone involved in the initiation of spermatogenesis in the pubescent male _____
129. dominant androgenic sex steroid secreted by the interstitial cells of Leydig _____

a. estradiol
b. testosterone
c. dihydrotestosterone
d. GnRH
e. FSH
f. LH
g. inhibin
h. melatonin
i. hCG
j. hCS
k. testis-determining factor (TDF)
l. Müllerian inhibition factor (MIF)
m. prolactin
n. prolactin-inhibiting hormone (PIH)
o. acrosome enzymes
p. oxytocin
q. prostaglandins

B. Crossword Puzzle — Reproduction

Across

1. anterior pituitary hormone that stimulates spermatogenesis in the seminiferous tubules
3. pineal gland hormone influenced by the light-dark cycle
8. labor and delivery (childbirth)
9. tubules, site of meiosis and the formation of sperm
10. male gamete
14. the active form of testosterone in male target cells
15. event influenced by oxytocin and prostaglandins
17. embryo cell layer that forms part of the placenta
20. formation of the male gamete
22. the dominant sex steroid in females
23. sperm travels through the _____ deferens during emission
25. combination of the chorion frondosum and decidua basalis
26. days one through five constitute the _____ phase of the uterus
27. the event that occurs as a result of a surge in plasma LH levels
28. the hypothalamic hormone that is secreted in a "pulsatile" fashion
30. the hypothalamic hormone that blocks the formation of milk
31. fingerlike extensions of the fallopian tubes in females
32. the dominant androgen in males

Down

2. fructose and citric acid flow into semen from the _____ vesicles
4. the sexual response in males that is regulated by activity in the sympathetic nervous system
5. after ovulation, the graafian follicle becomes a corpus _____
6. sperm or ovum
7. Sertoli cell secretion that inhibits FSH release from the anterior pituitary
11. the eight-cell ball of embryonic cells following fertilization
12. the sex chromosome genotype for a Turner's female
13. testis or ovary
15. the gonadotropin that stimulates testosterone secretion from Leydig cells
16. the hollow ball of cells that implants in the endometrium
18. the menstrual cycle event that may occur on about day twenty-one
19. formation of female gametes (ova) within the follicles of the ovary
21. nongerminal cells of the male seminiferous tubules
24. the inactive "heterochromatin" or X chromosome in female cells, known as a (an) _____ body
29. the chorionic hormone that mimics both growth hormone and prolactin

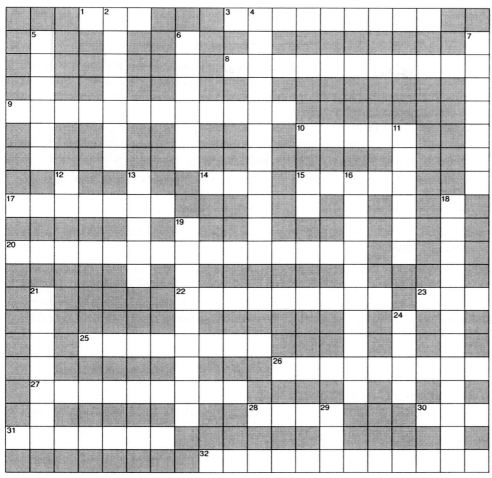

C. Essay

Essay Tutorial

This essay tutorial will answer the first essay question found in the "**Review Activities**" section of your *Human Physiology* textbook. Please look for *Essay Question* 1. at the end of chapter 20, read it carefully, and let me guide you through one possible answer. Watch for key terms in bold-face type, helpful tips and general suggestions on writing the essay or short-answer questions. Enjoy!

130. *Identify* the conversion **products** of testosterone and *describe* their **functions** in the brain, prostate, and seminiferous tubules.

Answer. As a nonpolar steroid molecule, *testosterone* enters all cells by simple diffusion from higher to lower concentrations. However, testosterone receptors are only present in those cells genetically programmed as "target" cells. Once inside the selective target cells, testosterone is converted by means of an enzyme called *5α-reductase* into the active hormone. Known as **dihydrotestosterone** (DHT), this activated hormone directly mediates the androgenic effect in these tissues. In the target neurons of the *brain,* DHT can, in turn, be changed by other enzymes into other 5α-reduced androgens — abbreviated **3α-diol** and **3β-diol**. Other brain cells make an enzyme called *aromatase*, which converts testosterone to **estradiol-17β**, the major estrogen sex steroid in females. This newly formed estradiol may mediate the negative feedback effect of testosterone on the secretion of *GnRH* from the hypothalamus and *LH* from the anterior pituitary gland, resulting in a decrease in blood levels of both hormones.

The stimulation of the *prostate* gland by testosterone, or its derivatives, is required for normal prostate growth and function. This is the "trophic," or "nourishing supportive" effect of testosterone. Without testosterone the prostate as well as other sex accessory organs atrophy ("lack nourishment"). The target cells within the *seminiferous tubules* of adult males are also able to convert incoming testosterone into 5α-reduced androgens, yet their significance is not well understood. The *Sertoli cell* of the seminiferous tubules must also be stimulated by testosterone, or its derivatives, for normal sperm production. During puberty, testosterone arrives to help initiate *spermatogenesis* and to maintain sperm production in the adult male thereafter.

Congratulations — by working through these essay questions with me in this study guide I hope you have learned a few tips for answering essay or short answer format questions. To summarize essay-writing techniques,

First, take time to read the question slowly, underline each critical word which will indicate the direction your answer should take and help you confine your discussion to the question.

Second, avoid rambling sentences that may lead you down a path that strays from the points you are trying to make. Remember, if words seem unnecessary they probably are, so don't use them.

Third, don't be afraid to express yourself since there is no perfect essay and most professors will give partial credit for honest efforts in the right direction. Here are a few more questions on the reproductive system. Good luck!

131. Draw a cross-section diagram of the *seminiferous tubule* and label each cell stage that occurs in meiosis during *spermatogenesis*. Include the important role of the *Sertoli cell* in this process.

132. Suppose a man is training for the Mr. Universe body-building contest and is abusing anabolic steroids. Discuss the possible effects these exogenous (out of the body) steroids would have on the negative feedback control of hormones from the hypothalamus, pituitary, and the testes. Include their possible effects on the sex accessory glands as well.

133. Divide the twenty-eight-day **menstrual** *cycle* into an *ovarian* cycle and a *uterine* cycle. Start with day one of the ovarian cycle, and describe the two phases of the ovarian cycle and the hormones involved. In a similar way, describe the *phases* and *hormones* characteristic of the uterine cycle.

134. Assuming ovulation and fertilization have occurred on day fourteen of the menstrual cycle, follow the growth and development of the embryo through implantation and formation of the *placenta*.

135. *Where* are the hormones human chorionic gonadotropin (hCG) and human chorionic somatomammotropin (hCS) produced, what are their *roles* in pregnancy, and which four hormones do they *mimic*?

Answers – Chapter 20

I. Sexual Reproduction
   A. 1. b, 2. e, 3. d, 4. e, 5. b, 6. a, 7. c, 8. d, 9. d, 10. c
   B. 11. T, 12. F—The Y chromosome is smaller and has different genes, 13. T, 14. T, 15. F—Replace "polar" with "Barr," 16. T, 17. F—Replace "before" with "after," 18. T, 19. T
II. Endocrine Regulation of Reproduction
   A. 20. d, 21. a, 22. c, 23. e, 24. a
   B. 25. T, 26. F—Replace "third" with "first," 27. F—Replace "lower" with "higher," 28. T, 29. F—Switch "LH" and "FSH," 30. T, 31. F—Replace "sooner" with "later," 32. T
III. Male Reproductive System
   A. 33. a, 34. b, 35. e, 36. a, 37. c, 38. c, 39. c
   B. 40. F—Switch "FSH" and "LH," 41. T, 42. F—Male hormone secretion declines gradually with age, 43. F—Estrogen is not considered an anabolic steroid, 44. T, 45. T, 46. T, 47. F—Replace "LH" with "FSH," 48. T, 49. F—In emission semen moves into the urethra; in ejaculation semen is expelled from the penis, 50. F—Replace "antagonistic" with "synergistic," 51. T
IV. Female Reproductive System
   A. 52. b, 53. a, 54. a, 55. d, 56. d, 57. b
   B. 58. T, 59. F—Replace "increases" with "decreases," 60. T, 61. T, 62. F—Switch "corpus luteum" and "ovarian follicles," 63. F—FSH and LH levels in the blood are influenced by other factors and do not rise and fall together
V. Menstrual Cycle
   A. 64. c, 65. e, 66. b, 67. d, 68. c, 69. b, 70. c, 71. b, 72. d, 73. c, 74. a, 75. c, 76. c
   B. 77. F—Many differences exist between estrous and menstruation, 78. T, 79. T, 80. F—The zona pellucida and corona radiata remain with the ovum, 81. T, 82. T, 83. F—Replace "luteal" with "follicular," 84. T, 85. F—Replace "implantation" with "ovulation"
   C. Label the figure — The Menstrual Cycle; See figure 20.36 in the text
VI. Fertilization, Pregnancy, and Parturition
   A. 86. b, 87. e, 88. b, 89. d, 90. d, 91. a, 92. b, 93. e, 94. d, 95. b, 96. a, 97. d, 98. d, 99. c
   B. 100. T, 101. F—Replace "prophase" with "metaphase," 102. T, 103. F—Replace "morula" with "blastocyst," 104. T, 105. T, 106. T, 107. F—Switch "artery" and "vein," 108. T, 109. T, 110. T, 111. T, 112. T
   C. Label the Figure — The Control of Mammary Gland Development During Pregnancy and Lactation; See figure 20.52 in the text
VII. Chapter Review

A. 113. k, 114. l, 115. c, 116. d, 117. g, 118. h, 119. f, 120. n, 121. p, 122. m, 123. q, 124. o, 125. j, 126. a, 127. i, 128. e, 129. b

B. Crossword Puzzle

			¹F	²S	H			³M	⁴E	L	A	T	O	N	I	N	
	⁵L			E		⁶G			J								⁷I
	U			M		A		⁸P	A	R	T	U	R	I	T	I	O	N
	T			I		M		C									H
⁹S	E	M	I	N	I	F	E	R	O	U	S						I
	U			A		T		L		¹⁰S	P	E	R	¹¹M		B
	M			L		E		A					O		I
		¹²X		¹³G		¹⁴D	H	T	¹⁵L	A	B	O	R		¹⁶	N
¹⁷C	H	O	R	I	O	N			I		H		L		U		¹⁸I
				N		¹⁹O			O			A		L		M
²⁰S	P	E	R	M	A	T	O	G	E	N	E	S	I	S		A	P
				D		G						T			L
²¹S				²²E	S	T	R	A	D	I	O	L		²³V	A	S
	E				N					C		²⁴B		N
	R		²⁵P	L	A	C	E	N	T	A		Y		A		T
	T				S			²⁶M	E	N	S	T	R	U	A	L
²⁷O	V	U	L	A	T	I	O	N			T		R		T
	L				S		²⁸G	N	R	²⁹H			³⁰P	I	H
³¹F	I	M	B	R	I	A			C			O
					³²T	E	S	T	O	S	T	E	R	O	N	E

NOTES

NOTES

NOTES

NOTES

NOTES

NOTES

NOTES

NOTES

NOTES

NOTES

NOTES

NOTES

NOTES

NOTES